Cancer Health Disparities

Chanita Hughes Halbert
Editor

Cancer Health Disparities

From Determinants of Disparities to Solutions for Equity

Springer

Editor
Chanita Hughes Halbert
University of Southern California
California, CA, USA

ISBN 978-3-031-37637-5 ISBN 978-3-031-37638-2 (eBook)
https://doi.org/10.1007/978-3-031-37638-2

This Springer imprint is published by the registered company Springer Nature Switzerland AG
The registered company address is: Gewerbestrasse 11, 6330 Cham, Switzerland

Paper in this product is recyclable.

Preface

After being involved in the one of the first scientific conferences that had a specific focus on cancer health disparities through the American Association for Cancer Research (AACR), I started attending AACR's Annual Meeting to increase my knowledge and understanding about basic science research in cancer and was inspired to integrate these concepts into my own behavioral science research program. It became clear to me that cancer risk and control behaviors had downstream effects on biological mechanisms that are important drivers of cancer outcomes, and that health promotion and disease prevention interventions could impact these behaviors as well as the biological pathways that contribute to the initiation and progression of disease and response to treatment. Around the same time, events were unfolding across the country that were raising awareness about the conditions in our communities that can contribute to cancer outcomes through multiple pathways. Specifically, Walter Scott was fatally shot by a police officer in North Charleston, SC, in 2015 after he was stopped for a tail light that was not working. After an investigation, it was determined that the policeman's account differed from the video recording of the event. Two years following the shooting, the policeman was sentenced to 20 years in prison for a second-degree murder. I was living in South Carolina and raising my two sons when Walter Scott was killed. I grew up in the South and knew about racism and discrimination, but this was the first time that *I really saw and felt* how pervasive racism and discrimination was, and witnessed the direct consequences these -isms have on health and well-being in my community. Professionally, I realized that if we continue to conduct cancer health disparities research in silos that are defined by our training in behavioral, basic, or clinical science, we would be doing a profound disservice to society, our communities, and all of those who came before us and paved the way for us to be in positions that allowed us to drive and sustain a change in cancer care for people of color and those who experience disadvantage because of their background, where they live, and where they receive cancer care services.

I was inspired to edit this book on solutions to cancer health disparities while establishing and leading the Transdisciplinary Center in Precision Medicine and Minority Men's Health at the Medical University of South Carolina. This center is funded by the National Institute on Minority Health and Health Disparities and the National Cancer Institute to conduct translational research to identify and address multilevel determinants of cancer risk and outcomes among racially diverse men. This center is based on emerging conceptual models of minority health and health disparities that are being developed to depict the linkages between basic biological processes, social factors, and psychological characteristics and guide studies that are being conducted to understand how these multilevel determinants interact and contribute to disparities in cancer risk and outcomes. Stress responses and reactivity to social, clinical, and psychological stressors are the focal areas for this center and, to my knowledge, is one of the first examples of a transdisciplinary translational research center that integrated the social context and lived experiences of racially diverse men into the conceptual framework and research design. The transdisciplinary focus of this center also illustrates the evolution of cancer health disparities research from descriptive studies on racial and ethnic differences in cancer risk and outcomes to multilevel investigations that examine the independent and interactive effects of biological, psychological, behavioral, and social determinants of cancer health disparities to develop and evaluate sustainable interventions for cancer prevention, control, and treatment.

Sixteen years after the first AACR Conference on the Science of Cancer Health Disparities, cancer health equity research has grown and evolved into a rigorous field of transdisciplinary science. This book was developed to: (1) provide an in-depth examination of the contribution of multilevel factors to cancer health disparities, (2) describe novel frameworks and approaches that are being used to understand and address cancer health disparities, and (3) describe interventions that have potential to promote equity in cancer risk and outcomes. The chapters in this book takes stock of where the field has been and highlights current and emerging priorities in cancer health disparities research with the hope that this content will contribute to the continued growth and evolution of this field while advancing and inspiring continued efforts and solutions for cancer health equity.

California, CA, USA Chanita Hughes Halbert

Acknowledgements

I am deeply grateful to all of the authors who contributed to this book. Each author's knowledge, expertise, and experiences as researchers and mentors made this book a reality. The chapters in this book were written during a global pandemic that had a profound impact on all aspects of our lives. I am indebted to each author who made space for this work and prioritized the development and completion of their chapters as we all adjusted to and managed our new normal. I am inspired by the commitment and passion of each author, and hope their experience contributing to this book was rewarding and helped to advance their research program and work in cancer health equity. I have tremendous respect for everyone who contributed directly or indirectly to this book and appreciate everyone's support and patience with me. Along those lines, I would like to thank the publisher for the opportunity to edit this book and for their accommodation with revisions to the production schedule. Editing this book was an important aspect of my professional development and I appreciate the guidance I received from my mentors and colleagues during each step of editing this book. We all stand on shoulders of those who came before us and I hope this book honors the pioneers and thought leaders in minority health and health disparities who came before me. Last, but not least, I would like to thank my family and pay special tribute to my late mother, Effie Hughes, whose journey with breast cancer became a blueprint for how I live my life and continues to give me the courage and strength to live my best day every day, even when faced with immense challenges. I love and miss you every day.

Contents

Multilevel Determinants of Cancer Health Disparities

Chanita Hughes Halbert

Introduction

Cancer, which is defined as the uncontrolled growth and spread of abnormal cells, affects individuals from all racial and ethnic backgrounds worldwide; this disease continues to be one of the leading causes of morbidity and mortality in the United States [1]. It is projected that more than 1.9 million new cancer cases will be diagnosed in 2022 and more than 609,360 deaths from cancer are expected [1]. Despite the improved strategies for cancer control, prevention, and treatment, racial and ethnic minorities in the United States continue to experience significant disparities in morbidity and mortality from this disease. Cancer health disparities are defined as differences in cancer risk and outcomes that occur among groups based on their racial/ethnic background, socioeconomic status, geographic location, and access to health care [2]; incidence, morbidity, morbidity, risk behaviors and exposures, and quality of survivorship are often used to measure cancer health disparities. Importantly, cancer health disparities research is intricately related to the broader field of minority health and health disparities and has a focus on understanding factors that contribute to disparities in the nature and distribution of cancer risk factors and disease, translating this evidence into interventions to reduce the burden of disease, and working with policy makers and other stakeholders to disseminate, implement, and sustain these strategies in diverse settings [2]. Early research on cancer health disparities focused on comparing African Americans and whites in terms of incidence, morbidity, and mortality [3]; understanding differences in these outcomes continues to be a priority for monitoring trends and identifying future opportunities to enhance cancer health equity. As a result of these efforts, racial/ethnic background, socioeconomic characteristics, access to high-quality cancer care, and psychological and social factors have emerged as important determinants

C. H. Halbert (✉)
University of Southern California, California, CA, USA
e-mail: hughesha@usc.edu

C. Hughes Halbert (ed.), *Cancer Health Disparities*,
https://doi.org/10.1007/978-3-031-37638-2_1

of cancer health disparities. This comparative work has been foundational for cancer health disparities research [2]; these first-generation studies laid the groundwork for this research to evolve into a transdisciplinary field that includes basic, clinical, and population-based researchers who collaborate to understand, prevent, and treat cancers among disparity populations that are defined based on race/ethnicity, socioeconomic resources, geographic location, and other variables that shape and influence the health-care experiences in the United States.

The evolution of cancer health disparities from descriptive investigations to transdisciplinary and translational studies has had a profound impact on how research in this area is conducted. For instance, early efforts to address cancer control strategies among disparity populations were developed to address cancer risk behaviors by targeting health beliefs and attitudes using health behavior theories (e.g., the health belief model, theory of reasoned action, and social networks) to guide the development and delivery of intervention content and strategies. However, limited progress and persistent disparities in cancer risk and outcomes among disparity populations and individuals from other medically underserved populations raised questions about the impact and relevance of these theory-based interventions. As a result, community-based participatory research (CBPR) is now recognized as a critical framework for developing, implementing, and evaluating cancer control interventions [4]; several academic-community partnerships have been established to enhance health promotion and disease prevention behaviors in disparity populations and medically underserved groups [5–7]. Many initiatives in cancer health disparities research now require that active and meaningful patient and community engagement be a focus of the research strategy. Relatedly, precision medicine and precision population health emphasize the translation of data on multilevel factors (e.g., biological, behavioral, and social characteristics) into personalized approaches; efforts are now being made to develop strategies and models for precision cancer prevention that emphasize equity and diversity [8].

Transdisciplinary research in cancer health disparities has created important opportunities to examine novel hypotheses that have the potential to transform cancer care delivery and research and enhance outcomes in all groups, especially those from disparity populations. Transdisciplinary and translational research is critical to cancer health equity; the development of novel concepts and methods during the past decade has been instrumental in transforming the scope and focus of translational research in cancer health disparities. For instance, genetic ancestry is now being integrated into basic science research in cancer health disparities to improve the precision of risk estimates and enable greater prediction of responses to treatment [9, 10]. Similarly, RNA sequence analysis is now being used to understand racial differences in cellular stress responses and molecular profiles among African American and white men undergoing prostate biopsy [11]. While these types of translational studies have traditionally focused on moving basic science discoveries into clinical care, recent reports emphasize the need to also translate these findings into population and public health practice [12], and key principles of basic science methods and approaches are being integrated into other disciplines. For instance, translational behavioral science research is now being conducted to examine the nature, distribution, and impact of stress reactivity among African American breast and prostate cancer patients [13–15]. Consistent with this, conceptual models of minority health and cancer health disparities now emphasize the importance of understanding and addressing multilevel determinants of cancer health disparities. Multilevel interventions are defined as those that address at least two levels of influence [16], and these types of interventions are being developed to target factors at the individual, community, health-care system, and sociopolitical levels to enhance cancer health equity [17] across the entire continuum from early detection, prevention, and treatment and cross-cutting issues that include recruitment and retention into clinical trials, biospecimens resources, and population-based research.

The first step to developing multilevel interventions, however, is to understand the contribution and effect of multilevel determinants within the context of cancer sites for which there are disparities in disease risk and outcomes. The Transdisciplinary Collaborative Center (TCC) in Precision Medicine and Minority Men's Health, for example, was designed to understand and address multilevel determinants of cancer health disparities among African American men using the principles of community-based participatory research and conceptual models of minority health and health disparities [14]. This TCC was developed based on previous research which demonstrated that (1) cancer is a priority for health promotion and disease prevention among African American men and women [7], (2) African American men are not likely to believe that they are at increased risk for developing prostate cancer despite African ancestry being an established risk factor for disease [18], and (3) empirical data showing that vitamin D supplementation may improve clinical outcomes among men who are diagnosed with low-risk disease [19]. Importantly, this TCC was established during a time of increased national coverage of the toxic social stressors (e.g., police violence, gun shootings) that African Americans experience as a result of systemic racism and discrimination. Based on previous conceptual frameworks and definitions of allostatic load [20] and studies showing racial differences in allostatic load [21], this TCC was designed to understand the association between allostatic load and disease processes and outcomes among clinically and racially diverse men [14]. Patient and community engagement was a requirement of the TCC consortium; therefore, CBPR provided the overarching framework to guide the research focus, study methods, and outreach and education strategies that were used to accomplish the specific aims of the center while engaging diverse stakeholders in the research activities and disseminating findings to community residents and other groups [14]. This TCC is one example of how transdisciplinary frameworks of minority health and health disparities were used to guide the objectives and methods in multilevel cancer health disparities research. This chapter uses conceptual models of minority health and cancer health disparities to describe multilevel determinants that are important to disparities, summarize key issues in examining these issues as part of transdisciplinary and translational research, and identify priorities for future research and opportunities to address these factors and enhance cancer health equity.

Multilevel Determinants of Cancer Health Disparities

Health-care System Factors Health-care systems, including those that are located in community settings, play a critical role in providing cancer care services that include screening tests and cancer treatment. As such, health-care systems and providers are important to cancer-related outcomes among all populations; reduced access to cancer care is a well-documented determinant of disparities [2]. Access to care has been conceptualized mostly in terms of health insurance coverage; however, access is multifactorial and is influenced by patient decisions to accept or decline cancer care services and treatment based on their beliefs, values, and preferences, if the services are easy or difficult to use, and if individuals can get to the facilities where care is offered. [22, 23] Recent research conducted by Halbert and colleagues illustrates the complexity of access to care. For instance, as part of demonstration study that was funded by the AHRQ to enhance the dissemination and implementation of evidence-based interventions for obesity prevention and reduction into primary care, this team found that 71% of obese or overweight primary care patients reported that they were ready to lose or manage their weight and 56% were confident in their ability to manage their weight. While 59% of these participants reported receiving provider advice to lose weight (e.g., ever advised by their provider to lose/manage weight) [24, 25], there was a disconnect between the level of support for obesity risk reduction and management that patients want and need and the resources and capacity that are available in primary care practices. That is to say, patients wanted intensive monitoring and ongoing support for behavioral risk management, but these resources were not readily available in the practice [26]. Further, providers reported that patients should have greater accountability for their own self-management [26].

Given the importance of health insurance status, considerable efforts have been made to increase health insurance coverage, and these efforts have had some beneficial outcomes. Following implementation of the Affordable Care Act (ACA), there were decreases in rates of being uninsured and in racial differences in health insurance coverage [27, 28]. Despite this, individuals from disparity populations who had private insurance coverage continue to have lower confidence in their ability to pay for medical costs and were less likely to have a usual source of care compared to whites [29]. Financial toxicity is a significant challenge among cancer patients [30], and financial strain is a barrier to health care regardless of one's personal history of disease. Recent research has shown that 36% of men who have access to high care through the Veterans Health Administration health-care system report financial strain [31]. The quality of cancer care services is also important to cancer health disparities. Quality metrics are based on whether or not patients receive screening and treatment according to guidelines; previous research has shown that the source of health insurance coverage plays an important role in receiving quality care. Patients who have Medicaid or no insurance may receive lower-quality care for many forms of cancer relative to patients who have private health insurance [32].

Environmental and Community Factors Environmental characteristics are now being recognized as important to cancer health disparities. Environmental factors have been conceptualized in different ways; the geographic location where individuals live is a fundamental component of the environment. This is because decisions about early detection, prevention, and cancer treatment are made within the general social, psychological, and behavioral context of an individual's life and community. Residency in a particular geographic region has implications for the types of cancer care services that individuals are able to access, the policies that govern when and how services are obtained, and the resources that exist for health promotion and disease control. Data are emerging on the association between geographic factors and cancer risk; for instance, Zeigler-Johnson et al. [33–35] found that census level neighborhood characteristics and self-reported socioeconomic factors were associated with the prostate cancer risk among African American and white prostate cancer patients. Specifically, greater neighborhood deprivation was associated with more aggressive disease among African American and white prostate cancer patients, but this association was most pronounced among African American men [34]. Similarly, studies in community-based samples of African Americans have shown that perceptions of the social environment (e.g., collective efficacy and neighborhood satisfaction) are associated significantly with decisions about cancer screening and adherence to recommendations for diet and physical activity [36, 37]. Recent work conducted by Babatunde et al. demonstrate that African American and white prostate cancer survivors differ in terms of living in geographic areas that have high social deprivation [38]. In a retrospective cohort of breast cancer patients, Babatunde and colleagues also found that greater social deprivation was associated with being diagnosed with a distant stage of diease [39]. African American race and being unmarried were also associated significantly with stage of higher stage of disease in this cohort [39].

Environmental factors also include the pollutants and carcinogens to which individuals are exposed based on where they live and work; geospatial methods are now being used to understand how these aspects of the built environment contribute to cancer risk, access to cancer control, and treatment outcomes [40–42]. However, perceptions of where one lives, and not just the geographic location and environmental exposures in these areas, are also important to cancer control behaviors among disparity populations. African Americans residents in a metropolitan area who reported greater collective efficacy were more likely to meet recommended guidelines for physical activity/diet relative to those who reported lower collective efficacy [43]. Similarly, African American smokers who reported more problems in their neighborhood and greater neighborhood vigilance had a higher likelihood for tobacco dependence [44].

Social Factors Social determinants are now recognized as being critical to cancer risk and outcomes. Social determinants of health (SDOH) are important to cancer health disparities because they reflect where and how care is delivered and the extent to which patients are able to manage acute and chronic conditions using community, clinical, and public health resources [45, 46]. Race and ethnicity are among the most important SDOHs of cancer care and outcomes in the United States; collecting race/ethnicity data and evaluating differences in cancer risk factors and outcomes based these variables is necessary, but not sufficient for identifying determinants and addressing these factors to improve outcomes and reduce disparities. More recent conceptual frameworks of SDOH include social isolation, financial stain, perceived stress, and geographic factors along existing variables such as race/ethnicity and health insurance coverage [47]. The CMS and other professional organizations now endorse the assessment of SDOHs among patients; the Institute of Medicine recommends that patients be asked about their education, income, marital status, stress levels, and financial strain as part of health care delivery [48]. Efforts have also been made to develop standardized tools to obtain this information from patients as part of research protocols [49] and clinical care [50], screen patients for social risk factors, and provide support to address unmet social needs. The empirical basis for screening patients for social risk factors is growing; recent research has shown that cancer control interventions may have limited effectiveness among patients who have unmet basic needs (e.g., housing, food insecurity) [51, 52].

Behavioral Factors Early detection, avoidance of cancer risk behaviors (e.g., cigarette smoking), and obtaining cancer treatment early are among the behavioral strategies that are important for reducing cancer morbidity and mortality in all populations. Despite this, many adults, especially those from racial/ethnic minority groups and other disparity populations, do not meet the recommended guidelines for healthy eating, are physically inactive, and smoke cigarettes [53]. For instance, Halbert et al. found that only 49% of African Americans in a community-based sample met the recommended guidelines for physical activity [43]. Similarly, only 34% of prostate cancer survivors in a retrospective cohort met recommended guidelines for moderate intensity physical activity [54]. Several interventions have been developed to enhance cancer control behaviors among disparity populations; this work has used community-based participatory approaches to develop and evaluate evidence-based interventions [55], applied patient navigation to address individual-level barriers to early detection and treatment [56, 57], and examined the effects of culturally-tailored interventions [58, 59]. Similarly, health beliefs and social factors have been addressed as part of theory-based interventions that were deployed in faith-based organizations [60] and community-based samples [55]. However, the effects of these health behavior change and cancer control interventions have been mixed. For instance, while there were small increases in the proportion of African Americans who met the recommended guidelines for physical activity in a recent comparative effectiveness trial, there were no differences in the proportion of residents who met the guidelines for vegetable intake between those who received integrated and standard risk education [55]. Similarly, previous research has shown that the effects of tailored letters about breast and cervical cancer screening are comparable to generic letters in terms of increasing mammography and Pap testing among low-income and minority women who are past due for these screening tests [61].

Biological Factors Following completion of the Human Genome Project, there has been a significant interest in understanding the association between cancer health disparities and biological factors. In addition to understanding the contribution of germline mutations in susceptibility genes, studies are now being conducted to identify molecular and genetic pathways that are important to the initiation and progression of disease. For instance, Hardiman and colleagues found that African American and white men differed in terms of their inflammatory and immune signatures using RNA sequence analysis [62]. Prostate tissue specimens from African American men were found to have overexpression of genes related to inflammatory processes. In other work, Davis et al. found that African American breast cancer patients had a greater proportion of DARC/ACKR1-negative tumors compared to white patients [63]. DARC/ACKR1 regulates immune responses; tumors that were positive for DARC/ACKR1 had a different immune response compared to those that were DARC/ACKR1 negative. Recent work has also shown an association between African ancestry and immunological profiles in an international cohort of African and African American women with triple negative breast cancer [64].

A Call to Action for Cancer Health Equity and Future Directions

The field of cancer health disparities research is at a critical juncture that is reflected in the movement from descriptive studies that characterized racial differences in cancer risk and outcomes to research that is designed to identify risk factors with greater precision. This evolution is due in part to the development of conceptual models and that describes multilevel determinants and ongoing efforts to improve their applicability and relevance to diverse groups. The Centers for Population Health and Health Disparities Model, for instance, was developed to identify and address disparities in cancer and cardiovascular disease and describe proximal, intermediate, and distal factors that span from biological to environmental characteristics [65]. More recently, the four levels of the socioecological model were expanded across five domains of influence (biological, behavioral, physical/built environment, sociocultural environment, and health-care system) using a life course perspective in the National Institute on Minority Health and Health Disparities Research Framework [34]. In addition to increasing the precision of these multilevel frameworks to reflect the mechanisms through which sociopolitical factors are linked with disparities in cancer risk and outcomes [66] and to guide research in specific domains (e.g., health-care systems) [67], these conceptual models highlight mechanisms, processes, and outcomes that are relevant to multiple drivers in cancer health disparities research.

For instance, stress and stress responses have been implicated as mechanisms that contribute to the initiation of cancer in animal studies [68], increase exposure to cancer risk behaviors (e.g., tobacco use and risk for relapse following cessation) [69], and reflect aspects of the sociopolitical environment that has implications for physical and mental exposures and barriers to health-care quality and access (e.g., structural racism, discrimination). Similarly, allostatic load was described several years ago as an indicator of biological dysregulation in response to psychological and social stress and has been used as a unifying framework to understand the ways in which physiological processes affect health outcomes [70–74]. Allostatic load was used as the overarching construct and focus in the TCC developed by Halbert and colleagues because it reflected the physiological consequences of upstream level determinants (e.g., structural racism and discrimination) and while also enabling examination and integration of biomarker data within and between organ sites for diseases that disproportionately affect minority men in terms of morbidity and mortality (e.g., prostate cancer, hypertension, diabetes). Consistent with this, recent reports have described allostatic load as a multidimensional factor that can be used to integrate and understand the effects of structural inequality due to multilevel determinants that include behavioral, social, and environmental factors [75]. However, research on allostatic load within the context of cancer health disparities is at an early stage; studies are just now beginning to characterize allostatic load in samples of cancer patients [76, 77] and individuals undergoing diagnostic procedures and treatment for cancer [78]. Continued efforts are needed to explore novel scientific questions and hypotheses about allostatic load as a biomarker of the effects of structural inequality and to identify the underlying biological pathways through which allostatic load and other stress responses contribute to cancer health disparities. Further, additional research is needed to identify the mechanisms through which psychological and social stressors influence cellular responses that are involved in the initiation and progression of disease and response to treatment among disparity populations [14] to build the evidence base about stress and stress responses as primary drivers of cancer risk and risk behaviors, disease initiation, and response to treatment among disparity populations.

This is also an important time in cancer health disparities research to continue to make progress in the methods that are used to characterize determinants of cancer risk and outcomes among disparity populations. For instance, the challenges and limitations associated with using self-reported races (SRR) in health services research and cancer health disparities have been described previously [79]. As a result of recent advances in genetic sciences, it is now possible to use genetic ancestry information to increase the precision of examining racial differences in biological mechanisms that are involved in the cancer process among diverse groups. This work is exciting and important, but the contribution of genetic factors has to be placed and prioritized within the context of the overarching health-care system, community, social, psychological, and behavioral factors. Following the police killing of George Floyd, considerable efforts have been made to increase the measurement of structural racism through funding supported by the National Institutes of Health. Relatedly, several place-based measures (e.g., redlining, segregation) have been described to characterize the distribution and impact of structural racism using geospatial methods [80]; epidemiological studies are now being conducted to integrate these approaches to understand cancer risk and outcomes in disparity populations. For instance, with funding from the National Cancer Institute, Cheng and colleagues will use data from two large cohorts to examine the associations between structural racism and smoking behaviors, lung cancer risk, and DNA methylation in blood leukocytes [81]. The examination of structural racism in current studies builds on previous investigations that explored the association between racial discrimination and cancer risk behaviors (e.g., cigarette smoking) and other outcomes; thus, it will be important for this research and other studies to build upon the existing evidence and generate new findings that can be used to guide the development of equity-focused interventions.

There continues to be a pressing need to translate findings on multilevel determinants of cancer health disparities into evidence-based equity-focused interventions. Equity-focused interventions are those that provide information, resources, and services that meet the specific needs of disparity populations. Multilevel interventions have an important role to play in addressing determinants across multiple levels of influence; there is considerable expectation that these approaches will enhance cancer equity because they are designed to address key drivers of disparities across individual, interpersonal, community, and health-care system levels. As data on the effects of multilevel interventions are being generated, it is important to acknowledge that all cancer care, including strategies and services for prevention, treatment, and control, occur within the overall context of an individual's life and circumstances. Accordingly, the effectiveness of interventions will be shaped by these factors. For instance, recent research has shown that after controlling for neighborhood socioeconomic status, genetic ancestry no longer had a significant association with all-cause mortality among African Americans enrolled in the Prostate, Lung, and Ovarian Cancer study [82]. Consistent with this, previous and ongoing efforts to integrate the community context into cancer health disparities research have used participatory strategies to engage diverse stakeholders in research efforts [7], and multilevel interventions are now being developed and evaluated to address multiple contexts simultaneously [83]. In light of emerging evidence about the impact of social risk factors on cancer treatment [84, 85] and the ability of unmet social needs to reduce the impact of cancer control interventions [52], greater efforts are needed to address social determinants of cancer risk and outcomes among disparity populations as part of equity-focused interventions. The Social and Health Care Integration Framework [86] was developed to guide the integration of social care into health-care systems. As we envision health-care systems that are able to address upstream level determinants through policies, programs, and practices, now is the time to focus on understanding how social care can be integrated into all domains of cancer care to achieve equity in disease risk and outcomes among disparity groups.

References

1. Siegel RL, Miller KD, Fuchs HE, Jemal A. Cancer statistics, 2022. CA Cancer J Clin. 2022;72:7–33. https://doi.org/10.3322/caac.21708.
2. American Association for Cancer Research. CancerDisparitiesProgressReport.org [Internet]. Philadelphia: American Association for Cancer Research; ©2022 [December 2022]. Available from http://www.CancerDisparitiesProgressReport.org/.
3. Thomas SB, Quinn SC, Butler J, Fryer CS, Garza MA. Toward a fourth generation of disparities research to achieve health equity. Annu Rev Public Health. 2011;32:399–416. https://doi.org/10.1146/annurev-publhealth-031210-101136.
4. Israel BA, Lichtenstein R, Lantz P, et al. The Detroit community-academic urban research center: development, implementation, and evaluation. J Public Health Manag Pract. 2001;7:1–19. https://doi.org/10.1097/00124784-200107050-00003.
5. Harvey I, Schulz A, Israel B, et al. The Healthy Connections project: a community-based participatory research project involving women at risk for diabetes and hypertension. Prog Community Health Partnersh. 2009;3:287–300. https://doi.org/10.1353/cpr.0.0088.
6. Schulz AJ, Israel BA, Coombe CM, et al. A community-based participatory planning process and multilevel intervention design: toward eliminating cardiovascular health inequities. Health Promot Pract. 2011;12:900–11. https://doi.org/10.1177/1524839909359156.
7. Weathers B, Barg FK, Bowman M, et al. Using a mixed-methods approach to identify health concerns in an African American community. Am J Public Health. 2011;101:2087–92. https://doi.org/10.2105/ajph.2010.191775.
8. Butler EN, Umar A, Heckman-Stoddard BM, Kundrod KA, Signorello LB, Castle PE. Redefining precision cancer prevention to promote health equity. Trends Cancer. 2022;8:295–302. https://doi.org/10.1016/j.trecan.2022.01.009.
9. Bonham VL, Green ED, Pérez-Stable EJ. Examining how race, ethnicity, and ancestry data are used in biomedical research. JAMA. 2018;16(320):1533–4. https://doi.org/10.1001/jama.2018.13609.
10. Borrell LN, Elhawary JR, Fuentes-Afflick E, et al. Race and genetic ancestry in medicine – a time for reckoning with racism. N Engl J Med. 2021;384(5):474–80. https://doi.org/10.1056/NEJMms2029562.
11. Hardiman G, Savage SJ, Hazard ES, et al. A systems approach to interrogate gene expression patterns in African American men presenting with clinically localized prostate cancer. Cancers (Basel). 2021;13:13. https://doi.org/10.3390/cancers13205143.
12. Dankwa-Mullan I, Rhee KB, Stoff DM, et al. Moving toward paradigm-shifting research in health disparities through translational, transformational, and transdisciplinary approaches. Am J Public Health. 2010;100:S19–24. https://doi.org/10.2105/ajph.2009.189167.
13. Halbert CH, Allen CG. Basic behavioral science research priorities in minority health and health disparities. Transl Behav Med. 2021;11:2033–42. https://doi.org/10.1093/tbm/ibab143.
14. Halbert CH, Allen CG, Jefferson M, et al. Lessons learned from the Medical University of South Carolina Transdisciplinary Collaborative Center (TCC) in precision medicine and minority men's health. Am J Mens Health. 2020;14:1557988320979236. https://doi.org/10.1177/1557988320979236.
15. Halbert CH, Jefferson MS, Danielson C, Froeliger B, Giordano A, Thaxton JE. An observational study and randomized trial of stress reactivity in cancer disparities. Health Psychol. 2020;39(9):745–57. https://doi.org/10.1037/hea0000882.
16. Agurs-Collins T, Persky S, Paskett ED, et al. Designing and assessing multilevel interventions to improve minority health and reduce health disparities. Am J Public Health. 2019;109:S86–s93. https://doi.org/10.2105/ajph.2018.304730.
17. Paskett E, Thompson B, Ammerman AS, Ortega AN, Marsteller J, Richardson D. Multilevel interventions to address health disparities show promise in improving population health. Health Aff. 2016;35:1429–34. https://doi.org/10.1377/hlthaff.2015.1360.

18. Rice LJ, Jefferson M, Briggs V, et al. Discordance in perceived risk and epidemiological outcomes of prostate cancer among African American men. Prev Med Rep. 2017;7:1–6. https://doi.org/10.1016/j.pmedr.2017.04.010.
19. Marshall DT, Savage SJ, Garrett-Mayer E, et al. Vitamin D3 supplementation at 4000 international units per day for one year results in a decrease of positive cores at repeat biopsy in subjects with low-risk prostate cancer under active surveillance. J Clin Endocrinol Metab. 2012;97:2315–24. https://doi.org/10.1210/jc.2012-1451.
20. Seeman T, Epel E, Gruenewald T, Karlamangla A, McEwen BS. Socio-economic differentials in peripheral biology: cumulative allostatic load. Ann N Y Acad Sci. 2010;1186:223–39. https://doi.org/10.1111/j.1749-6632.2009.05341.x.
21. Duru OK, Harawa NT, Kermah D, Norris KC. Allostatic load burden and racial disparities in mortality. J Natl Med Assoc. 2012;104:89–95. https://doi.org/10.1016/s0027-9684(15)30120-6.
22. Saurman E. Improving access: modifying Penchansky and Thomas's Theory of Access. J Health Serv Res Policy. 2015;21:36. https://doi.org/10.1177/1355819615600001.
23. Penchansky R, Thomas JW. The concept of access: definition and relationship to consumer satisfaction. Med Care. 1981;19(2):127–40. https://doi.org/10.1097/00005650-198102000-00001.
24. Halbert CH, Jefferson M, Melvin CL, Rice L, Chukwuka KM. Provider advice about weight loss in a primary care sample of obese and overweight patients. J Prim Care Community Health. 2017;8:239–46. https://doi.org/10.1177/2150131917715336.
25. Halbert CH, Jefferson M, Nemeth L, et al. Weight loss attempts in a racially diverse sample of primary care patients. Prev Med Rep. 2018;10:167–71. https://doi.org/10.1016/j.pmedr.2017.11.009.
26. Nemeth LS, Rice LJ, Potts M, Melvin C, Jefferson M, Hughes-Halbert C. Priorities and preferences for weight management and cardiovascular risk reduction in primary care. Fam Community Health. 2017;40:245–52. https://doi.org/10.1097/fch.0000000000000155.
27. Crowley RA, Bornstein SS. Improving the patient protection and affordable care act's insurance coverage provisions: a position paper from the American College of Physicians. Ann Intern Med. 2019;170(9):651–3. https://doi.org/10.7326/M18-3401.
28. Artiga S, Orgera K, Damico A. Health coverage by race and ethnicity, 2010–2019. Kaiser Family Foundation; 2021. Available at: https://www.kff.org/racial-equity-and-health-policy/issue-brief/health-coverage-by-race-and-ethnicity/.
29. Artiga S, Young K, Garfield R, Majerol M. Racial and ethnic disparities in access to and utilization of care among insured adults. Kaiser Family Foundation; 2015. Available at: https://files.kff.org/attachment/issue-brief-racial-and-ethnic-disparities-in-access-to-and-utilization-of-care-among-insured-adults.
30. National Cancer Institute. Financial Toxicity and Cancer Treatment (PDQ®)–Health Professional Version. Available at: https://www.cancer.gov/about-cancer/managing-care/track-care-costs/financial-toxicity-hp-pdq
31. Bauer AG, Jefferson M, Nahhas GJ, et al. Financial toxicity and strain among men receiving prostate cancer care in an equal access healthcare system. Cancer Med. 2020;9:8765–71. https://doi.org/10.1002/cam4.3484.
32. Parikh-Patel A, Morris CR, Kizer KW. Disparities in quality of cancer care: the role of health insurance and population demographics. Medicine (Baltimore). 2017;96:e9125. https://doi.org/10.1097/md.0000000000009125.
33. Zeigler-Johnson C, Morales KH, Glanz K, Spangler E, Mitchell J, Rebbeck TR. Individual- and neighborhood-level education influences the effect of obesity on prostate cancer treatment failure after prostatectomy. Cancer Causes Control. 2015;26:1329–37.
34. Zeigler-Johnson CM, Tierney A, Rebbeck TR, Rundle A. Prostate cancer severity associations with neighborhood deprivation. Prostate Cancer. 2011;2011:846263. https://doi.org/10.1155/2011/846263.
35. McIntire RK, Keith SW, Boamah M, Leader AE, Glanz K, Klassen AC, Zeigler-Johnson CM. A prostate cancer composite score to identify high burden neighborhoods. Prev Med. 2018;112:47–53. https://doi.org/10.1016/j.ypmed.2018.04.003.

36. Halbert CH, Bellamy S, Briggs V, et al. Collective efficacy and obesity-related health behaviors in a community sample of African Americans. J Community Health. 2014;39(1):124–31.
37. Halbert CH, Melvin C, Briggs V, et al. Neighborhood satisfaction and colorectal cancer screening in a community sample of African Americans. J Community Health. 2015;1–8:38.
38. Babatunde OA, Pearce JL, Jefferson MS, et al. Racial distribution of neighborhood-level social deprivation in a retrospective cohort of prostate cancer survivors. Diseases. 2022;10:10. https://doi.org/10.3390/diseases10040075.
39. Babatunde OA, Zahnd WE, Eberth JM, et al. Association between neighborhood social deprivation and stage at diagnosis among breast cancer patients in South Carolina. Int J Environ Res Public Health. 2021;18(22). https://doi.org/10.3390/ijerph182211824.
40. Erhunmwunsee L, Wing SE, Shen J, et al. The association between polluted neighborhoods and TP53-mutated non-small cell lung cancer. Cancer Epidemiol Biomark Prev. 2021;30(8):1498–505. https://doi.org/10.1158/1055-9965.Epi-20-1555.
41. Letellier N, Wing SE, Yang JA, et al. The role of neighborhood air pollution exposure on somatic non-small cell lung cancer mutations in the Los Angeles basin (2013–2018). Int J Environ Res Public Health. 2022;19. https://doi.org/10.3390/ijerph191711027.
42. Sosa E, D'Souza G, Akhtar A, et al. Racial and socioeconomic disparities in lung cancer screening in the United States: a systematic review. CA Cancer J Clin. 2021;71:299–314. https://doi.org/10.3322/caac.21671.
43. Halbert CH, Bellamy S, Briggs V, et al. Collective efficacy and obesity-related health behaviors in a community sample of African Americans. J Community Health. 2014;39:124–31. https://doi.org/10.1007/s10900-013-9748-z.
44. Reitzel LR, Vidrine JI, Businelle MS, et al. Neighborhood perceptions are associated with tobacco dependence among African American smokers. Nicotine Tob Res. 2012;14:786–93. https://doi.org/10.1093/ntr/ntr285.
45. Braveman P, Gottlieb L. The social determinants of health: it's time to consider the causes of the causes. Public Health Rep. 2014;129:19–31. https://doi.org/10.1177/00333549141291s206.
46. Adler NE, Glymour MM, Fielding J. Addressing social determinants of health and health inequalities. JAMA. 2016;316:1641–2. https://doi.org/10.1001/jama.2016.14058.
47. Javed Z, Haisum Maqsood M, Yahya T, et al. Race, racism, and cardiovascular health: applying a social determinants of health framework to racial/ethnic disparities in cardiovascular disease. Circ Cardiovasc Qual Outcomes. 2022;15:e007917. https://doi.org/10.1161/circoutcomes.121.007917.
48. Institute of Medicine. Capturing social and behavioral domains and measures in electronic health records: phase 2. The National Academies Press; 2014. p. 374.
49. Hamilton CM, Strader LC, Pratt JG, et al. The PhenX Toolkit: get the most from your measures. Am J Epidemiol. 2011;174(3):253–60. [Social determinants of health collection available at: https://www.phenxtoolkit.org/collections/view/6] https://doi.org/10.1093/aje/kwr193.
50. Centers for Medicare and Medicaid. The accountable health communities health-related social needs screening tool. Available at: https://innovation.cms.gov/files/worksheets/ahcm-screeningtool.pdf
51. Kreuter MW, McQueen A, Boyum S, Fu Q. Unmet basic needs and health intervention effectiveness in low-income populations. Prev Med. 2016;91:70–5. https://doi.org/10.1016/j.ypmed.2016.08.006.
52. Cappelletti ER, Kreuter MW, Boyum S, Thompson T. Basic needs, stress and the effects of tailored health communication in vulnerable populations. Health Educ Res. 2015;30:591–8. https://doi.org/10.1093/her/cyv033.
53. American Cancer Society. Cancer prevention & early detection facts & figures tables and figures 2022. Atlanta: American Cancer Society; 2022.
54. Halbert CH, Jefferson MS, Drake R, et al. Social and clinical determinants of physical activity in prostate cancer survivors. Support Care Cancer. 2021;29:459–65. https://doi.org/10.1007/s00520-020-05482-1.

55. Halbert CH, Bellamy S, Briggs V, et al. A comparative effectiveness education trial for lifestyle health behavior change in African Americans. Health Educ Res. 2017;32:207–18. https://doi.org/10.1093/her/cyx039.
56. Graboyes EM, Sterba KR, Li H, et al. Development and evaluation of a navigation-based, multilevel intervention to improve the delivery of timely, guideline-adherent adjuvant therapy for patients with head and neck cancer. JCO Oncol Pract. 2021;17:e1512–23. https://doi.org/10.1200/op.20.00943.
57. Ko NY, Snyder FR, Raich PC, et al. Racial and ethnic differences in patient navigation: results from the Patient Navigation Research Program. Cancer. 2016;122:2715–22. https://doi.org/10.1002/cncr.30109.
58. Halbert CH, Kessler L, Troxel AB, Stopfer JE, Domchek S. Effect of genetic counseling and testing for BRCA1 and BRCA2 mutations in African American women: a randomized trial. Public Health Genomics. 2010;13:440–8. https://doi.org/10.1159/000293990.
59. Kreuter MW, Sugg-Skinner C, Holt CL, et al. Cultural tailoring for mammography and fruit and vegetable intake among low-income African-American women in urban public health centers. Prev Med. 2005;41:53–62. https://doi.org/10.1016/j.ypmed.2004.10.013.
60. Resnicow K, Jackson A, Wang T, et al. A motivational interviewing intervention to increase fruit and vegetable intake through Black churches: results of the eat for life trial. Am J Public Health. 2001;91:1686–93. https://doi.org/10.2105/ajph.91.10.1686.
61. Jibaja-Weiss ML, Volk RJ, Kingery P, Smith QW, Holcomb JD. Tailored messages for breast and cervical cancer screening of low-income and minority women using medical records data. Patient Educ Couns. 2003;50:123–32. https://doi.org/10.1016/s0738-3991(02)00119-2.
62. Hardiman G, Savage SJ, Hazard ES, et al. Systems analysis of the prostate transcriptome in African-American men compared with European-American men. Pharmacogenomics. 2016;17:1129–43. https://doi.org/10.2217/pgs-2016-0025.
63. Jenkins BD, Martini RN, Hire R, et al. Atypical chemokine receptor 1 (DARC/ACKR1) in breast tumors is associated with survival, circulating chemokines, tumor-infiltrating immune cells, and African ancestry. Cancer Epidemiol Biomark Prev. 2019;28:690–700. https://doi.org/10.1158/1055-9965.Epi-18-0955.
64. Martini R, Delpe P, Chu TR, et al. African ancestry-associated gene expression profiles in triple-negative breast cancer underlie altered tumor biology and clinical outcome in women of African descent. Cancer Discov. 2022;12:2530–51. https://doi.org/10.1158/2159-8290.Cd-22-0138.
65. Warnecke RB, Oh A, Breen N, et al. Approaching health disparities from a population perspective: the National Institutes of Health Centers for Population Health and Health Disparities. Am J Public Health. 2008;98:1608–15. https://doi.org/10.2105/ajph.2006.102525.
66. Linnenbringer E, Gehlert S, Geronimus AT. Black-white disparities in breast cancer subtype: the intersection of socially patterned stress and genetic expression. AIMS Public Health. 2017;4:526–56. https://doi.org/10.3934/publichealth.2017.5.526.
67. Kilbourne AM, Switzer G, Hyman K, Crowley-Matoka M, Fine MJ. Advancing health disparities research within the health care system: a conceptual framework. Am J Public Health. 2006;96:2113–21. https://doi.org/10.2105/ajph.2005.077628.
68. Hermes GL, Delgado B, Tretiakova M, et al. Social isolation dysregulates endocrine and behavioral stress while increasing malignant burden of spontaneous mammary tumors. Proc Natl Acad Sci U S A. 2009;106:22393–8. https://doi.org/10.1073/pnas.0910753106.
69. U.S. National Cancer Institute. A socioecological approach to addressing tobacco-related health disparities. National Cancer Institute Tobacco Control Monograph 22. NIH Publication No. 17-CA-8035A. Bethesda: U.S. Department of Health and Human Services, National Institutes of Health, National Cancer Institute; 2017.
70. Juster RP, McEwen BS, Lupien SJ. Allostatic load biomarkers of chronic stress and impact on health and cognition. Neurosci Biobehav Rev. 2010;35:2–16. https://doi.org/10.1016/j.neubiorev.2009.10.002.

71. McEwen BS. Stress, adaptation, and disease. Allostasis and allostatic load. Ann N Y Acad Sci. 1998;840:33–44.
72. McEwen BS. Biomarkers for assessing population and individual health and disease related to stress and adaptation. Metab Clin Exp. 2015;64:S2–S10. https://doi.org/10.1016/j.metabol.2014.10.029.
73. McEwen BS, Gianaros PJ. Central role of the brain in stress and adaptation: links to socioeconomic status, health, and disease. Ann N Y Acad Sci. 2010;1186:190–222. https://doi.org/10.1111/j.1749-6632.2009.05331.x.
74. Logan JG, Barksdale DJ. Allostasis and allostatic load: expanding the discourse on stress and cardiovascular disease. J Clin Nurs. 2008;17(7b):201–8.
75. Obeng-Gyasi S, Tarver W, Carlos RC, Andersen BL. Allostatic load: a framework to understand breast cancer outcomes in Black women. NPJ Breast Cancer. 2021;7:100. https://doi.org/10.1038/s41523-021-00309-6.
76. Xing CY, Doose M, Qin B, et al. Pre-diagnostic allostatic load and health-related quality of life in a cohort of Black breast cancer survivors. Breast Cancer Res Treat. 2020;184:901–14. https://doi.org/10.1007/s10549-020-05901-1.
77. Parente V, Hale L, Palermo T. Association between breast cancer and allostatic load by race: National Health and Nutrition Examination Survey 1999–2008. Psychooncology. 2013;22(3):621–8. https://doi.org/10.1002/pon.3044.
78. Halbert CH, Jefferson M, Ambrose L, Caulder S, Savage SJ. Resiliency and allostatic load among Veterans at risk for adverse prostate cancer outcomes. Ethn Dis. 2020;30:177–84. https://doi.org/10.18865/ed.30.S1.177.
79. Rebbeck TR, Halbert CH, Sankar P. Genetics, epidemiology, and cancer disparities: is it black and white? J Clin Oncol. 2006;24:2164–9. https://doi.org/10.1200/jco.2005.05.1656.
80. Dean LT, Thorpe RJ. What structural racism is (or is not) and how to measure it: clarity for public health and medical researchers. Am J Epidemiol. 2022;191:1521–6. https://doi.org/10.1093/aje/kwac112.
81. Cheng IC. Understanding the role of structural racism on racial/ethnic inequities in lung cancer risk. Available at: https://reporter.nih.gov/search/jv_4LEb4XE-1_nD2cXWTqg/project-details/10450374
82. Iyer HS, Gomez SL, Cheng I, Rebbeck TR. Relative impact of genetic ancestry and neighborhood socioeconomic status on all-cause mortality in self-identified African Americans. PLoS One. 2022;17:e0273735. https://doi.org/10.1371/journal.pone.0273735.
83. Paskett ED, Pennell ML, Ruffin MT, et al. A multi-level model to understand cervical cancer disparities in Appalachia. Cancer Prev Res. 2020;13:223–8. https://doi.org/10.1158/1940-6207.Capr-19-0239.
84. Raber M, Jackson A, Basen-Engquist K, et al. Food insecurity among people with cancer: nutritional needs as an essential component of care. J Natl Cancer Inst. 2022;114:1577. https://doi.org/10.1093/jnci/djac135.
85. Fan Q, Keene DE, Banegas MP, et al. Housing insecurity among patients with cancer. J Natl Cancer Inst. 2022;114:1584. https://doi.org/10.1093/jnci/djac136.
86. The National Academies of Sciences, Engineering, and Medicine. Integrating social care into the delivery of health care: moving upstream to improve the nation's health. The National Academies Press; 2019. p. 194.

Basic Science Research in Cancer Health Disparities

Ted Obi and Robert A. Winn

Introduction

Overall, the incidence and mortality related to cancer continue to decrease over time; however, some communities remain at increased risk of having or dying from certain cancers [1]. According to the National Cancer Institute (NCI), Blacks continue to have higher death rates than all other races for many cancer types. For instance, although fatalities from prostate cancer have dropped in recent decades, Black men continue to be twice as likely to die from prostate cancer compared to their White male counterparts. Using a lens of health equity, a better understanding of the historical context of the ways in which racism in medicine is needed to identify and prioritize future research and clinical efforts to achieve equity and justice in cancer care. Similar to the racial injustices in law, housing, and economic opportunity, medicine is tainted with a myriad of historical examples that contribute to the health disparities that exist today. For instance, J. Marion Sims is often considered the "Father of Modern Gynecology," but he used Black slaves to conduct experimental surgeries to treat vescicovaginal and rectovaginal fistulas without using anesthesia. One particular slave named Anarcha Westcott endured at least 30 painful procedures until Sims perfected his technique in 1845. Shortly after this, Sims moved to New York City, where he opened a women's hospital to treat White women with gynecological disorders using anesthesia. Today, Black women continue to experience worse outcomes in maternal health, where they are two to six times more likely than women from other backgrounds to die from pregnancy complications. In this chapter, we review key historical events that set the stage for basic

T. Obi
Mt Sinai School of Medicine, New York, NY, USA

R. A. Winn (✉)
Massey Cancer Center, Virginia Commonwealth University, Richmond, VA, USA
e-mail: robert.winn@vcuhealth.org

C. Hughes Halbert (ed.), *Cancer Health Disparities*,
https://doi.org/10.1007/978-3-031-37638-2_2

and translational research in cancer, describe ongoing efforts to apply these methods to address cancer health disparities and identify future priorities for basic science research in cancer health disparities.

Foundations of Basic Science Research in Cancer

Human cancer-derived cell lines are fundamental models used in the investigation of mechanisms that underlie cancer biology as well as in testing the therapeutic efficacy of anticancer agents [2]. Nearly 70 years ago, cancer-research scientists across the globe competed to be the first to develop human cancer in vitro [3]. At the time, no scientists could grow human cells in the laboratory for more than a few weeks [3]. This paradigm shifted on February 8, 1951, when a 31-year-old, young, Black woman and mother of five living in Baltimore by the name of Henrietta Lacks stepped into Johns Hopkins [3]. According to gynecologist Howard Jones, Lacks presented with no ordinary cervical cancer. Her cancer was found to be a rare, aggressive adenocarcinoma and glandular in nature [3]. During the visit, a culture from her cervical cancer was taken to the laboratory of George Gey, where he discovered the first continuous cancer cell line, which would be dubbed HeLa cells [3]. Within a few years, HeLa cells became the foundation upon which cancer biology research and innovation stood (and continues to stands today). But what about HeLa cells made them so explosive throughout the scientific community and lauded at the time to be the key to curing cancer?

The utility of cancer cell lines is linked to their ability to provide an indefinite source of biological material for experimental purposes. The HeLa cells created a standard model to study the pathophysiology of cancer, avoiding differences between samples and allowing the reproducibility of experimental data [3, 4]. In essence, cancer-research scientists were able to apply standard quality control measures to an endless supply of cells from the same cancer type. Henrietta Lacks' contribution to the scientific and medical communities was hardly confined to cancer. In 1953, George Gey and his colleagues detailed one of the first applications of HeLa cells. They showed that the Polio virus grew easily and could kill HeLa cells. Their finding revealed the diagnostic utility of HeLa cells in the fight against Polio [5]. In 1964, HeLa cells were used to study potential treatment benefits of a drug called hydroxyurea, which is currently the standard of care for patients with sickle cell anemia. During the same year, these cells were taken to outer space and used to study how irradiation and space travel impact astronauts. The range in which HeLa cells were used for investigation was wide. Decades later, Harald Zur Hausen used HeLa cells to discover how the presence of HPV leads to cervical cancer which resulted in the HPV vaccine. In 1985, a drug called camptothecin was found to slow cancer growth after being treated on HeLa cells [6]. In the turn of the century, scientists used HeLa cells to understand how HIV and Ebola infect people [7]. Although passing away just 8 months after her cervical cancer diagnosis, Henrietta Lacks' impact on medical research and innovation remains immortal [3]. To date, her cells have led to over 110,000 research publications [7].

Although the oldest and most commonly used cell lines, HeLa cells are not the only cell lines used today in basic science research in cancer. Since 1951, scientists have discovered other cell lines and used them to advance our understanding of cancer biology and to test how therapeutic agents interact with different cells. A pioneer in cancer cell line discovery, Adi Gazdar is responsible for establishing and characterizing more than 400 human tumor cell lines. His work to create and distribute cell lines and models helped characterize the retroviral particles in patients with T-cell lymphoma, investigate anticancer therapies on lung cancer, and define molecular subtypes of small and non-small cell lung cancers that assist with diagnosis today. The groundwork that Gazdar and his colleagues laid has informed current biomedical research and innovation. Today, cell lines are available from major suppliers like American Type Culture Collection (ATCC), which is a global bioresource center that maintains nearly 4000 human cell lines to support global scientific research [8]. These commercially available cell lines represent various tissue and disease states. However, a significant proportion of samples are from patients of European ancestry. One study searched the ATCC database for cell lines derived from normal and malignant breast tissue and found 59 specimens designated as Caucasian/White. Further investigation revealed that there were only 14 non-Caucasian/White cell lines and of these, 11 were designated as Black, 1 was designated as Hispanic, and 1 was designated as East Indian [9]. Similarly, of 32 listed prostate cell lines available from major suppliers (e.g., ATCC, Sigma Aldrich, and the European Collection of Authenticated Cell Cultures), 97% are of European origin even though men of African ancestry have the highest incidence of prostate cancer worldwide [10]. The scarcity of racial and ethnic minorities is preserved in tissue microarray technology [11]. Tissue microarray technology was developed by J. Kononen and collaborators in 1998. It is an effective tool used for high-throughput molecular analysis of tissue samples, allowing for the identification of diagnostic and prognostic markers and therapeutics in cancer. Prior to tissue microarray, the validation of these markers was time-consuming, labor-intensive, and costly [12].

Patient-derived xenografts (PDXs) are also commonly used in basic science research in cancer. PDXs are tumor tissues that have been taken from a patient and implanted into immunodeficient mice. PDX models are used to create an environment that allows for the natural growth of the tumor, which has enabled cancer researchers to test anticancer agents, plan treatment, and learn what treatments may be best for patients [13]. A major advantage of using PDX instead of cancer cell lines is the preserved heterogeneity of the human stromal cell microenvironment. Unlike cancer cell lines, PDX models grow in physiologically relevant tumor microenvironments as the primary tumor site which translates into similar responses to anticancer agents [14]. However, similar to cancer cell lines, PDX biospecimens lack racial and ethnic diversity. In the repository of NCI patient-derived models, 62.86% and the majority of specimens are missing racial/ethnic data. Of those with racial/ethnic data, 36.19% were obtained from Whites and only 0.95% were obtained from African Americans [15]. To accelerate translational research using PDX, the NCI launched PDXNet in 2017. To specifically address the scarcity of racial/ethnic minority PDXs, NCI added two PDX Development and Trial Centers (PDTC) at

University of California Davis and Baylor College of Medicine with the goal of establishing 200 minority-derived PDXs to guide precision medicine decision-making in racial/ethnically diverse patients in California and Texas, respectively [16]. Results have been forthcoming from these and other established initiatives in enhancing the diversity of biospecimens and other resources to support basic science research in cancer. However, recent research has shown that a variety of factors contribute to the overall desicion-making and willingness of racial/ethnically diverse populations to participate in and donate to these studies [17–19]. Thus, several barriers may need to be addressed to enhance the diversity of resources that are used to collect, store, and use biospecimens from these diverse populations.

Current Efforts in Basic Science Research to Address Cancer Health Disparities

Similar to the advances that have been made to create cell lines and use PDX models to understand cancer initiation, progression, and response to treatment, basic science research in cancer health disparities focuses on developing and applying innovative tools and methods to increase the precision of cancer care across the continuum of prevention, early detection, and treatment by understanding pathways and mechanisms involved in cancer risk and treatment outcomes. Tumor markers, or cancer biomarkers, for instance, can potentially work independently or together with evidence-based screening strategies to enhance early detection. However, in most cases, patients are identified and prioritized for early detection based on self-reported behaviors (e.g., cigarette smoking for lung cancer screening) and risk factors without consideration of how these factors are shaped by and expressed in social and clinical contexts.

Epigenetics is a research area that integrates biological, clinical, and social mechanisms that are involved in disease risk and outcomes [20] and is now being used to develop cancer biomarkers. Within the context of cancer health disparities, epigenetics has several important advantages that include integrating multiple types (e.g., social, genetic) of determinants into the research paradigm to understand disease processes and outcomes [21–23]. Epigenetic processes control normal growth and development; epigenetic mechanisms are important to epigenetic programming that include DNA methylation and histone modification in altering gene expression and function [21, 24, 25]. Previous research has demonstrated that cancer is associated with a global reduction in DNA methylation [25, 26]. Hypermethylation of cytosine bases in promoter regions overlapping CpG islands in some tumor suppressor genes has also been shown to be associated with cancer [25, 27, 28]. Previous epigenetics research has demonstrated that African Americans have lower methylation levels compared to Whites [29–31]; however, limited empirical data are available on racial differences in methylation changes related to cancer sites that disproportionately affect African Americans in terms of morbidity and mortality (e.g., lung cancer) [32, 33]. Further, epigenetic-based therapeutic targeting in cancers using DNA hypomethylating agents have largely been unsuccessful in clinical trials. Thus, there remains a significant need to identify additional epigenetic processes that may inform the development of new therapeutic agents and early detection strategies that can be used in diverse populations.

Accordingly, research is now being done to understand how epigenetic changes and methylation status are expressed and influenced by social and environmental factors among medically underserved groups. These social and environmental factors could result in acquired biomolecular epigenetic changes that ultimately affect the initiation and progression of cancer by modulating gene transcription due to inappropriate gene silencing [34–38]. For instance, Winn and colleagues have identified protein arginine methylation as a potential biomarker for detecting lung cancer and a possible drug target for this disease. Although protein methylation was first described in 1968, the importance of this posttranslational modification is just now being recognized [39]. Protein arginine methylation is one of the most abundant posttranslational modifications [40]. Nitrogens of arginine within the protein can be posttranslationally modified via the addition of a methyl group, a process known as arginine methylation. The process of adding methyl groups to arginine is catalyzed by a class of enzymes: protein arginine methyl transferases (PRMT). Of the eight functional PRMTs identified to date, only PRMT1 and PRMT6 are associated with lung cancer. Moreover, in silico analysis of the cancer genome atlas (TCGA) revealed that only PRMT6 is associated with increased expression in African American men compared to White men. Strikingly, lung targeted expression of PRMT6 in an in vivo mouse model, which mimics PRMT6 amplification events in human lung tumors, resulted in increased lung tumor development. Furthermore, tobacco smoke also induces PRMT6 expression, and other works have shown that PRMT6 is associated with inflammatory response [41–43]. Together with chronic and prolonged exposure to environmental social stressors (e.g., neighborhood crime, poverty), these epigenetic changes and activation of pro-inflammatory pathways may explain why African American men have a greater risk for lung cancer morbidity and mortality despite having a later age at smoking initiation. With the support of the NCI's P20 Specialized Program of Research Excellence (SPORE) grant in lung cancer disparities, research is now being conducted to (1) understand and compare the interactive effects of environmental stressors, smoking, and PRMT6 expression between African American/Black and non-Hispanic White men, (2) examine PRMT6/protein expression profiles in relation to environmental stressors and smoking among African American and White men, and (3) determine if PRMT6 promoter hypomethylation can be detected in liquid biopsies. Ultimately, this work could reduce lung cancer disparities by improving the precision of lung cancer risk prediction and increasing early detection using a biomarker (PRMT6) that captures both individual and community risks. None of the current risk models (LCRAT, Bach, etc.) have included significant numbers of African American men in their validation, nor have ever considered the community context of stress.

Future Directions and Conclusions

As new discoveries and advancements are being made for cancer treatment and early detection through basic science research, it is becoming increasingly apparent that observed disparities in cancer risk and outcomes are due to complex factors. That is to say, individuals who reside in poor, segregated neighborhoods are likely to have greater morbidity and mortality from cancer [44–46]. Neighborhood and community context are important to the expression of genetic factors; in the case of lung cancer, it is increasingly evident that disparities between African American and White men in survival from this disease are likely being driven by a complex and poorly understood interaction between unequal access to care, social determinants of health, community stress, tobacco exposure, and molecular determinants [47, 48]. At the same time, it is important to recognize that all research and clinical care has a historical context that is continuously being shaped by current event. Lived experiences continue to inform patient behavior and clinical practices. In the field of pulmonology, for instance, the historical belief that Blacks have 15% less lung capacities than Whites continues to perpetuate inequitable care. Spirometers used to measure lung volume and the rate of flow through airways as an indicator of pulmonary disease inaccurately measure lung function and may result in the misclassification of disease severity in racial and ethnic minorities [49].

To address cancer health disparities, some leaders believe that an increased representation of scientists and clinicians from disparity population is the key to cancer health equity and justice. Relatedly, the National Institutes of Health (NIH) has identified the lack of diversity in the physician-scientist workforce as the primary challenge to clinical and scientific research, acknowledging that researchers and providers from different backgrounds bring a diversity of experiences and ideas to the laboratory setting to solve complex problems [50]. The NIH employs over 1000 scientists in its research program; however, of those, only 5% were Black, Hispanic, American Indian, or Native American in 2018 [51]. A diverse workforce is the bedrock for biomedical innovation and can also serve as a conduit for increasing racial and ethnic minority representation in clinical trials and other types of cancer research. Throughout the clinical research design and implementation stages, there have been missed opportunities to innovate on what we have historically known. Additionally, because of decades of de-prioritization of minority health and unethical research practices, communities of color are less likely to participate in clinical trials. Clinical trials have been used to ensure the safety and efficacy of novel drug treatments and medical devices for the general public. In the field of oncology, limited diversity in clinical trials reduces output and yields treatment, prevention, and early detection strategies that do not speak to the heterogeneity of cancer and its impact on minority populations. Disparity populations often do not participate in clinical trials and other types of cancer research because of distrust of the medical system, lack of awareness of the clinical trials and other studies, and the logistical burdens of study participation [52–54]. Diverse investigators who have lived experiences that are similar to the those of the patients and communities that they wish to engage with are important for addressing cancer health disparities through greater representation of disparity populations.

Increasing the diversity of the biomedical research and clinical workforce is critical, but it is also important for basic science research in cancer health disparities to incorporate and analyze measures that capture the social and environmental context through which biological pathways and mechanisms are expressed. To do this, policies and guidelines are needed to ensure that data on social drivers of health (SDOH) are collected and harmonized in studies. As data on SDOH are collected as part of basic science studies, novel methods will be needed to evaluate the intersectionality between biological, social, and behavioral determinants so that translational efforts are informed by the complex ways in which these factors contribute to cancer risk and outcomes.

References

1. https://www.cancer.gov/about-cancer/understanding/disparities.
2. Sharma SV, Haber DA, Settleman J. Cell line-based platforms to evaluate the therapeutic efficacy of candidate anticancer agents. Nat Rev Cancer. 2010;10(4):241–53.
3. Masters J. HeLa cells 50 years on: the good, the bad and the ugly. Nat Rev Cancer. 2002;2:315–9.
4. Neve RM, Chin K, Fridlyand J, Yeh J, Baehner FL, Fevr T, Clark L, Bayani N, Coppe JP, Tong F, et al. A collection of breast cancer cell lines for the study of functionally distinct cancer subtypes. Cancer Cell. 2006;10:515–27.
5. Scherer WF, Syverton JT, Gey GO. Studies on the propagation *in vitro* of poliomyelitis viruses. J Exp Med. 1953;97:695–709.
6. Hsiang YH, Hertzberg R, Hecht S, Liu LF. Camptothecin induces protein-linked DNA breaks via mammalian DNA topoisomerase I. J Biol Chem. 1985;260(27):14873–8.
7. National Institutes of Health. Significant research advances enabled by HeLa cells. Available at: https://osp.od.nih.gov/scientific-sharing/hela-cells-timeline.
8. American type culture collection. Available at: https://www.atcc.org/.
9. Hooker SE Jr, Woods-Burnham L, Bathina M, Lloyd S, Gorjala P, Mitra R, Nonn L, Kimbro KS, Kittles RA. Genetic ancestry analysis reveals misclassification of commonly used cancer cell lines. Cancer Epidemiol Biomark Prev. 2019;28(6):1003–9.
10. Badal S, Campbell KS, Valentine H, Ragin C. The need for cell lines from diverse ethnic backgrounds for prostate cancer research. Nat Rev Urol. 2019;16(12):691–2.
11. Seijo E, Lima D, Iriabho E, Almeida J, Monico J, Echeverri M, Gutierrez S, Flores I, Lee JH, Fisher K, Grizzle WE, Sica GL, Butler C, Hicks C, Meade CD, Sodeke SO, Moroz K, Coppola D, Munoz-Antonia T. Construction and validation of a multi-institutional tissue microarray of invasive ductal carcinoma from racially and ethnically diverse populations. Cancer Control. 2016;23(4):383–9.
12. Jawhar NM. Tissue microarray: a rapidly evolving diagnostic and research tool. Ann Saudi Med. 2009;29(2):123–7.
13. National Cancer Institute. NCI dictionaries. Available at: https://www.cancer.gov/publications/dictionaries/cancer-terms/def/patient-derived-xenograft.
14. Kerbel RS. Human tumor xenografts as predictive preclinical models for anticancer drug activity in humans: better than commonly perceived-but they can be improved. Cancer Biol Ther. 2003;2:S134–9.
15. Guerrero S, López-Cortés A, Indacochea A, et al. Analysis of racial/ethnic representation in select basic and applied cancer research studies. Sci Rep. 2018;8:13978.

16. University of California-Davis. University of California Minority Patient-Derived Xenograft Development and Trial Center (UCaMP) to reduce cancer health disparities. Available at: https://www.pdxnetwork.org/new-page.
17. McDonald JA, Vadaparampil S, Bowen D, Magwood G, Obeid JS, Jefferson M, Drake R, Gebregziabher M, Hughes HC. Intentions to donate to a biobank in a national sample of African Americans. Public Health Genomics. 2014;17(3):173–82.
18. McDonald JA, Weathers B, Barg FK, Troxel AB, Shea JA, Bowen D, Guerra CE, Halbert CH. Donation intentions for cancer genetics research among African Americans. Genet Test Mol Biomarkers. 2012;16(4):252–8.
19. McDonald JA, Barg FK, Weathers B, Guerra CE, Troxel AB, Domchek S, Bowen D, Shea JA, Halbert CH. Understanding participation by African Americans in cancer genetics research. J Natl Med Assoc. 2012;104(7–8):324–30.
20. Pickersgill M, Niewohner J, Muller R, Martin P, Cunningham-Burley S. Mapping the new molecular landscape: social dimensions of epigenetics. New Genet Soc. 2013;32:429–47.
21. National Cancer Institute. Epigenomics and epigenetics research. Washington, DC: National Cancer Institute; 2018.
22. Aranda-Anzaldo A, Dent MAR. Landscaping the epigenetic landscape of cancer. Prog Biophys Mol Biol. 2018;140:155–74.
23. Mohammed SI, Springfield S, Das R. Role of epigenetics in cancer health disparities. Methods Mol Biol. 2012;863:395–410.
24. Yehuda R, Daskalakis NP, Desarnaud F, et al. Epigenetic biomarkers as predictors and correlates of symptom improvement following psychotherapy in combat veterans with PTSD. Front Psych. 2013;4:118.
25. Radley JJ, Kabbaj M, Jacobson L, Heydendael W, Yehuda R, Herman JP. Stress risk factors and stress-related pathology: neuroplasticity, epigenetics and endophenotypes. Stress. 2011;14:481–97.
26. Ehrlich M, Lacey M. DNA methylation and differentiation: silencing, upregulation and modulation of gene expression. Epigenomics. 2013;5:553–68.
27. Pfeifer GP. Defining driver DNA methylation changes in human cancer. Int J Mol Sci. 2018;19
28. Costello JF, Fruhwald MC, Smiraglia DJ, et al. Aberrant CpG-Island methylation has non-random and tumour-type-specific patterns. Nat Genet. 2000;24:132–8.
29. Esteller M, Corn PG, Baylin SB, Herman JG. A gene hypermethylation profile of human cancer. Cancer Res. 2001;61:3225–9.
30. Figueiredo JC, Grau MV, Wallace K, et al. Global DNA hypomethylation (LINE-1) in the normal colon and lifestyle characteristics and dietary and genetic factors. Cancer Epidemiol Biomark Prev. 2009;18:1041–9.
31. Terry MB, Ferris JS, Pilsner R, et al. Genomic DNA methylation among women in a multiethnic New York City birth cohort. Cancer Epidemiol Biomark Prev. 2008;17:2306–10.
32. Hulbert A, Jusue-Torres I, Stark A, et al. Early detection of lung cancer using DNA promoter hypermethylation in plasma and sputum. Clin Cancer Res. 2017;23:1998–2005.
33. Wrangle J, Machida EO, Danilova L, et al. Functional identification of cancer-specific methylation of CDO1, HOXA9, and TAC1 for the diagnosis of lung cancer. Clin Cancer Res. 2014;20:1856–64.
34. Herman JG, Graff JR, Myohanen S, Nelkin BD, Baylin SB. Methylation-specific pcr: a novel pcr assay for methylation status of cpg islands. Proc Natl Acad Sci U S A. 1996;93(18):9821–6.
35. Belinsky SA, Nikula KJ, Palmisano WA, Michels R, Saccomanno G, Gabrielson E, Baylin SB, Herman JG. Aberrant methylation of p16(ink4a) is an early event in lung cancer and a potential biomarker for early diagnosis. Proc Natl Acad Sci U S A. 1998;95(20):11891–6.
36. Palmisano WA, Divine KK, Saccomanno G, Gilliland FD, Baylin SB, Herman JG, Belinsky SA. Predicting lung cancer by detecting aberrant promoter methylation in sputum. Cancer Res. 2000;60(21):5954–8.
37. Herman JG, Baylin SB. Gene silencing in cancer in association with promoter hypermethylation. N Engl J Med. 2003;349(21):2042–54.

38. Belinsky SA. Gene-promoter hypermethylation as a biomarker in lung cancer. Nat Rev Cancer. 2004;4(9):707–17.
39. Paik WK, Kim S. Protein methylase I. Purification and properties of the enzyme. J Biol Chem. 1968;243(9):2108–14.
40. Lin WJ, Gary JD, Yang MC, Clarke S, Herschman HR. The mammalian immediate-early TIS21 protein and the leukemia-associated BTG1 protein interact with a protein-arginine n-methyltransferase. J Biol Chem. 1996;271(25):15034–44.
41. Kim JH, Yoo BC, Yang WS, Kim E, Hong S, Cho JY. The role of protein arginine methyltransferases in inflammatory responses. Mediat Inflamm. 2016;2016:4028353.
42. Zhang H, Han C, Li T, Li N, Cao X. The methyltransferase prmt6 attenuates antiviral innate immunity by blocking TBK1-IRF3 signaling. Cell Mol Immunol. 2019;16(10):800–9.
43. Blanc RS, Richard S. Arginine methylation: the coming of age. Mol Cell. 2017;65(1):8–24.
44. Clegg LX, Reichman ME, Miller BA, Hankey BF, Singh GK, Lin YD, Goodman MT, Lynch CF, Schwartz SM, Chen VW, Bernstein L, Gomez SL, Graff JJ, Lin CC, Johnson NJ, Edwards BK. Impact of socioeconomic status on cancer incidence and stage at diagnosis: selected findings from the surveillance, epidemiology, and end results: national longitudinal mortality study. Cancer Causes Control. 2009;20(4):417–35.
45. Hayanga AJ, Zeliadt SB, Backhus LM. Residential segregation and lung cancer mortality in the United States. JAMA Surg. 2013;148(1):37–42.
46. Annesi CA, Poulson MR, Mak KS, Tapan U, Dechert TA, Litle VR, Suzuki K. The impact of residential racial segregation on non-small cell lung cancer treatment and outcomes. Ann Thorac Surg. 2022;113(4):1291–8.
47. Vidrine JI, Reitzel LR, Wetter DW. The role of tobacco in cancer health disparities. Curr Oncol Rep. 2009;11:475.
48. American Lung Association. State of lung cancer. Available at: https://www.lung.org/research/state-of-lung-cancer
49. Vyas DA, Eisenstein LG, Jones DS. Hidden in plain sight – reconsidering the use of race correction in clinical algorithms. N Engl J Med. 2020;383(9):874–82.
50. National Institutes of Health. Physician-scientist workforce working group report. Bethesda, MD: National Institutes of Health; 2014. Available at: https://report.nih.gov/workforce/psw/index.aspx.
51. Mervis J. NIH hopes 'cluster hiring' will improve diversity. Science. 6479;367. Available at: https://www.sciencemag.org/news/2020/01/nih-s-new-cluster-hiring-program-aims-help-schools-attract-diverse-faculty.
52. Clark LT, Watkins L, Piña IL, Elmer M, Akinboboye O, Gorham M, Jamerson B, McCullough C, Pierre C, Polis AB, Puckrein G, Regnante JM. Increasing diversity in clinical trials: overcoming critical barriers. Curr Probl Cardiol. 2019;44(5):148–72.
53. Scharff DP, Mathews KJ, Jackson P, Hoffsuemmer J, Martin E, Edwards D. More than Tuskegee: understanding mistrust about research participation. J Health Care Poor Underserved. 2010;21(3):879–97.
54. Halbert CH, McDonald J, Vadaparampil S, Rice L, Jefferson M. Conducting precision medicine research with African Americans. PLoS One. 2016;11(7):e0154850.

Chronic Stress, Biobehavioral Processes and Health Implications in Understanding Disparities

Joshua P. Kronenfeld, Michael H. Antoni, and Frank J. Penedo

Integrated Biopsychosocial Models of Stress, Adversity, and Disparities in Health Outcomes

In everyday life, stress and adversity provide significant challenges that must be overcome in order to successfully navigate through daily activities [1]. In the healthcare arena, additional stressors including access to healthcare, health maintenance and disease prevention, and availability of curative treatments provide further barriers to patients and their families [2]. Psychological stress and mental adversity can significantly affect physical health, so it is critical that these factors be ameliorated in patients suffering with them [3]. Profound healthcare disparities, often seen across racial, ethnic, or sociodemographic minorities, also contribute to the stress and adversity felt by many patients [4, 5]. Physicians and other care providers have a duty to help these patients overcome these challenges in an effort to provide equitable care to all patients and improve the health of communities [6].

Before discussing interventions designed to dampen the stress response and promote overall wellness, a thorough understanding of factors contributing to this response must be ascertained [7]. Stress has evolved to provide a mechanism for successful adaptation to external stimuli encountered throughout the life span [8].

J. P. Kronenfeld
Department of Surgery, University of Miami Miller School of Medicine, Miami, FL, USA
e-mail: j.kronenfeld@umiami.edu

M. H. Antoni
Department of Psychology & Sylvester Comprehensive Cancer Center, University of Miami, Coral Gables, FL, USA
e-mail: mantoni@miami.edu

F. J. Penedo (✉)
Departments of Medicine and Psychology & Sylvester Comprehensive Cancer Center, University of Miami, Coral Gables, FL, USA
e-mail: Frank.Penedo@miami.edu

C. Hughes Halbert (ed.), *Cancer Health Disparities*,
https://doi.org/10.1007/978-3-031-37638-2_3

When challenges are encountered, and stress is brought on, a person naturally adapts to the stressor and carries the experience with them as they progress through life [9]. Stress triggers the hypothalamic-pituitary-adrenal (HPA) axis to release glucocorticoids that activate short-term responses to individual stressors [10]. Although the hormonal release is short-lived, the stressors may have implications in all facets of life, and Myers et al. have demonstrated, through the *life time model*, that from birth to death, stress can impart its effects on physical well-being [11]. In fact, long-term stress can lead to declines in immune health and neurodegenerative dysregulation linked to HPA-axis dysfunction [10, 12]. Stressors may begin with challenging experiences in childhood (e.g., childhood adversity, experiences of bullying or discrimination, childhood trauma, etc.), and when combined with adult traumas and chronic life stressors, the burden may be too great and overwhelm the individual [13, 14]. Chronic psychosocial stress, including living in low-income neighborhoods, has even been linked to low birthweight children in African American women [15, 16]. As individuals progress through life, decreased functional physical status, increased pain, and cognitive decline all contribute to additional stressors. Finally, biological and genetic factors, many not yet identified, can contribute to a predisposition of an increased stressed state [17].

An individual will often point to a single event as a trigger for their stress response, but the stress appreciated is likely an overall accumulation of multiple stressors throughout various aspects of life [18]. A patient only has so much reserve capacity before they can no longer sustain themselves and a breaking point is reached, an idea originally described by Gallo et al. [19] The model entitled *reserve capacity model* incorporates three fundamental psychosocial pathways: low socioeconomic status, increased negative (or reduced positive) emotions, and increased physiological and emotional reactivity to stress [19, 20]. Patients who experience one, or all three, psychosocial pathway(s) will be predisposed to the deleterious effects of stress for a variety of reasons. Individuals of low socioeconomic status often have decreased available resources (e.g., reserve capacity) to cope with and manage stress, which, in turn, may lead to further increases in stress [19]. Additionally, patients with increased negative emotions or reactivity to stress may also not possess the ability (e.g., reserve capacity) to cope with stressors before feeling overwhelmed [21]. Over time, a dearth of adequate coping resources can generate adverse physical and emotional outcomes, as described above, and can lead to systemic ill effects of stress [22]. This never-ending cycle of stress, inadequate resources, and further stress described in this model explains the challenges that some individuals face with chronic, debilitating, and unrelenting stress.

Another model detailing the interconnection of stress and environment, particularly when the environment surrounding a person includes discrimination and societal injustice, is the *ecosocial and interpersonal model* described by Krieger et al. [23–25] Although many studies focus on the impact of interpersonal discrimination, the impacts of structural discrimination cannot be overlooked as its effects can also have significant negative implications to the health of an individual [26]. The model discusses five key factors that contribute to stress and adversity, namely, economic and social deprivation (e.g., residential or occupational segregation leading to economic and financial inequities), toxic substances and hazardous conditions (e.g., older housing that may contain lead paints which leads to renal failure), socially inflicted trauma (e.g., interpersonal racial discrimination promoting fear and anger), targeted marketing of commodities (e.g., high-alcohol beverages advertised to poor communities that can lead to liver disease or hypertension), and inadequate healthcare (e.g., decreased screening and early detection of illness leading to untreated disease) [27]. The stressors felt by individuals are derived from daily interactions between people but also are experienced through daily challenges faced by community and societal inequities. While the correction of interpersonal challenges may palliate the stress experienced, systemic ecosocial changes throughout the community must be incorporated to fully eradicate the issue.

Jackson et al. have described yet another model detailing sources of stress and adversity through the investigation of *biobehavioral mechanisms* [28]. In cancer survivors, patients often suffer from persistent deleterious symptoms, including stress, anxiety, fatigue, and pain, long after the cessation of treatment [29, 30]. One explanation for this persistence of symptoms is that biological factors have been irreversibly altered during the intense treatment regimen prescribed for a malignancy [31]. Alterations to chromosomal telomeric length are just one example of genomic-wide changes that occur when a person is exposed to significant stressors [29]. Additional epigenetic changes, such as deoxyribonucleic acid (DNA) methylation and histone modifications, have also been attributed to prolonged psychosocial distress [28, 32]. These epigenetic changes may also lead to chronic fatigue and memory loss, two factors that can also increase the stress and adversity appreciated by an individual [33]. The biological factors, combined with the aforementioned lifetime, reserve capacity, and ecosocial factors, contribute to the challenges experienced by many patients.

The final model to discuss has been proposed by Yanez et al. and combines the previously described models to understand the full complement of factors that influence stress and adversity [34]. The model, focusing on cancer-specific stressors, details the interactions between social, cultural, psychosocial, disease-specific, healthcare, and medical factors that determine health outcomes and may contribute to disparities [34]. Socioeconomic factors (e.g., limited access to care, poor economic status, etc.) form the basis of stressors that may negatively impact cancer health outcomes [34–36]. Psychosocial (e.g., coping mechanisms) and behavioral (e.g., substance use) factors can also have implications in the overall well-being of an individual, which, in turn, may affect the stress and adversity experienced by individuals [37, 38]. Finally, medical factors including infectious diseases, malignancies, or other comorbidities contribute to the overall stressors encountered by an individual [34, 39]. As discussed in the above models, without adequate resources to cope and ameliorate these stressors, an individual will succumb to their experiences and have challenges in daily function [18, 19]. In order to identify the utility of these various models, a discussion is required of the many stressors and interpersonal challenges patients face that contribute to negative stress responses.

Prevalent Chronic Stressors and Processes in Specific Communities

Disparities and inequities contribute to chronic stressors that affect minority patients and contribute to chronic psychosocial distress. In minority racial, ethnic, or other minority communities sociodemographic status may play a particular role in stress and adversity. Although the mantra that cancer does not discriminate based on an individual's socioeconomic status holds true, poorer cancer outcomes are well-documented among individuals with lower income, less education, and lower rates of health insurance. For instance, among Hispanics and Blacks, socioeconomic status is related to poor cardiometabolic health (e.g., high blood pressure, dyslipidemia, insulin resistance, etc.), which can adversely affect overall health, stress, and cancer outcomes [40, 41]. Education level is perhaps one of the most influential components in determining an individual's socioeconomic status [42]. According to the US Census Bureau, less than 70% of Hispanics and 86% of Blacks have attained a high-school diploma, compared to 93% of non-Hispanic Whites (NHW) [43]. Only 16% of Hispanics and 21% of Blacks have a bachelor's degree and 5% of Hispanics and 8% of Blacks have a graduate or advanced professional degree compared to 36% and 14%, respectively, in NHWs [43, 44]. These disparities in education limit financial opportunities and create resource gaps. Additionally, schools in areas with large minority populations receive less funding, a disparity that influences social determinants of health and may impact stress, oncologic, and health outcomes [11, 45, 46]. A scarcity of resources for individuals and their families who have recently migrated to the United States also may lead to challenges in learning English and securing dependable employment with suitable health insurance benefits [47]. Finally, without adequate language programs for Hispanics and their families, health literacy also becomes an important issue driving the healthcare disparities [48].

The combination of education and literacy barriers faced by minority patients contributes to decreased household income levels. This income inequality, another prominent disparity in minority communities, has been independently associated with poorer health outcomes and increased stress [49]. In 2017, median household income among Hispanics ($50.4 k) and Blacks ($40.3 k) was significantly less than median household income for NHWs ($68.1 k) [50]. Hispanics and Blacks have historically been disproportionately clustered in low-skilled and low-paying jobs which can be attributed to the previously described disparities (e.g., inadequate funding for quality education, underdeveloped programs to promote literacy, etc.) [51, 52]. Individuals with lower incomes have been shown to have a decreased life expectancy when compared to individuals of higher economic status, an alarming statistic that shows how the lack of income equality in Hispanics and Blacks can actually lead to earlier mortality [53]. Low income and socioeconomic status have been linked to an increased stress state which negatively affects health outcomes in these patients as well [54].

Material deprivation, more common in communities of racial and ethnic minorities, is another potential source of significant stress among individuals and their families [55]. These patients perceive that they have a decreased social standing due to their limited resources, monetary savings, and material possessions [56]. These feelings cause stress on parents and family leaders as they strive to provide for their families. It also leads to stress on children and other dependents as they may recognize the hardships experienced by their caretakers [57]. Dependents often tend to mirror the behavior of their parents or family leaders, so a perception of hardship felt by these individuals will lead to significant stress and adversity on children and other dependents [58]. While a lack of material possessions does not intuitively explain an increase in stress, the factors surrounding this dearth of resources can lead to further understanding of the challenges these individuals face [57, 59].

Hispanics and Blacks also have the lowest health insurance rates of any racial or ethnic groups with 34% and 21%, respectively, reportedly without health insurance, more than twice the uninsured rate of NHW [60, 61]. Educational gaps drive the lack of health insurance as individuals with lower levels of education often hold jobs that do not provide insurance coverage or offer limited plans with significant deductibles or out of pocket expenses. Additional factors that determine an individual's type of work further exacerbate disparities in health insurance including language barriers and discrimination. First-generation Hispanics may primarily speak Spanish or other non-English languages at home, and nearly 30% report that they are not fluent in English [43]. Careers and jobs that will provide an individual and their family with health insurance may be less attainable for individuals who do not demonstrate fluency and/or literacy in English [62]. In some instances, Hispanics or Blacks are even deliberately discriminated against, due to their race or ethnicity, and are not hired by employers [63, 64]. Poor health literacy and inadequate health insurance in Hispanics and Blacks result, in part, from disparate resource allocation that yields fewer educational opportunities that subsequently limits job opportunities [65]. These factors contribute significant stress to individuals as patients are often unable to seek medical care [66]. Patients are more likely to present with later-stage cancers in emergency settings without access to adequate health services, and these barriers contribute to a significant feeling of stress and adversity in these patients [67–69].

Perceived discrimination among racial and ethnic minorities is another factor contributing to stress [70]. In communities where group-based or systemic discrimination is noted, individuals report feelings of a lack of security in one's home as well as an anger toward individuals perceived to be the oppressors [71]. This anger perpetuates a hostile and stressful environment for all parties and can have negative implications such as increased feelings of adversity [72]. In addition, unconscious biases may play a role in disparate care delivered to minority patients in healthcare settings. Unconscious or implicit bias is defined as biases that are activated unintentionally but silently exert influence on a person's perception or behavior toward another individual; these biases can affect interactions between patients and healthcare professionals [73, 74]. For instance, physicians caring for minorities may be less likely to arrive at serious diagnoses or refer the patient to a specialist relative to

NHW patients [75]. Providers may even be less likely to refer minorities to specialty services due to an implicit bias that the patient may not be able to pay for the additional services [76, 77]. These disparate approaches to care lead to significant feelings of anger and stress as patients perceive that they may not be receiving equitable care.

Additionally, neighborhood factors such as food insecurity or violence can contribute to significant stressors. Food deserts, or neighborhoods where access to healthy and affordable nutrition, remain a constant challenge for minority patients [78, 79]. The US Department of Agriculture has demonstrated that low-income and minority populations, including Hispanics and Blacks, are more likely to live further from supermarkets and access to quality produce when compared to NHW [80]. Additionally, individuals who live in areas with increased neighborhood violence may be less able to access these supermarkets, even if they are close to home, due to an inability to safely walk through their neighborhood to these markets [81]. The paucity of healthy, affordable, and accessible food leads to an increased intake of high fat, high carbohydrate, and low fruit/vegetable meals and a reliance on fast-food restaurants [82]. This, in turn, can lead to adverse health effects including increased cardiovascular disease, decreased wound healing, increased stress, and poorer oncologic outcomes [83, 84]. Investment in community nutrition education and improved access to supermarkets and healthy food options is imperative to alleviating the stress associated with inadequate access to healthy and affordable foods.

Neighborhood violence can contribute to significant ongoing stress with implications on health outcomes as well [85]. Financial inequities and inadequate school funding, as discussed above, contribute to an increase in violent behaviors in some, but certainly not all, minority communities [86]. With limited available extracurricular activities in underfunded public schools, minority youth may associate with gangs or other dangerous organizations for camaraderie and social acceptance [87]. This burden reaches further than just to the minority youth as the neighborhood violence and crime that stem from these activities lead to an increased stress burden of all individuals in the community due to a lack of security in one's home or public places [88].

As mentioned above, the continuous stress activation in patients can have negative health and oncologic consequences, which can all be traced back to a need for investment in equitable schools and educational programs for all children. The increase in neighborhood violence also impacts the ability of minorities to remain physical active and exercise outside [89]. While nonviolent neighborhoods are conducive to going on walks or engaging in exercise or community activities in local parks, violent neighborhoods tend to yield a more sedentary population with an increased body mass index (BMI) [90]. This sedentary lifestyle, and increase in BMI, contributes to poor cardiovascular, pulmonary, and general health, and it has poor prognostic implications for patients undergoing treatment for malignancies [91]. Additionally, poor health outcomes, as noted above, lead to increased stress, decreased ability to overcome illness, and poorer outcomes in various cancers [92–95].

While patients of racial and ethnic minorities have many challenges, as discussed above, additional groups of patients are subjected to stressors that can lead to deleterious effects as well. One such group of patients are those identifying as lesbian, gay, bisexual, transgender, or queer (LGBTQ) [96]. These patients are at an increased risk of experiencing distal minority stress processes, or stressors from discrimination and violence that disproportionately affect LGBTQ individuals [97, 98]. Additionally, LGBTQ patients often experience proximal minority stress processes, or internal stressors, due to internalized concealment with one's sexual orientation or gender identity [97, 99]. While public support has increased in recent years, LGBTQ patients continue to be at a high risk for stress, depression, and compromised mental health [100]. These feelings often begin during childhood or adolescence and can contribute to the other stressors experienced throughout their lives [101].

Patients at the extremes of age also experience significant stressors. In children and adolescents, these stressors may be particularly harmful due to heightened sensitivity during development and maturation [102]. In children, these stressors can be driven by interpersonal relationships with others, difficulty assimilating to ever-changing environments, and challenges establishing individuality and independence [103]. If exposed to persistent stress from an early age, children and adolescents can develop long-term neurologic, metabolic, immunogenic, and cardiac alterations [102, 104]. In older or elderly adults, stressors can also be present that affect long-term health and well-being [105]. Adults may carry stressors about providing for dependents and succeeding in careers, while elderly patients may begin to suffer from physical and cognitive decline that can wear on a them emotionally [106, 107]. In addition to a baseline cognitive impairment often seen in an aging patient, those receiving treatment for malignancies, more often seen in adults and elderly patients, can have an increased incidence of cognitive decline [108]. While the mechanisms behind cancer-related cognitive impairment, commonly referred to as "chemo-brain," remain unclear, many patients face challenges as a result of their chemotherapy treatment regimen [109]. Among other symptoms, patients may experience problems with concentration and memory, decreased occupational performance, and alterations to their overall quality of life [110, 111]. These physical and cognitive derangements make it difficult for these patients to function independently, often requiring the assistance of family or other caregivers to perform activities of daily living [112]. All of these factors contribute to increases stress in the individual as they may feel burdensome to those around them [113].

In addition to older adults and elderly patients experiencing stressors due to medical treatments, patients with illnesses or comorbidities are at an increased risk from experiencing stressors [114]. Patients with more serious illnesses such as severe traumas, complex malignancies, or permanent disabilities are likely to have prolonged stressors that can affect other aspects of their lives [115, 116]. Patients with other illnesses (e.g., hypertension, diabetes, chronic kidney disease, etc.) will still experience stress and adversity often related to the need for frequent medical visits, complex medication regimen, or feelings of depression due to a perceived poor health [117, 118]. As many people (up to 60%) have medical comorbidities, these stressors are pervasive and affect many individuals [119].

Finally, in rural communities, there are additional challenges faced by patients that may contribute to stress and adversity. Emergency services or referral centers may not be easily accessible to patients should a healthcare provider discover a condition requiring immediate assistance [120]. In rural areas, this may pose challenges including increased healthcare transportation costs as well as increased transportation times that may lead to adverse outcomes for patients [121]. Patients living in these areas with limited healthcare access face additional stressors as they often feel cutoff from their providers without a suitable way to seek care if needed [122]. While all the aforementioned conditions generate chronic stressors in specific communities, cancer-specific-related stressors also present unique challenges for patients and their families.

Impact of Chronic Stressors and Intra- and Interpersonal Processes on Biobehavioral Mechanisms in Cancer in Specific Communities

Health-related quality of life (HRQoL) is significantly affected by the diagnosis, treatment, and outcomes of malignancies [123]. At the time of diagnosis, patients often experience a wide range of feelings and emotions and are concerned about prognostic and treatment information [124]. While the stress and anxiety may differ based on malignancy, and malignancies with notoriously poorer prognoses (e.g., pancreatic cancer) may elicit a more profound stress response, the diagnosis of any malignancies will provoke feelings of stress in a patient [125–127]. After diagnosis, patients will begin their treatment regimen. Depending on the malignancy, treatment may include chemotherapy, radiation therapy, endocrine treatment, surgical excisions, or a combination of two or more modalities [128]. Patients may suffer deleterious side effects from treatments (e.g., neurocognitive decline from chemotherapy, pain or cutaneous symptoms from radiation therapy, decreased libido from endocrine treatments, scarring or persistent discomfort from surgical excisions, etc.) that may trigger stress [129–131]. Following treatment, patients often continue to fear progression or recurrence of their malignancy [132]. In addition, cancer survivors are required to maintain close follow-up with providers and often are subjected to continued screenings with laboratory and radiologic examinations as well [117]. In all facets of malignancy care, patients are subjected to stressful moments, and the chronic stress felt by these patients is often challenging to cope with.

For patients of sociodemographic minorities, additional challenges are faced when undergoing treatment for a malignancy. Hispanic and Black patients are often subjected to disparate cancer-related outcomes and poorer prognoses [133]. These disparities may be attributed to later-stage diagnoses due to decreased access to health screening services, limited availability of curative therapies due to a paucity of health insurance plans that cover these treatments, and inadequate follow-up due to poor health literacy or limited understanding of recommendations [68]. Increased morbidity and mortality are experienced by these patients which contribute to decreased HRQoL and increased chronic stressors [34].

In specific cancers, patients experience stress through a variety of biobehavioral mechanisms. In breast cancer, the most common cancer among women, patients suffer from significant stressors despite often having a favorable prognosis [134]. Surgery for breast cancer may leave a woman with decreased body image and self-esteem, a significant source of stress for survivors [135]. Strategies have been implemented to overcome these challenges, such as breast conservation therapy or breast reconstruction options, but many women report continued stress and decreased self-esteem despite these options [136]. Additionally, surgery and radiation therapy for breast cancer are risk factors for chronic upper extremity lymphedema, a condition with persistent pain and swelling of the arms due to inadequate drainage of lymphatic vessels. This condition leads to chronic discomfort, frequent visits to the doctor, and chronic stress.

In prostate cancer, males face a variety of challenges when undergoing treatment. Surgical resection of the prostate can lead to chronic pain and discomfort at surgical sites, urinary incontinence, and sexual dysfunction [137]. Many male patients (up to 70%) report decreased HRQoL due to an inability to attain an erection and be intimate with their partners [138]. Despite medications and other invasive treatments, many male patients report a continued inability to attain an erection for years after their cancer treatment has been completed [139]. Additionally, hormonal therapies (e.g., androgen deprivation therapy), often prescribed for prostate cancer survivors, can cause cognitive decline, depression, osteoporosis, and sexual dysfunction [140, 141]. These chronic side effects lead to stressors causing significant decreases in HRQoL and general well-being [142].

In cancers of the ovaries, often an oophorectomy is required which can have significant biochemical side effects [143]. Without adequate hormone secretion, women may experience fatigue, depression or anxiety, cognitive decline, osteoporosis, and decreased libido [144]. Patients often will take hormone supplementation to counteract these side effects, but significant stress is increased in post-oophorectomy patients [145, 146]. In cervical cancer, side effects of treatment may include painful intercourse, irregular menses, increased urinary frequency or incontinence, or inability to conceive [147]. These treatment side effects lead to profound stress in cancer survivors and pose unique challenges and stressors to clinicians, patients, and their families [148].

Pancreatic cancer is the leading cause of cancer-related mortality in the United States with a 5-year overall survival of only 10% [149–151]. Only 15–20% of patients are eligible to undergo potentially curative surgical resection, as most tumors are deemed unresectable due to locally advanced disease or distant metastases at the time of diagnosis [152, 153]. The advanced stage of presentation necessitates treatment with toxic chemotherapy and radiation therapy regimens that lead to significant, often long-term side effects. Even curative surgery for most pancreatic cancer patients involves a complex procedure, which is associated with significant postoperative morbidity in many patients [154, 155]. These treatments and particularly surgery may lead to prolonged hospital stays, treatment-related dysfunction, and chronic and debilitating side effects that persist well beyond the treatment and perioperative period and impact all aspects of HRQoL [156, 157].

Finally, colon cancer, the second leading cause of cancer-related death when male and female patients are combined, contributes to significant psychosocial distress [158]. Patients undergoing treatment for colorectal cancers may require complex surgical and medical treatments [159]. Chemotherapy side effects, including fatigue, hair loss, and cognitive impairments, lead to increased stress, but surgical interventions pose unique challenges. After surgery to remove all or part of the colon, patients may experience changes to bowel habits and require frequent trips to the bathroom [160]. Patients may also be required to have a colostomy, ileostomy, or other means for stool diversion. These aspects of colon cancer treatment make it particularly challenging for patients to cope with their disease and can provide significant chronic stressors [161, 162]. While some of these challenges can be overcome through medical or surgical therapies (e.g., increased fiber intake, reversal of a colostomy, etc.), the stressors may have already led to systemic changes and deleterious effects [163]. The discussion of negative symptomatology leading to decreased HRQoL and chronic stressors can be exhaustive, so it is imperative that psychosocial interventions be developed to assist in patient coping and stress management.

Psychosocial Intervention Effects on Stress, Biobehavioral Processes, and Outcomes in Cancer Patients

Interventions designed to reduce the effects of stress or teach patients to cope with challenges in their lives are paramount to minimizing the long-term hazards of chronic stressors. One such strategy is through the use of cognitive behavioral therapy (CBT). CBT is defined as a psychosocial intervention that combines the principles of behavioral and cognitive psychology to promote mindfulness and wellness [164]. Maladaptive and avoidance behaviors are often targeted to assist in patients overcoming their fears and avoidance of stress-provoking situations [165]. This method of stress reduction is one of the most broadly utilized, and evidence of its efficacy has been shown for breast, prostate, colon, and many other cancers [164–167]. A similar model, cognitive-behavioral stress management (CBSM), focuses on a patient's emotions and behaviors in an attempt to identify irrational thoughts and change behaviors through repetitive patterns. This model has been utilized to increase adherence to medications or treatment regimen, decrease depressive symptoms, and decrease systemic symptoms of inflammation [168, 169].

Supportive expressive therapy (SET) is another intervention utilized to improve HRQoL in cancer survivors. The intervention works to facilitate the building of bonds with family members and healthcare professionals to forge a strong social support system for patients [170]. Patients are encouraged to express their emotions and cope with challenges during treatment, including potential end-of-life discussions [170, 171]. SET has been utilized in a variety of malignancies but has been most extensively studied in localized and metastatic breast cancer [171, 172]. In addition to SET, acceptance and commitment therapy (ACT) has been shown to increase HRQoL and decrease stress in cancer survivors [173]. ACT works to reduce or eliminate avoidance of deleterious behaviors and increase a patient's commitment to behaviors that are positive or helpful to their well-being or treatment regimen [174]. Studies have shown that through the use of ACT, patients have decreased emotional distress, anxiety, and depression while increasing treatment adherence, psychological flexibility, and overall quality of life [173, 174]. Finally, mindfulness-based stress reduction (MBSR) has been shown to decrease stress and improve cognitive function in cancer survivors [175]. MBSR is typically a structured group-based program that incorporates meditation, yoga, and walking meditation [176]. Patients are encouraged to utilize these calming skills in their everyday lives, after the group sessions have finished [176]. Through the use of MBSR, patients have reported improvements in stress, depression, anxiety, and overall quality-of-life [177].

Although mentioned above, it is important to highlight the benefits self-reflection, meditation, and yoga can have on a patient's stress response and overall well-being [178]. In randomized control trials, yoga has been found to have beneficial effects on both physical and psychosocial symptoms [179]. Yoga can be quickly learned and practiced in both individual and group-based settings, and patients report feeling decreased stress and anxiety after each session [180]. Additionally, other forms of complementary and alternative medicine, such as acupuncture, may provide stress relief to some patients [181]. In addition to interventions designed to target individuals, programs that target systemic changes, especially in underserved communities, are also needed and extremely beneficial to imparting positive outcomes in stress reduction for cancer survivors.

Inadequate access to oncologic care is a fundamental challenge for minority communities and can lead to significant feelings of stress and anxiety in patients. Ensuring adequate access requires trust in the healthcare system and trust that physicians and other providers will provide exemplary and equitable care for all patients [182]. Gaining the trust of sociodemographic minorities often requires engaging community leaders to discuss specific actions the healthcare providers in the community can take to earn (and sustain) trust [183]. Minority patients often have strong bonds within their communities and look to their mentors and leaders for sources of support and guidance [184]. Community organizations such churches, civic groups, sporting venues, or other areas of community gathering places provide a platform to meet with and discuss available services [185]. Minority patients may not have always had access to available or affordable healthcare, so an effort must be made to inform these populations of available preventative, health-maintenance, and treatment resources [186]. Through programs that increase community outreach and patient understanding of available services, sociodemographic minorities may be able to access the healthcare system and decrease stress and anxiety.

Once a community is engaged and begins to trust the healthcare infrastructure, it is important to work with these community leaders to identify perceived areas of need in the minority communities [187]. Studies have shown that patients in underserved communities, including those of Hispanic and Black race/ethnicity, appreciate being engaged in discussions about their healthcare needs [188, 189]. For instance, in some communities, patients may be interested in smoking cessation programs or screening for malignancies, while other communities may be concerned with sexually transmitted infections and preventing their spread [188, 190]. Through discussions with community leaders, healthcare providers can empower patients to take an interest in their healthcare while also gaining the trust of these patients as discussed above [185]. Only through community partnerships, and establishment of community advisory boards, can minority patients and providers achieve a healthcare system trusted by all and engaged with providing the needed services in a given community [191]. Additionally, sustained community-based engagement and investment in education and other programs have a mutual and reciprocal benefit for providers and hospital systems as well [192]. By engaging with minority communities, patients will feel more comfortable accessing the healthcare system, a step that will work toward quelling the fears, stress, and anxiety associated with visiting a doctor's office, hospital, or clinic.

In specific underserved communities, additional actions must be taken to design targeted programs to alleviate stress and anxiety, and several examples of such interventions are detailed below. In Hispanic and Latino prostate cancer survivors, culturally adapted interventions have been designed to improve the quality-of-life in Spanish monolingual patients with prostate cancer [193]. An intervention, *Encuentros de Salud*, includes CBSM models to decrease symptom burden and improve HRQoL in patients with localized prostate cancer [194]. In Hispanic and Latina breast cancer survivors, peer-developed stress management interventions have been introduced to improve quality-of-life [195]. The CBSM program, *Nuevo Amanecer*, was translated into Spanish, adjusted to adhere to the unique cultural considerations, and shown to reduce psychosocial health disparities in Latina breast cancer survivors [196].

In African American and Caribbean Black breast cancer survivors, culturally informed interventions have been designed to address the unique needs of these patients [197, 198]. One such psychosocial intervention integrated weekly group-based therapy sessions and promoted improved survival in this specific population [199]. A more recent intervention, *Project CARE*, integrated a CBSM intervention for underserved African American breast cancer survivors that integrated group-based weekly sessions [200]. The sessions were designed to reduce anxiety, promote cognitive restructuring, provide coping skills training, build interpersonal skills, and enhance social networks and were shown to improve psychosocial well-being and quality-of-life [201].

For LGBTQ cancer survivors, interventions have been designed to integrate the unique challenges faced by these patients in an effort to reduce psychosocial distress as well. An intervention, *EXCAP*, was designed to integrate a home-based exercise program into the usual cancer management for lesbian and gay cancer survivors and was found to reduce psychosocial distress [202]. While this population of patients has unique challenges, few interventions have been designed to alleviate distress during cancer treatments, and a call to action has been issued to develop new interventions [203].

In patients with human immunodeficiency virus (HIV) or acquired immunodeficiency syndrome (AIDS), CBSM interventions have been utilized to decrease depression and anxiety symptoms [204]. These group-based interventions, tailored toward the unique needs of patients with HIV/AIDS, were also noted to decrease systemic levels of stress hormones, objectively mitigating the psychosocial burden brought on by their disease [205]. While the tailored interventions described above are of great benefit to patients, additional interventions are always needed to target specific underserved populations. Due to differences in cultural upbringing and belief systems, patients of different races, ethnicities, sexual orientation, or other demographics require modulated interventions to target their specific needs.

A novel strategy, currently being tested and developed, is the use of electronic (eHealth) and mobile (mHealth) platforms to deliver targeted interventions to patients [206]. These interventions target a variety of psychosocial and physicals domains in an effort to decrease stress and improve HRQoL. Pain is a pervasive symptom of cancer and its treatments and is prevalent in more than half of cancer patients during active treatment [207]. Researchers have led eHealth and mHealth programs for cancer pain management using a brief pain coping skill trainings [208]. Delivered over tablet videoconferencing, the intervention is both feasible and acceptable to cancer patients with persistent cancer- and treatment-related pain with benefits comparable to a traditional in-person intervention (e.g., decreased pain sensitivity, increased self-efficacy for pain management) [209, 210]. Fatigue has also been targeted by eHealth and mHealth interventions, and in patients with chronic myeloid leukemia, and via tablet videoconference platform, patients had improvements in fatigue and overall HRQoL [211]. Finally, in the psychosocial distress domain, tablet-based mHealth ACT interventions have been established to reduced cancer-specific distress in patients [212]. There are many other examples in the literature and numerous additional studies currently underway to facilitate at-home and mobile psychosocial interventions aimed at decreasing stress.

Conclusions and Future Directions

As more is learned about the biologic and psychologic pathways that trigger and manifest stress, continued innovation is needed. While many underserved and minority populations requiring special attention and tailored interventions are discussed above, there are many more understudied and at-risk communities. Patients in these vulnerable groups may benefit from targeted interventions, and investigation is needed to identify these populations and develop suitable platforms. While much is now understood in this field, the biologic and biochemical pathways must be further understood in order to truly quantify the efficacy of interventions. Finally, we need to engage patients in helping to tailor their own psychosocial interventions. As healthcare providers, we must work with each patient to better understand their stressors and how they cope. Through these discussions, and clinical trials, interventions can be constructed to reach as broad an audience as possible, working to create a stress-free environment for all who seek it.

To conclude, chronic stress can be generated from many different facets of life, and patients with cancer diagnoses have additional challenges due to poor prognoses, rigorous treatment regimen, and frequent medical visits. As psychosocial stress builds, systemic physical and mental effects can manifest such as cognitive decline, cardiovascular disease, immunologic deficiencies, and many others. In specific underserved communities, such as minority Black/Hispanic, or LGBTQ communities, additional stressors must be considered when evaluating patients and identifying the sources of psychosocial distress. These stressors may be due to barriers to equitable healthcare, language/cultural differences, decreased educational opportunities, neighborhood violence and food insecurity, social discrimination, or other challenges. Interventions designed to ameliorate chronic stressors and psychosocial burden must be cognizant of these unique challenges and tailor their content to address these unique considerations. Stress is a pervasive challenge for all patients, and healthcare providers must remain vigilant when caring for individuals as managing psychosocial stress can be just as important as managing medical illness as well.

References

1. Slavich GM. Life stress and health: a review of conceptual issues and recent findings. Teach Psychol. 2016;43(4):346–55.
2. Rodriguez EM, Smith L. Provider perspectives on stressors, support, and access to mental health care for Latinx youth. Qual Health Res. 2020;30(4):547–59.
3. Ahmad AH, Zakaria R. Pain in times of stress. Malays J Med Sci. 2015;22(Spec Issue):52–61.
4. Williams DR, Mohammed SA. Discrimination and racial disparities in health: evidence and needed research. J Behav Med. 2009;32(1):20–47.
5. Baciu A, Negussie Y, Geller A, Weinstein JN, editors. Communities in action: pathways to health equity. Washington, DC: National Academies Press; 2017.
6. Jordan TR, Khubchandani J, Wiblishauser M. The impact of perceived stress and coping adequacy on the health of nurses: a pilot investigation. Nurs Res Pract. 2016;2016:5843256.
7. Myers HF, Taylor S, Alvy KT, Arrington A, Richardson MA. Parental and family predictors of behavior problems in inner-city black children. Am J Community Psychol. 1992;20(5):557–76.
8. Meyer SE, Chrousos GP, Gold PW. Major depression and the stress system: a life span perspective. Dev Psychopathol. 2001;13(3):565–80.
9. Cameron HA, Schoenfeld TJ. Behavioral and structural adaptations to stress. Front Neuroendocrinol. 2018;49:106–13.
10. Dunlavey CJ. Introduction to the hypothalamic-pituitary-adrenal axis: healthy and dysregulated stress responses, developmental stress and neurodegeneration. J Undergrad Neurosci Educ. 2018;16(2):R59–60.

11. Anderson NB, Bulatao RA, Cohen B, editors. Critical perspectives on racial and ethnic differences in health in late life. Washington, DC: National Academies Press; 2004.
12. Esch T, Stefano GB, Fricchione GL, Benson H. The role of stress in neurodegenerative diseases and mental disorders. Neuro Endocrinol Lett. 2002;23(3):199–208.
13. Myers HF. Ethnicity- and socio-economic status-related stresses in context: an integrative review and conceptual model. J Behav Med. 2009;32(1):9–19.
14. Myers HF, Wyatt GE, Ullman JB, et al. Cumulative burden of lifetime adversities: trauma and mental health in low-SES African Americans and Latino/as. Psychol Trauma. 2015;7(3):243–51.
15. Orr ST, James SA, Miller CA, et al. Psychosocial stressors and low birthweight in an urban population. Am J Prev Med. 1996;12(6):459–66.
16. Holland ML, Kitzman H, Veazie P. The effects of stress on birth weight in low-income, unmarried black women. Womens Health Issues. 2009;19(6):390–7.
17. Sharma S, Powers A, Bradley B, Ressler KJ. Gene X environment determinants of stress- and anxiety-related disorders. Annu Rev Psychol. 2016;67:239–61.
18. Toussaint L, Shields GS, Dorn G, Slavich GM. Effects of lifetime stress exposure on mental and physical health in young adulthood: how stress degrades and forgiveness protects health. J Health Psychol. 2016;21(6):1004–14.
19. Gallo LC, de Los Monteros KE, Shivpuri S. Socioeconomic status and health: what is the role of reserve capacity? Curr Dir Psychol Sci. 2009;18(5):269–74.
20. Gallo LC, Bogart LM, Vranceanu AM, Matthews KA. Socioeconomic status, resources, psychological experiences, and emotional responses: a test of the reserve capacity model. J Pers Soc Psychol. 2005;88(2):386–99.
21. Matthews KA, Gallo LC, Taylor SE. Are psychosocial factors mediators of socioeconomic status and health connections? A progress report and blueprint for the future. Ann N Y Acad Sci. 2010;1186:146–73.
22. Gallo LC, Matthews KA. Understanding the association between socioeconomic status and physical health: do negative emotions play a role? Psychol Bull. 2003;129(1):10–51.
23. Krieger N. Methods for the scientific study of discrimination and health: an ecosocial approach. Am J Public Health. 2012;102(5):936–44.
24. Krieger N. Embodying inequality: a review of concepts, measures, and methods for studying health consequences of discrimination. Int J Health Serv. 1999;29(2):295–352.
25. Williams DR, Collins C. US socioeconomic and racial differences in health: patterns and explanations. Annu Rev Sociol. 1995;21(1):349–86.
26. Krieger N. Discrimination and health inequities. Int J Health Serv. 2014;44(4):643–710.
27. Krieger N. Theories for social epidemiology in the 21st century: an ecosocial perspective. Int J Epidemiol. 2001;30(4):668–77.
28. Starkweather AR, Alhaeeri AA, Montpetit A, et al. An integrative review of factors associated with telomere length and implications for biobehavioral research. Nurs Res. 2014;63(1):36–50.
29. Alhareeri AA, Archer KJ, Fu H, et al. Telomere lengths in women treated for breast cancer show associations with chemotherapy, pain symptoms, and cognitive domain measures: a longitudinal study. Breast Cancer Res. 2020;22(1):137.
30. Corbett T, Groarke A, Walsh JC, McGuire BE. Cancer-related fatigue in post-treatment cancer survivors: application of the common sense model of illness representations. BMC Cancer. 2016;16(1):919.
31. Bower JE. Cancer-related fatigue – mechanisms, risk factors, and treatments. Nat Rev Clin Oncol. 2014;11(10):597–609.
32. Lyon D, Elmore L, Aboalela N, et al. Potential epigenetic mechanism(s) associated with the persistence of psychoneurological symptoms in women receiving chemotherapy for breast cancer: a hypothesis. Biol Res Nurs. 2014;16(2):160–74.

33. Yang GS, Mi X, Jackson-Cook CK, et al. Differential DNA methylation following chemotherapy for breast cancer is associated with lack of memory improvement at one year. Epigenetics. 2020;15(5):499–510.
34. Yanez B, McGinty HL, Buitrago D, Ramirez AG, Penedo FJ. Cancer outcomes in Hispanics/Latinos in the United States: an integrative review and conceptual model of determinants of health. J Lat Psychol. 2016;4(2):114–29.
35. Ward E, Jemal A, Cokkinides V, et al. Cancer disparities by race/ethnicity and socioeconomic status. CA Cancer J Clin. 2004;54(2):78–93.
36. Ashing-Giwa KT, Padilla GV, Bohorquez DE, Tejero JS, Garcia M. Understanding the breast cancer experience of Latina women. J Psychosoc Oncol. 2006;24(3):19–52.
37. Kahende JW, Malarcher AM, Teplinskaya A, Asman KJ. Quit attempt correlates among smokers by race/ethnicity. Int J Environ Res Public Health. 2011;8(10):3871–88.
38. Yanez B, Thompson EH, Stanton AL. Quality of life among Latina breast cancer patients: a systematic review of the literature. J Cancer Surviv. 2011;5(2):191–207.
39. Cokkinides VE, Bandi P, Siegel RL, Jemal A. Cancer-related risk factors and preventive measures in US Hispanics/Latinos. CA Cancer J Clin. 2012;62(6):353–63.
40. McCurley JL, Penedo F, Roesch SC, et al. Psychosocial factors in the relationship between socioeconomic status and cardiometabolic risk: the HCHS/SOL sociocultural ancillary study. Ann Behav Med. 2017;51(4):477–88.
41. Williams DR, Mohammed SA, Leavell J, Collins C. Race, socioeconomic status, and health: complexities, ongoing challenges, and research opportunities. Ann N Y Acad Sci. 2010;1186:69–101.
42. Winkleby MA, Jatulis DE, Frank E, Fortmann SP. Socioeconomic status and health: how education, income, and occupation contribute to risk factors for cardiovascular disease. Am J Public Health. 1992;82(6):816–20.
43. OMH. Profile: Hispanic/Latino Americans. US Department of Health and Human Services. https://minorityhealth.hhs.gov/omh/browse.aspx?lvl=3&lvlid=64. Published 2019. Accessed 29 Sept 2020.
44. OMH. Profile: Black/African Americans. US Department of Health and Human Services. https://minorityhealth.hhs.gov/omh/browse.aspx?lvl=3&lvlid=61. Published 2019. Accessed 8 Dec 2020.
45. Tienda M, Mitchell F, National Research Council (U.S.). Panel on Hispanics in the United States, National Research Council (U.S.). Committee on Population. Hispanics and the future of America. Washington, DC: National Academies Press; 2006.
46. Singh GK, Jemal A. Socioeconomic and racial/ethnic disparities in cancer mortality, incidence, and survival in the United States, 1950–2014: over six decades of changing patterns and widening inequalities. J Environ Public Health. 2017;2017:2819372.
47. Jacobson HE, Hund L, Soto MF. Predictors of English health literacy among U.S. Hispanic immigrants: the importance of language, bilingualism and sociolinguistic environment. Lit Numer Stud. 2016;24(1):43–64.
48. Santos MG, Handley MA, Omark K, Schillinger D. ESL participation as a mechanism for advancing health literacy in immigrant communities. J Health Commun. 2014;19(Suppl 2):89–105.
49. Lynch J, Smith GD, Harper S, et al. Is income inequality a determinant of population health? Part 1. A systematic review. Milbank Q. 2004;82(1):5–99.
50. Census. Real median household income by race and Hispanic origin: 1967 to 2017. US Department of Commerce. https://www.census.gov/content/dam/Census/library/visualizations/2018/demo/p60-263/figure1.pdf. Published 2018. Accessed 29 Sept 2020.
51. Monnat SM, Raffalovich LE, Tsao HS. Trends in the family income distribution by race/ethnicity and income source, 1988–2009. Popul Rev. 2012;51(1):85–115.
52. Pager D, Pedulla DS. Race, self-selection, and the job search process. AJS. 2015;120(4):1005–54.

53. National Research Council (U.S.), Committee on Future Directions for Behavioral and Social Sciences Research at the National Institutes of Health, Singer B, Ryff CD. New horizons in health: an integrative approach. Washington, DC: National Academy Press; 2001.
54. Schneiderman N, Ironson G, Siegel SD. Stress and health: psychological, behavioral, and biological determinants. Annu Rev Clin Psychol. 2005;1:607–28.
55. Lipovcan LK, Prizmic-Larsen Z, Brkljacic T. Materialism, affective states, and life satisfaction: case of Croatia. Springerplus. 2015;4:699.
56. Baum A, Garofalo JP, Yali AM. Socioeconomic status and chronic stress. Does stress account for SES effects on health? Ann N Y Acad Sci. 1999;896:131–44.
57. Neece CL, Green SA, Baker BL. Parenting stress and child behavior problems: a transactional relationship across time. Am J Intellect Dev Disabil. 2012;117(1):48–66.
58. Barroso NE, Mendez L, Graziano PA, Bagner DM. Parenting stress through the lens of different clinical groups: a systematic review & meta-analysis. J Abnorm Child Psychol. 2018;46(3):449–61.
59. Luthar SS. The culture of affluence: psychological costs of material wealth. Child Dev. 2003;74(6):1581–93.
60. Monnat SM. The new destination disadvantage: disparities in Hispanic health insurance coverage rates in metropolitan and nonmetropolitan new and established destinations. Rural Sociol. 2017;82(1):3–43.
61. Sohn H. Racial and ethnic disparities in health insurance coverage: dynamics of gaining and losing coverage over the life-course. Popul Res Policy Rev. 2017;36(2):181–201.
62. Steinberg EM, Valenzuela-Araujo D, Zickafoose JS, Kieffer E, DeCamp LR. The "battle" of managing language barriers in health care. Clin Pediatr (Phila). 2016;55(14):1318–27.
63. Chavez LJ, Ornelas IJ, Lyles CR, Williams EC. Racial/ethnic workplace discrimination: association with tobacco and alcohol use. Am J Prev Med. 2015;48(1):42–9.
64. Couch KA, Fairlie R. Last hired, first fired? Black-white unemployment and the business cycle. Demography. 2010;47(1):227–47.
65. Todorovic N, Jovic-Vranes A, Djikanovic B, Pilipovic-Broceta N, Vasiljevic N, Racic M. Health literacy: current status and challenges in the work of family doctors in Bosnia and Herzegovina. Int J Environ Res Public Health. 2019;16(8):1324.
66. Devoe JE, Baez A, Angier H, Krois L, Edlund C, Carney PA. Insurance + access not equal to health care: typology of barriers to health care access for low-income families. Ann Fam Med. 2007;5(6):511–8.
67. McGee R. Does stress cause cancer? There's no good evidence of a relation between stressful events and cancer. BMJ. 1999;319(7216):1015–6.
68. Kronenfeld JP, Ryon EL, Goldberg D, et al. Disparities in presentation at time of hepatocellular carcinoma diagnosis: a United States safety-net collaborative study. Ann Surg Oncol. 2020;28(4):1929–36.
69. Kronenfeld JP, Goel N. ASO author reflections: access to care and screening inequities for patients at risk for hepatocellular carcinoma. Ann Surg Oncol. 2020;28(4):1937–8.
70. Pascoe EA, Smart Richman L. Perceived discrimination and health: a meta-analytic review. Psychol Bull. 2009;135(4):531–54.
71. Smart Richman L, Leary MR. Reactions to discrimination, stigmatization, ostracism, and other forms of interpersonal rejection: a multimotive model. Psychol Rev. 2009;116(2):365–83.
72. Hill LK, Sherwood A, McNeilly M, Anderson NB, Blumenthal JA, Hinderliter AL. Impact of racial discrimination and hostility on adrenergic receptor responsiveness in African American adults. Psychosom Med. 2018;80(2):208–15.
73. Blair IV, Steiner JF, Havranek EP. Unconscious (implicit) bias and health disparities: where do we go from here? Perm J. 2011;15(2):71–8.
74. FitzGerald C, Hurst S. Implicit bias in healthcare professionals: a systematic review. BMC Med Ethics. 2017;18(1):19.
75. Stepanikova I. Racial-ethnic biases, time pressure, and medical decisions. J Health Soc Behav. 2012;53(3):329–43.

76. Weiner S. "I can't afford that!": dilemmas in the care of the uninsured and underinsured. J Gen Intern Med. 2001;16(6):412–8.
77. Reschovsky JD, O'Malley AS. Do primary care physicians treating minority patients report problems delivering high-quality care? Health Aff (Millwood). 2008;27(3):w222–31.
78. Burner ERE, Menchine MD, Kubicek K, Robles M, Kagawa Singer M, Arora S. Perceptions of family among low-income patients with diabetes in a text-based mobile health intervention. J Diabetes Sci Technol. 2018;12(6):1203–10.
79. Gailey S, Bruckner TA. Obesity among black women in food deserts: an "omnibus" test of differential risk. SSM Popul Health. 2019;7:100363.
80. USDA. Characteristics and influential factors of food deserts. US Department of Agriculture. https://www.ers.usda.gov/webdocs/publications/45014/30940_err140.pdf. Published 2012. Accessed 29 Sept 2020.
81. Wilbur J, Zenk S, Wang E, et al. Neighborhood characteristics, adherence to walking, and depressive symptoms in midlife African American women. J Womens Health (Larchmt). 2009;18(8):1201–10.
82. Institute of Medicine (U.S.), Committee on Childhood Obesity Prevention Actions for Local Governments, Parker L, Burns AC, Sanchez E. Local government actions to prevent childhood obesity. Washington, DC: National Academies Press; 2009.
83. Kelli HM, Kim JH, Samman Tahhan A, et al. Living in food deserts and adverse cardiovascular outcomes in patients with cardiovascular disease. J Am Heart Assoc. 2019;8(4):e010694.
84. Kim DH. Nutritional issues in patients with cancer. Intest Res. 2019;17(4):455–62.
85. Cutrona CE, Wallace G, Wesner KA. Neighborhood characteristics and depression: an examination of stress processes. Curr Dir Psychol Sci. 2006;15(4):188–92.
86. Estrada-Martinez LM, Cantrell C, Sewell W, Butler-Barnes S, Cabrera-Nguyen EP. Adolescent neighborhood environments and Latino intraethnic disparities in trajectories of serious violent behaviors. Hisp J Behav Sci. 2017;39(4):504–27.
87. Martinez CR, Degarmo DS, Eddy JM. Promoting academic success among Latino youth. Hisp J Behav Sci. 2004;26(2):128–51.
88. McGill TM, Self-Brown SR, Lai BS, et al. Effects of exposure to community violence and family violence on school functioning problems among urban youth: the potential mediating role of posttraumatic stress symptoms. Front Public Health. 2014;2:8.
89. Cooley-Strickland M, Quille TJ, Griffin RS, Stuart EA, Bradshaw CP, Furr-Holden D. Community violence and youth: affect, behavior, substance use, and academics. Clin Child Fam Psychol Rev. 2009;12(2):127–56.
90. Theall KP, Chaparro MP, Denstel K, Bilfield A, Drury SS. Childhood obesity and the associated roles of neighborhood and biologic stress. Prev Med Rep. 2019;14:100849.
91. Kerr J, Anderson C, Lippman SM. Physical activity, sedentary behaviour, diet, and cancer: an update and emerging new evidence. Lancet Oncol. 2017;18(8):e457–71.
92. Sun L, Zhu Y, Qian Q, Tang L. Body mass index and prognosis of breast cancer: an analysis by menstruation status when breast cancer diagnosis. Medicine (Baltimore). 2018;97(26):e11220.
93. Arem H, Irwin ML. Obesity and endometrial cancer survival: a systematic review. Int J Obes. 2013;37(5):634–9.
94. Yu YD, Byun SS, Lee SE, Hong SK. Impact of body mass index on oncological outcomes of prostate cancer patients after radical prostatectomy. Sci Rep. 2018;8(1):11962.
95. Salleh MR. Life event, stress and illness. Malays J Med Sci. 2008;15(4):9–18.
96. Rowe D, Ng YC, O'Keefe L, Crawford D. Providers' attitudes and knowledge of lesbian, gay, bisexual, and transgender health. Fed Pract. 2017;34(11):28–34.
97. Mays VM, Juster RP, Williamson TJ, Seeman TE, Cochran SD. Chronic physiologic effects of stress among lesbian, gay, and bisexual adults: results from the National Health and Nutrition Examination Survey. Psychosom Med. 2018;80(6):551–63.
98. White Hughto JM, Reisner SL, Pachankis JE. Transgender stigma and health: a critical review of stigma determinants, mechanisms, and interventions. Soc Sci Med. 2015;147:222–31.

99. Herek GM. Sexual stigma and sexual prejudice in the United States: a conceptual framework. Neb Symp Motiv. 2009;54:65–111.
100. Russell ST, Fish JN. Mental health in lesbian, gay, bisexual, and transgender (LGBT) youth. Annu Rev Clin Psychol. 2016;12:465–87.
101. Floyd FJ, Bakeman R. Coming-out across the life course: implications of age and historical context. Arch Sex Behav. 2006;35(3):287–96.
102. Condon EM. Chronic stress in children and adolescents: a review of biomarkers for use in pediatric research. Biol Res Nurs. 2018;20(5):473–96.
103. Wolke D, Lereya ST. Long-term effects of bullying. Arch Dis Child. 2015;100(9):879–85.
104. Simmons JG, Badcock PB, Whittle SL, et al. The lifetime experience of traumatic events is associated with hair cortisol concentrations in community-based children. Psychoneuroendocrinology. 2016;63:276–81.
105. de Frias CM, Whyne E. Stress on health-related quality of life in older adults: the protective nature of mindfulness. Aging Ment Health. 2015;19(3):201–6.
106. Thomas PA, Liu H, Umberson D. Family Relationships and Well-Being. Innov Aging. 2017;1(3):igx025.
107. Dickinson WJ, Potter GG, Hybels CF, McQuoid DR, Steffens DC. Change in stress and social support as predictors of cognitive decline in older adults with and without depression. Int J Geriatr Psychiatry. 2011;26(12):1267–74.
108. Vardy J. Cognitive function in breast cancer survivors. Cancer Treat Res. 2009;151:387–419.
109. Zhang Q, Gao X, Liu S, Yu L, Zhu J, Qiu S. Therapies for cognitive impairment in breast cancer survivors treated with chemotherapy: a protocol for systematic review. Medicine (Baltimore). 2020;99(19):e20092.
110. Piacentine LB, Miller JF, Haberlein S, Bloom AS. Perceived cognitive changes with chemotherapy for breast cancer: a pilot study. Appl Nurs Res. 2016;29:9–11.
111. Ahles TA, Root JC, Ryan EL. Cancer- and cancer treatment-associated cognitive change: an update on the state of the science. J Clin Oncol. 2012;30(30):3675–86.
112. Selamat MH, Loh SY, Mackenzie L, Vardy J. Chemobrain experienced by breast cancer survivors: a meta-ethnography study investigating research and care implications. PLoS One. 2014;9(9):e108002.
113. Cahill E, Lewis LM, Barg FK, Bogner HR. "You don't want to burden them": older adults' views on family involvement in care. J Fam Nurs. 2009;15(3):295–317.
114. Duric V, Clayton S, Leong ML, Yuan LL. Comorbidity factors and brain mechanisms linking chronic stress and systemic illness. Neural Plast. 2016;2016:5460732.
115. Schelling G. Post-traumatic stress disorder in somatic disease: lessons from critically ill patients. Prog Brain Res. 2008;167:229–37.
116. Barre PV, Padmaja G, Rana S, Tiamongla. Stress and quality of life in cancer patients: medical and psychological intervention. Indian J Psychol Med. 2018;40(3):232–8.
117. Roohafza H, Kabir A, Sadeghi M, et al. Stress as a risk factor for noncompliance with treatment regimens in patients with diabetes and hypertension. ARYA Atheroscler. 2016;12(4):166–71.
118. Williamson AE, Ellis DA, Wilson P, McQueenie R, McConnachie A. Understanding repeated non-attendance in health services: a pilot analysis of administrative data and full study protocol for a national retrospective cohort. BMJ Open. 2017;7(2):e014120.
119. CDC. Chronic diseases in America. US Department of Health and Human Services. https://www.cdc.gov/chronicdisease/resources/infographic/chronic-diseases.htm. Published 2020. Accessed 9 Dec 2020.
120. Jong M, Mendez I, Jong R. Enhancing access to care in northern rural communities via telehealth. Int J Circumpolar Health. 2019;78(2):1554174.
121. Varela C, Young S, Mkandawire N, Groen RS, Banza L, Viste A. Transportation barriers to access health care for surgical conditions in Malawi a cross sectional nationwide household survey. BMC Public Health. 2019;19(1):264.
122. Cyr ME, Etchin AG, Guthrie BJ, Benneyan JC. Access to specialty healthcare in urban versus rural US populations: a systematic literature review. BMC Health Serv Res. 2019;19(1):974.

123. Sitlinger A, Zafar SY. Health-related quality of life: the impact on morbidity and mortality. Surg Oncol Clin N Am. 2018;27(4):675–84.
124. Osoba D. Health-related quality of life and cancer clinical trials. Ther Adv Med Oncol. 2011;3(2):57–71.
125. Kruk J, Aboul-Enein BH, Bernstein J, Gronostaj M. Psychological stress and cellular aging in cancer: a meta-analysis. Oxidative Med Cell Longev. 2019;2019:1270397.
126. Passik SD, Roth AJ. Anxiety symptoms and panic attacks preceding pancreatic cancer diagnosis. Psychooncology. 1999;8(3):268–72.
127. Park HY. Emotional support and palliative care for distressed patients suffering from pancreatic cancer. Korean J Gastroenterol. 2019;74(2):95–100.
128. Zhang XY, Zhang PY. Combinations in multimodality treatments and clinical outcomes during cancer. Oncol Lett. 2016;12(6):4301–4.
129. Kovalchuk A, Kolb B. Chemo brain: from discerning mechanisms to lifting the brain fog-an aging connection. Cell Cycle. 2017;16(14):1345–9.
130. Doo AR, Shin YS, Yoo S, Park JK. Radiation-induced neuropathic pain successfully treated with systemic lidocaine administration. J Pain Res. 2018;11:545–8.
131. Van Loey NE, Van Son MJ. Psychopathology and psychological problems in patients with burn scars: epidemiology and management. Am J Clin Dermatol. 2003;4(4):245–72.
132. Dinkel A, Herschbach P. Fear of progression in cancer patients and survivors. Recent Results Cancer Res. 2018;210:13–33.
133. Ozdemir BC, Dotto GP. Racial differences in cancer susceptibility and survival: more than the color of the skin? Trends Cancer. 2017;3(3):181–97.
134. Baqutayan SM. The effect of anxiety on breast cancer patients. Indian J Psychol Med. 2012;34(2):119–23.
135. Guedes TSR, Dantas de Oliveira NP, Holanda AM, et al. Body image of women submitted to breast cancer treatment. Asian Pac J Cancer Prev. 2018;19(6):1487–93.
136. Archangelo SCV, Sabino Neto M, Veiga DF, Garcia EB, Ferreira LM. Sexuality, depression and body image after breast reconstruction. Clinics (Sao Paulo). 2019;74:e883.
137. Singla N, Singla AK. Post-prostatectomy incontinence: etiology, evaluation, and management. Turk J Urol. 2014;40(1):1–8.
138. Chung E, Gillman M. Prostate cancer survivorship: a review of erectile dysfunction and penile rehabilitation after prostate cancer therapy. Med J Aust. 2014;200(10):582–5.
139. Kim JH, Lee SW. Current status of penile rehabilitation after radical prostatectomy. Korean J Urol. 2015;56(2):99–108.
140. Rhee H, Gunter JH, Heathcote P, et al. Adverse effects of androgen-deprivation therapy in prostate cancer and their management. BJU Int. 2015;115(Suppl 5):3–13.
141. Penedo FJ, Fox RS, Oswald LB, et al. Technology-based psychosocial intervention to improve quality of life and reduce symptom burden in men with advanced prostate cancer: results from a randomized controlled trial. Int J Behav Med. 2020;27(5):490–505.
142. Victorson D, Schalet BD, Kundu S, et al. Establishing a common metric for self-reported anxiety in patients with prostate cancer: linking the memorial anxiety scale for prostate cancer with PROMIS anxiety. Cancer. 2019;125(18):3249–58.
143. Rocca WA, Grossardt BR, Maraganore DM. The long-term effects of oophorectomy on cognitive and motor aging are age dependent. Neurodegener Dis. 2008;5(3–4):257–60.
144. Erekson EA, Martin DK, Zhu K, et al. Sexual function in older women after oophorectomy. Obstet Gynecol. 2012;120(4):833–42.
145. Rocca WA, Shuster LT, Grossardt BR, et al. Long-term effects of bilateral oophorectomy on brain aging: unanswered questions from the Mayo Clinic Cohort Study of Oophorectomy and Aging. Womens Health (Lond). 2009;5(1):39–48.
146. Ethokovic DD, Jovic JJ, Ethokovic JD, Knezevic MZ, Djukic-Dejanovic S, Ristic-Ignjatovic DI. Effects of hormone replacement therapy on depressive and anxiety symptoms after oophorectomy. Med Glas (Zenica). 2015;12(1):79–85.

147. Ros C, Espuna M. Impact of cervical cancer treatment on micturition and sexual function. Actas Urol Esp. 2013;37(1):40–6.
148. Andersen BL. Stress and quality of life following cervical cancer. J Natl Cancer Inst Monogr. 1996;21:65–70.
149. Society AC. Cancer facts & figures 2019. American Cancer Society. https://www.cancer.org/content/dam/cancer-org/research/cancer-facts-and-statistics/annual-cancer-facts-and-figures/2019/cancer-facts-and-figures-2019.pdf. Published 2019. Accessed 20 June 2020.
150. Research HFfPC. Pancreatic cancer facts. http://pancreatic.org/pancreatic-cancer/pancreatic-cancer-facts/. Published 2019. Accessed 20 June 2020.
151. NIH. Cancer stat facts: common cancer sites. United States Department of Health and Human Services. https://seer.cancer.gov/statfacts/html/common.html. Published 2020. Accessed 20 June 2020.
152. Bilimoria KY, Bentrem DJ, Ko CY, Stewart AK, Winchester DP, Talamonti MS. National failure to operate on early stage pancreatic cancer. Ann Surg. 2007;246(2):173–80.
153. Badger SA, Brant JL, Jones C, et al. The role of surgery for pancreatic cancer: a 12-year review of patient outcome. Ulster Med J. 2010;79(2):70–5.
154. Artinyan A, Soriano PA, Prendergast C, Low T, Ellenhorn JD, Kim J. The anatomic location of pancreatic cancer is a prognostic factor for survival. HPB (Oxford). 2008;10(5):371–6.
155. Kim CB, Ahmed S, Hsueh EC. Current surgical management of pancreatic cancer. J Gastrointest Oncol. 2011;2(3):126–35.
156. Borges EL, Franceschini J, Costa LH, Fernandes AL, Jamnik S, Santoro IL. Family caregiver burden: the burden of caring for lung cancer patients according to the cancer stage and patient quality of life. J Bras Pneumol. 2017;43(1):18–23.
157. Adler NE, Page A, Institute of Medicine (U.S.), Committee on Psychosocial Services to Cancer Patients/Families in a Community Setting. Cancer care for the whole patient: meeting psychosocial health needs. Washington, DC: National Academies Press; 2008.
158. ACS. Key statistics for colorectal cancer. American Cancer Society. https://www.cancer.org/cancer/colon-rectal-cancer/about/key-statistics.html#:~:text=Deaths%20from%20colorectal%20cancer,about%2053%2C200%20deaths%20during%202020. Published 2020. Accessed 9 Dec 2020.
159. Zhang GQ, Taylor JP, Stem M, et al. Aggressive multimodal treatment and metastatic colorectal cancer survival. J Am Coll Surg. 2020;230(4):689–98.
160. Adachi Y, Kakisako K, Sato K, Shiraishi N, Miyahara M, Kitano S. Factors influencing bowel function after low anterior resection and sigmoid colectomy. Hepato-Gastroenterology. 2000;47(31):155–8.
161. Dabirian A, Yaghmaei F, Rassouli M, Tafreshi MZ. Quality of life in ostomy patients: a qualitative study. Patient Prefer Adherence. 2010;5:1–5.
162. Silva NM, Santos MAD, Rosado SR, Galvao CM, Sonobe HM. Psychological aspects of patients with intestinal stoma: integrative review. Rev Lat Am Enfermagem. 2017;25:e2950.
163. Ang SG, Chen HC, Siah RJ, He HG, Klainin-Yobas P. Stressors relating to patient psychological health following stoma surgery: an integrated literature review. Oncol Nurs Forum. 2013;40(6):587–94.
164. Sun H, Huang H, Ji S, et al. The efficacy of cognitive behavioral therapy to treat depression and anxiety and improve quality of life among early-stage breast cancer patients. Integr Cancer Ther. 2019;18:1534735419829573.
165. Greer JA, Traeger L, Bemis H, et al. A pilot randomized controlled trial of brief cognitive-behavioral therapy for anxiety in patients with terminal cancer. Oncologist. 2012;17(10):1337–45.
166. Penedo FJ, Molton I, Dahn JR, et al. A randomized clinical trial of group-based cognitive-behavioral stress management in localized prostate cancer: development of stress management skills improves quality of life and benefit finding. Ann Behav Med. 2006;31(3):261–70.

167. Moonsammy SH, Guglietti CL, Santa Mina D, et al. A pilot study of an exercise & cognitive behavioral therapy intervention for epithelial ovarian cancer patients. J Ovarian Res. 2013;6(1):21.
168. Antoni MH, Lutgendorf SK, Blomberg B, et al. Cognitive-behavioral stress management reverses anxiety-related leukocyte transcriptional dynamics. Biol Psychiatry. 2012;71(4):366–72.
169. Schneiderman N, Antoni M, Ironson G. Cognitive behavioral stress management and secondary prevention in HIV/AIDS. American Psychological Association. https://www.apa.org/pi/aids/resources/research/schneiderman. Published 2011. Accessed 9 Dec 2020.
170. Spiegel D, Butler LD, Giese-Davis J, et al. Effects of supportive-expressive group therapy on survival of patients with metastatic breast cancer: a randomized prospective trial. Cancer. 2007;110(5):1130–8.
171. Giese-Davis J, Koopman C, Butler LD, et al. Change in emotion-regulation strategy for women with metastatic breast cancer following supportive-expressive group therapy. J Consult Clin Psychol. 2002;70(4):916–25.
172. Spiegel D, Cordova M. Supportive-expressive group therapy and life extension of breast cancer patients: Spiegel et al. (1989). Adv Mind Body Med. 2001;17(1):38–41.
173. Feros DL, Lane L, Ciarrochi J, Blackledge JT. Acceptance and commitment therapy (ACT) for improving the lives of cancer patients: a preliminary study. Psychooncology. 2013;22(2):459–64.
174. Gonzalez-Fernandez S, Fernandez-Rodriguez C. Acceptance and commitment therapy in cancer: review of applications and findings. Behav Med. 2019;45(3):255–69.
175. Rush SE, Sharma M. Mindfulness-based stress reduction as a stress management intervention for cancer care: a systematic review. J Evid Based Complementary Altern Med. 2017;22(2):348–60.
176. Cramer H, Lauche R, Paul A, Dobos G. Mindfulness-based stress reduction for breast cancer-a systematic review and meta-analysis. Curr Oncol. 2012;19(5):e343–52.
177. Zhang Q, Zhao H, Zheng Y. Effectiveness of mindfulness-based stress reduction (MBSR) on symptom variables and health-related quality of life in breast cancer patients – a systematic review and meta-analysis. Support Care Cancer. 2019;27(3):771–81.
178. Agarwal RP, Maroko-Afek A. Yoga into cancer care: a review of the evidence-based research. Int J Yoga. 2018;11(1):3–29.
179. Buffart LM, van Uffelen JG, Riphagen II, et al. Physical and psychosocial benefits of yoga in cancer patients and survivors, a systematic review and meta-analysis of randomized controlled trials. BMC Cancer. 2012;12:559.
180. Banerjee B, Vadiraj HS, Ram A, et al. Effects of an integrated yoga program in modulating psychological stress and radiation-induced genotoxic stress in breast cancer patients undergoing radiotherapy. Integr Cancer Ther. 2007;6(3):242–50.
181. Birch S, Lee MS, Alraek T, Kim TH. Evidence, safety and recommendations for when to use acupuncture for treating cancer related symptoms: a narrative review. Integr Med Res. 2019;8(3):160–6.
182. Birkhauer J, Gaab J, Kossowsky J, et al. Trust in the health care professional and health outcome: a meta-analysis. PLoS One. 2017;12(2):e0170988.
183. Ramirez AG, Choi BY, Munoz E, et al. Assessing the effect of patient navigator assistance for psychosocial support services on health-related quality of life in a randomized clinical trial in Latino breast, prostate, and colorectal cancer survivors. Cancer. 2020;126(5):1112–23.
184. Hernandez R, Carnethon M, Penedo FJ, Martinez L, Boehm J, Schueller SM. Exploring well-being among US Hispanics/Latinos in a church-based institution: a qualitative study. J Posit Psychol. 2016;11(5):511–21.
185. Rivera-Hernandez M. The role of religious leaders in health promotion for older Mexicans with diabetes. J Relig Health. 2015;54(1):303–15.

186. Amirehsani KA, Hu J, Wallace DC, et al. US healthcare experiences of Hispanic patients with diabetes and family members: a qualitative analysis. J Community Health Nurs. 2017;34(3):126–35.
187. Cyril S, Smith BJ, Possamai-Inesedy A, Renzaho AM. Exploring the role of community engagement in improving the health of disadvantaged populations: a systematic review. Glob Health Action. 2015;8:29842.
188. Hebert JR, Braun KL, Meade CD, Bloom J, Kobetz E. Community-based participatory research adds value to the National Cancer Institute's research portfolio. Prog Community Health Partnersh. 2015;9(Suppl):1–4.
189. Eaton LA, Driffin DD, Kegler C, et al. The role of stigma and medical mistrust in the routine health care engagement of black men who have sex with men. Am J Public Health. 2015;105(2):e75–82.
190. Graves KD, Jensen RE, Canar J, et al. Through the lens of culture: quality of life among Latina breast cancer survivors. Breast Cancer Res Treat. 2012;136(2):603–13.
191. Fingrut W, Beck LA, Lo D. Building an oncology community of practice to improve cancer care. Curr Oncol. 2018;25(6):371–7.
192. Kimminau KS, Jernigan C, LeMaster J, et al. Patient vs. community engagement: emerging issues. Med Care. 2018;56(Suppl 10 Suppl 1):S53–7.
193. Penedo FJ, Traeger L, Dahn J, et al. Cognitive behavioral stress management intervention improves quality of life in Spanish monolingual Hispanic men treated for localized prostate cancer: results of a randomized controlled trial. Int J Behav Med. 2007;14(3):164–72.
194. Penedo FJ, Antoni MH, Moreno PI, et al. Study design and protocol for a culturally adapted cognitive behavioral stress and self-management intervention for localized prostate cancer: the Encuentros de Salud study. Contemp Clin Trials. 2018;71:173–80.
195. Napoles AM, Santoyo-Olsson J, Ortiz C, et al. Randomized controlled trial of Nuevo Amanecer: a peer-delivered stress management intervention for Spanish-speaking Latinas with breast cancer. Clin Trials. 2014;11(2):230–8.
196. Napoles AM, Ortiz C, Santoyo-Olsson J, et al. Nuevo Amanecer: results of a randomized controlled trial of a community-based, peer-delivered stress management intervention to improve quality of life in Latinas with breast cancer. Am J Public Health. 2015;105(Suppl 3):e55–63.
197. Whitehead NE, Hearn LE. Psychosocial interventions addressing the needs of Black women diagnosed with breast cancer: a review of the current landscape. Psychooncology. 2015;24(5):497–507.
198. Wang AW, Bouchard LC, Gudenkauf LM, et al. Differential psychological effects of cognitive-behavioral stress management among breast cancer patients with high and low initial cancer-specific distress. J Psychosom Res. 2018;113:52–7.
199. Spiegel D, Bloom JR, Kraemer HC, Gottheil E. Effect of psychosocial treatment on survival of patients with metastatic breast cancer. Lancet. 1989;2(8668):888–91.
200. Lechner SC, Ennis-Whitehead N, Robertson BR, et al. Adaptation of a psycho-oncology intervention for black breast cancer survivors: project CARE. Couns Psychol. 2012;41(2):286–312.
201. Lechner SC, Whitehead NE, Vargas S, et al. Does a community-based stress management intervention affect psychological adaptation among underserved black breast cancer survivors? J Natl Cancer Inst Monogr. 2014;2014(50):315–22.
202. Kamen C, Heckler C, Janelsins MC, et al. A dyadic exercise intervention to reduce psychological distress among lesbian, gay, and heterosexual cancer survivors. LGBT Health. 2016;3(1):57–64.
203. Kamen C, Mustian KM, Dozier A, Bowen DJ, Li Y. Disparities in psychological distress impacting lesbian, gay, bisexual and transgender cancer survivors. Psychooncology. 2015;24(11):1384–91.
204. Antoni MH, Baggett L, Ironson G, et al. Cognitive-behavioral stress management intervention buffers distress responses and immunologic changes following notification of HIV-1 seropositivity. J Consult Clin Psychol. 1991;59(6):906–15.

205. Lutgendorf SK, Antoni MH, Ironson G, et al. Changes in cognitive coping skills and social support during cognitive behavioral stress management intervention and distress outcomes in symptomatic human immunodeficiency virus (HIV)-seropositive gay men. Psychosom Med. 1998;60(2):204–14.
206. Penedo FJ, Oswald LB, Kronenfeld JP, Garcia SF, Cella D, Yanez B. The increasing value of eHealth in the delivery of patient-centred cancer care. Lancet Oncol. 2020;21(5):e240–51.
207. van den Beuken-van Everdingen MHH, Hochstenbach LM, Joosten EA, Tjan-Heijnen VC, Janssen DJ. Update on prevalence of pain in patients with cancer: systematic review and meta-analysis. J Pain Symptom Manag. 2016;51(6):21.
208. Somers TJ, Abernethy AP, Edmond SN, et al. A pilot study of a mobile health pain coping skills training protocol for patients with persistent cancer pain. J Pain Symptom Manag. 2015;50(4):6.
209. Somers TJ, Kelleher SA, Westbrook KW, et al. A small randomized controlled pilot trial comparing mobile and traditional pain coping skills training protocols for cancer patients with pain. Pain Res Treat. 2016;2016:2473629.
210. Kelleher SA, Winger JG, Dorfman CS, et al. A behavioral cancer pain intervention: a randomized noninferiority trial comparing in-person with videoconference delivery. Psychooncology. 2019;28(8):1671–8.
211. Jim HSL, Hyland KA, Nelson AM, et al. Internet-assisted cognitive behavioral intervention for targeted therapy-related fatigue in chronic myeloid leukemia: results from a pilot randomized trial. Cancer. 2019;126(1):174–80.
212. Bouchard LC, Yanez B, Dahn JR, et al. Brief report of a tablet-delivered psychosocial intervention for men with advanced prostate cancer: acceptability and efficacy by race. Transl Behav Med. 2018;9(4):8.

Translational Efforts in Precision Medicine to Address Disparities

Melissa B. Davis, Meagan Ford, Rachel Martini, and Lisa A. Newman

Overview of Translational Research

Translational research, defined as the application of scientific knowledge into a novel or modified medical practice, is hinged upon the concept of evidence-based medicine [1]. Translational research is the foundational avenue to strategically focus efforts toward improving the health and well-being in the USA and beyond. Within the context of minority health and racial cancer health disparities, translational research could elevate fundamental discovery science that defines biological mechanisms that contribute to differences in disease risk and outcomes and translates these discoveries into strategies for disease prevention and treatment in clinical settings. To be meaningful and effective at addressing cancer health disparities, additional investments in outreach and dissemination of translational research are needed to enhance uptake and application of findings from fundamental science at the bedside and the ultimate translation of these discoveries into general adoption and implementation of strategies through healthcare policies and professional guidelines [2]. Translational research is one of the cornerstones of clinical interventions and healthcare delivery, but not all populations have benefited from these research efforts. The current guidelines for genetic counseling and testing for BRCA1 and BRCA2 mutations are key examples of the translation of research findings from discovery/basic science into a clinical intervention. Following the initial discovery of cancer susceptibility genes through preclinical and clinical association studies [3–5], large genome-wide association studies helped to determine the relative risks associated with specific deleterious alternations [6–9]. Ultimately, these

M. B. Davis (✉)
Morehouse School of Medicine, Atlanta, GA, USA
e-mail: mbd4001@med.cornell.edu

M. Ford · R. Martini · L. A. Newman
Weill Cornell Medicine, New York, NY, USA

C. Hughes Halbert (ed.), *Cancer Health Disparities*,
https://doi.org/10.1007/978-3-031-37638-2_4

associations were translated into specific genetic testing tools, which provide patients with genetic risk information for clinical interventions and genetic counseling [10, 11]. It is now standard practice for high-risk patients to be referred to genetic testing, typically reserved for those who have a family history of cancer and, interestingly, who have an *ancestry* associated with BRCA1/2 gene mutations [12, 13]. High-risk patients subsequently have access to preventive strategies, as indicated based on their BRCA1/2 genetic test result. However, women of color are less likely than white women to be referred to genetic counseling [14–16] largely due to lack of evidence that it would be of equal benefit [17, 18], as well as emerging evidence that genetic risk alleles are not the same in all ancestral backgrounds [16] but also due to bias and accessibility [16]. Further, non-white patients are more likely to harbor mutations in BRCA1/2 genes that are "variants of unknown significance" (VUS) [19–21]. The inability to determine the significance of these mutations is a consequence of the underrepresentation of non-white women (and men) in the GWAS and genetic risk studies that serve as the empirical data underlying these genetic tests [22, 23]. An additional consequence of homogenous GWAS populations is manifested in the recent application of combinatorial GWAS risk alleles, a calculation of polygenic risk scores (PRS). Although PRS has been proven to be a better translation of GWAS findings [24], similar to VUS in panel testing, PRS calculations do not perform well in non-white populations [25]. As a result of the lack of diversity in GWAS cohorts, genetic modifiers, which are harbored in genetic ancestry, are still widely unknown.

The Arc of Health Justice: Overcoming a History of Medical Abuse and Neglect

The first step of changing the trajectory of poor clinical outcomes in racial disparities through translational research is to understand the history of disparities and the problems that need to be addressed. Over 30 years ago, the Heckler Report, generated by a Task Force on Black and Minority Health, produced a nine-volume document [26] giving a bleak account of the perpetual disparities of minority health that has existed since the beginning of recorded US history. Racial inequality has had a pervasive impact on the general well-being and survival of Black/African American (B/AA) communities [27, 28], a persistent state of minority since the abolishment of slavery [29]. Adding to health disparities driven by limited access to care are the grave injustices of mistreatment of minority groups for the supposed cause of medical advancements. The combined neglect, marginalization, and unethical actions of the medical community have undermined the trust Black/African American communities have in both the health system and the healthcare providers, reified by ongoing racism and bias in health care [30–32]. The shift from racial discrimination to financial discriminations continues to limit health access across social strata associated with race; however, even with full access to all that is available in clinical settings to treat cancers, treatment options may still not be equitable and suitable for the specific clinicopathology of cancer in minoritized populations.

Recent evidence in breast and prostate cancers indicate that racial disparities persist even in affluent communities where quality and access to care should not contribute to or influence survival [33, 34]. This suggests that treatment is not equally effective across race groups. Indisputable evidence indicates that certain drivers, or root causes, of disparities of incidence and survival are consequences of social determinants of health (SDOH); however, biological factors, which might interact with social intermediaries, also impact disease risks and outcomes [35]. These factors, and the effect of each, must be characterized across the diverse population of cancer patients. Studies that compare the biological determinants and tumor phenotypes across race groups have uncovered several tumorigenic mechanisms that are significantly different among self-reported race groups [36–39]. With these discoveries comes a growing acceptance that inclusion of diverse populations in clinical research is pivotal to ensure broad applications and translation of findings into treatments and strategies for health promotion and disease control [40]. Without inclusion of diverse populations in clinical research, there is a lack of scientific rigor that lessens the significance of scientific discovery, leading to clinical inefficiencies. The deprioritization of minority groups has allowed this negligence to pervade scientific research in numerous ways, including lack of funding and dampened enthusiasm of publication, therefore limiting impact through gatekeeping and policies that permit exclusion of these populations in population-based studies.

The Transformative Power of Precision Medicine on Disparities with Diversity in Translational Research

Precision medicine is one of the newest iterations of translational research that is hinged upon forward-thinking and technologically advanced research findings to tailor treatment regimens based on patient-derived data. Precision medicine refers to a personalized approach to curative treatments, tailored to fit the specific cause and drivers of disease progression. The promise of personalized medicine as first defined in NIH's "Healthy People 2000" was that, by this decade, there would be an individualized approach to disease diagnosis and treatment, hinged upon a precise understanding of pathogenic genetic drivers and a deeper characterization of individual health and genetic background. This was a laudable goal that required leaps of advancement in technology and broad applications of these technologies in clinic. Further, it was anticipated that doctors would become prophetic and could implement preventative measures to circumvent the outcome of disease diagnosis altogether as a result of personalized or precision medicine prognostic tools. Precision medicine has certainly advanced, and our understanding of genetic drivers, genetic risk, and the intermediaries of that risk have improved exponentially. However, we continue to fall short of the ultimate goal [40].

The utilization of precision medicine technologies in disparities research aims to strategically utilize population diversity to develop targeted therapeutics, prognostics, or diagnostics that leverage distinctions in disease drivers that vary among individuals, rather than perpetuating the one-size-fits-all paradigm [37, 40, 41]. When we consider the constellation of causes that align when patients acquire a malignancy, it is not a far stretch to consider every cancer case as a unique disease. Because every individual is unique in genetic makeup, in lived experiences, and in a lifetime of environmental exposures, it is therefore feasible to consider that the tumors' microenvironment, the patient's system, is unique for each case as well. Current investigations that compare the tumor microenvironments of patients in multiethnic cohorts have begun to uncover a vast array of differences that could be exploited for therapies and diagnostics, particularly related to immune phenotypes, in several types of cancers [42–48].

In the wake of personalized medicine, genomic tools have revealed biological variation across patient populations in nearly all diseases that investigate multiethnic cohorts [49–56]. For instance, nearly a decade ago, prostate cancer risk studies identified a region of chromosome 8 (8q24) as a high-risk locus with copy number variation that occurs more frequently in men of African descent [57–61]. A single variant at the same genomic locus has also been reported as an African-specific variant, attributing nearly 32% of familial prostate cancer risk in African Americans [57]. This study was the culmination of more than four different consortia that included over 17K men of African descent. Studies of with cohorts of such magnitude, comprised solely of minorities, were not considered a feasible or even necessary endeavor a decade ago. Ultimately, in order to translate into clinical applications that impact disparities, results such as these must align with the evolving concepts of diverse genomic platforms for precision medicine.

Bridging the Clinical Gap of Cancer Survival Disparities with Translational Research

Despite advancements in basic science, the impact and value of precision medicine has been slow to reach underserved communities, potentially because of the way in which early race and racial group membership were conceptualized and measured in early translational studies. The cure for cancer is not a single drug but combinations of treatment strategies that address specific details of each patient. And for some patients, these personalized approaches can be curative. For other patients, however, precision tools have proven to be much less effective, and the exclusion of racial/ethnic minorities in precision medicine research actually worsens the disparities gap. By incorporating diversity in the patient cohorts that are used in precision medicine research, there would be greater opportunity for translational research to overcome racial disparities in cancer survival.

Traditionally, research on racial disparities has been viewed mainly through a lens of socioeconomic consequences that drive inequality in marginalized race groups. Because race is embedded in the history of political social constructs, race-based research and race-modified medical applications can still be met with substantial resistance [2]. Concerns have been raised about linking race with immutable biological and genetic features; early manifestations of "race-based medicine" were met with considerable skepticism among communities, healthcare providers, and researchers [62–64]. These early iterations of race-based medicine resulted in what would be considered irresponsible conjecture and racist science by creating treatment paradigms, or clinical decision-tree branches based only on self-reported race.

To uncover the potential of population-level genetics to power precision medicine tools, large longitudinal cohort studies are needed to improve our understanding of variation in biological mechanisms of risk and disease progression across diverse patient populations. The precision medicine movement, however, has created opportunities to examine the direct and indirect contribution of biological factors to cancer health disparities. A potentially appeasing option that has been developed through precision medicine initiatives is to utilize genetic ancestry to characterize patient groups and remove self-reported/self-identified race groups from translational research altogether [39, 65–69].

At the same time, however, race captures the social and cultural exposures of individuals, and these factors do have biological implications [70]. Imperative to our plight of overcoming disparities is utilizing all of the information available and include both genetic ancestry and social race constructs as part of translational studies. If we are to overcome the multifaceted causes, we have to quantify them. There are concerted efforts to target recruitment and enrollment of diverse ethnic groups to address our gaps of knowledge where race/ethnicity specific health risks are concerned. The PolyEthnic-1000 [71] project is a prime example of an initiative providing public access to genomic data from targeted diverse populations. In addition, cancer site specific consortia, such as the International Center for the Study of Breast Cancer Subtypes (ICSBCS) [72] and the Prostate Cancer Transatlantic Consortium (CaPTC) [73] are synergizing collaborative efforts, in partnership with minoritized communities and international networks of investigators to provide unprecedented insights in biological determinants related to genetic ancestry. These efforts also recognize that generational differences in social experiences may also be modified over time and are connected to the physical or geographical residence of individuals. The neighborhood effect of social constructs is also an imperative factor to consider in translational research in cancer health disparities. Harnessing the convergence of social and biological determinants will empower our ability to truly be precise with patient needs and predictive algorithms to intervene and reduce disease risk. Effectively, this is the primary goal of translational research: to improve outcomes by applying new knowledge from scientific research. While the field has fallen short of this vision thus far, incredible capacity has been developed to interrogate the human genome, transcriptome, proteome, etc. at increasingly accessible clinical interfaces. Along the way, we have also established that there is a tremendous amount of genetic variation across the human species, which should not always be interpreted as deleterious in nature, but rather a modified or evolved/adapted version of a canonical mechanism. Translating these revelations requires a reframing of clinical genomics, which is still in process that involves resetting the standard of a "healthy genome," or even a "reference genome." The delay of translating genomic findings is largely due to a severe lack of genetic data in diverse populations. As indicated previously, most of the initial disparity studies were underpowered due to lack of ethnic minority representation in public data [22] and lack of programmatic funding to support new initiatives to increase minority representation. However, now led by the very minority communities that are stakeholders for better outcomes, there is renewed interest in disparities research, particularly those employing ancestry measurements as opposed to race-group proxies. Importantly, this new surge of interest can empower better clinical tools to improve disparate outcomes.

As it relates to cancer, many of the most promising precision medicine endeavors involve understanding the dynamics of tumor biology to uncover drivers of tumor progression. The paucity of data from non-white populations is an example of how studies with limited racial/ethnic diversity perpetuate gaps in our knowledge about cancer biology in these groups. Of the largest consortiums of cancer databases (e.g., the CRUK, AACR-GENIE [74], TCGA [74], and Metabric), there is growing representation of non-white ethnicity in the newer iterations of these initiatives [75]. However, the non-white populations in these cohorts remain disproportionately lower, compared to their actual percentage in the general population [76, 77]. Despite a dearth of diversity in data, the contrasting differences among race groups in recent consortia are robust enough to be detected, replicated, and validated.

When genomic studies include quantified genetic ancestry as a variable in statistical models, the analyses can uncover novel findings appropriate for the broader population. Most recent GWAS are reframing study designs to include substantial numbers of non-European participants, such as the RESPOND study [78] and the AMBER consortium [79]. The resulting investigations include discoveries of population-specific risk alleles [80], shared structural variants that are conserved in patients of African descent [81], and validation of these findings in populations across the African diaspora [82–84]. Indeed, the differential prevalence of specific genetic changes among race groups began a new conversation about heritable genetic drivers in race groups that may reflect shared genetic ancestry. This postulation then made genome sequencing across admixed populations, with better representation of the world population, an imperative next step. However, not all genetic mechanisms derive from ancestral heritage, but rather the impact of the environment. Unraveling the intrinsic from extrinsic would require a convergence of data elements that were typically only investigated in siloes. The indisputable influence of social determinants was soon linked to the translation of these factors into genetic alterations [65, 85–92]. To truly find causation and inflection points of these observed differences, statistical power has to be improved, through increase in numbers of diverse ethnic/race groups.

The genomics era brought our initial mountainous puzzle of how to handle "Big Data," and it is equally challenging to integrate these terabytes of genomic information per patient with a lifetime of dynamic clinical information and medical history that is captured in the medical record [93–99]. As these processes are vetted and benchmarked for suitability and accuracy, once feasibly deployed in clinic, data science could be transformational in disparities research. Having equal access to all patient data could eliminate the continuous issue of patient population accessibility in medical research. This has already been seen during the COVID-19 pandemic, where health systems were able to report the specific factors that were shared among patients who suffered severe or fatal outcomes [100, 101]. Research conducted to understand risk factors for adverse outcomes among COVID-19 patients can serve as a model for other disease disparities to identify both clinical and social determinants of population-level disparities. The next step will be translating these data models into actionable clinical goals.

Race-Conscious Data Science and Artificial Intelligence

Considered to be part of precision medicine, computational approaches such as machine learning, neural network simulation, and spatial statistics have opened many doors and generated new opportunities to improve clinical diagnostics and simulate the effects of therapeutics [102–104]. This adds another aspect of precision medicine, the use of artificial intelligence, and the increasingly common utility of data science [105–107]. In the current environment where data is plentiful and accessible through innovative approaches, we are poised to make exceptional progress in cancer health disparities, if the technologies are deployed and applied broadly [107, 108]. Algorithms for data science research have the capacity to integrate multimodal data sources, such as digital footprints, electronic medical records, and social media to build automated databases and chart review dashboards with language processing methods. Further, real-world data (RWD) predictive models have emerged and can identify at-risk patients within a health system. One benefit to RWD research is that it is inherently cross-sectional. While some research designs/studies require significant effort on the part of the subjects, data science does not require anything, outside of consent, as the data acquired is self-accruing through automated systems. The actual data are the real-world events, test results, and clinical and demographic variables that are already captured through the course of health care. With the mandate of all medical serving institutions to convert to electronic medical records came a tsunami of information, in the form of personal health information (PHI) data. This data could be mined to power clinical studies and translating scientific findings into applicable knowledge to treat patients.

In addition to PHI, reframing clinical pathology into computational tools also presents new opportunities to learn phenotypic distinctions across the diverse patient population. Artificial intelligence (AI) has been proffered as a method of transcending subjective bias in human observations or preconceived notions of clinical relevance. Data-driven predictions can trigger novel hypotheses that would not have otherwise been derived. Similar to GWAS and genomic research, AI is built upon deep learning algorithms by training on large subsets of patient data, and the source of these data have been homogenous populations. This results in algorithms that are not transferrable or generalizable to the broader diverse population. Therefore, inappropriate application/interpretation of AI can be detrimental rather than beneficial, by contriving distinctions among diverse ethnic groups that are actually biases in the algorithm's performance rather than biology. Therefore, we must consider modifications to AI training sets and adjustments to account for racial bias. This all hinges on the equitable resources of minority-serving healthcare institutions to ensure comprehensive RWD is captured and harmonized in a standardized way. So, we are again at a precipice of improving disparities within the context of structural barriers that lead to reduced access to telehealth and other electronic healthcare resources (e.g., patient portals) [41].

Emerging Opportunities and Priorities for the Future Translational Research

In 2015, a pivotal and historical announcement was made by then Vice President Joseph Biden, to accelerate the momentum of cancer research and achieve a decade's worth of advances in a 5-year span – the "Cancer Moonshot Initiative." A Blue Ribbon Panel was assembled and produced several assessments [109–111] to outline the current state of cancer knowledge and identify research opportunities that could propel technology and achieve the Moonshot goals. In their assessment, the panel conveyed cancer disparities as a thematic aspect of needed research, to be threaded through all levels of the cancer continuum research agenda, from prevention, diagnostics, and therapeutics to survivorship [109, 110, 112]. The panel boldly suggested that rather than specific studies focused on disparities, that all proposed research would include some aspect of disparities investigation included in either the study design or in recruitment of the minority populations. The moonshot investigators who were awarded these coveted grants are currently reporting findings related to new aspects of cancer, such as tumor atlases and evolution maps that track mutational accumulation over time. A few of these are starting to report findings that support long-standing theories on biological determinants of disparities, which had previously not received adequate funding to address in larger populations [113–121]. While several small cohort and pilot studies first introduced the concepts of biological mechanisms driving higher prevalence of aggressive tumor phenotypes in racially disparate mortality [120, 122, 123], current research trends seek to utilize genetic ancestry, which consistently went unacknowledged, untested, and underpresented in the breadth of previous primary literature. Prior to the advent of ancestry studies, population ancestry was under-appreciated for its capacity to harbor genetic risk and genomic anomalies that are important for risk management [124] diagnostic and therapeutic research platforms [23, 125]. Among these include genomic structural changes in the 8q24 genomic region related to African Ancestry in prostate cancer risk [61, 126, 127], cancer risk alleles associated with Asian ancestry in lung cancer [124, 128, 129], and several distinctions in ancestry-associated tumor expression signatures regulated by signaling pathways that are typical therapeutic targets [43, 130–132]. The Cancer Moonshot Initiative is another example of the future directions and strategies that are needed for translational research to advance cancer health equity. However, several critical issues still need to be addressed as part of the Cancer Moonshot and similar types of programs. That is to say, the inclusion of disparity populations in discovery science has to be increased, and the adequate representation of these groups should be considered as a criterion of scientific rigor. Relatedly, precision medicine approaches should be applied to clinical research studies to determine causes and identify potential intervention targets. Lastly, these strategies have to be available and accessible in community-serving clinics to have the greatest reach and impact on cancer health disparities. If all of the planned enrollment and integrated analyses occur across the evolving landscape of disparities research in translational medicine, we will certainly see the mitigation of several aspects of bias in cancer outcomes. As we have increased awareness and modified research policies to require inclusion of minority populations, and we utilize novel approaches to harness diversity in genomic background and social factors in translational research, the field of disparities research is poised to transform the culture of race-based research. Translational research can finally become transformative, and health justice can be achieved – in our lifetime (Figs. 1, 2, 3, 4, and 5).

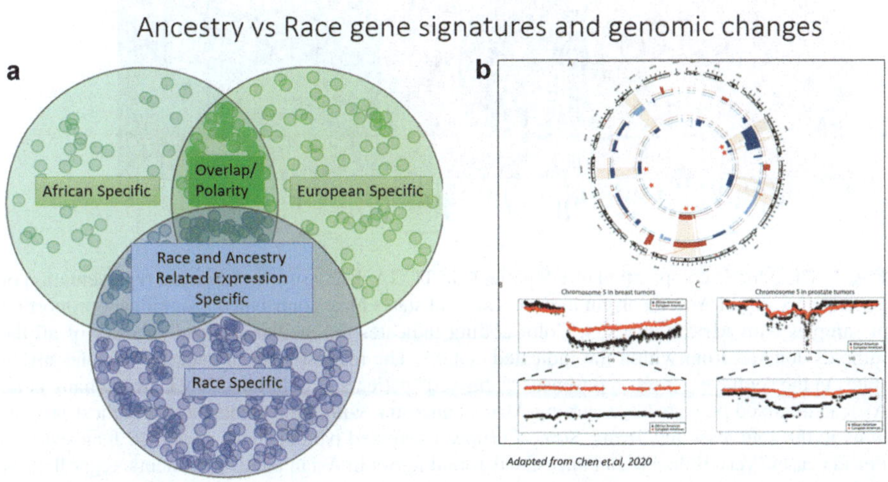

Fig. 1 The role of race versus ancestry in gene expression of tumors. (**a**) In breast cancer RNAseq analyses of triple-negative breast cancer (TNBC), gene expression has been associated with genetic ancestry of African and European origin. In addition, gene expression is also associated exclusively with self-reported race. This indicates there are factors in both genetic/inherited traits and social factors correlated with racial constructs. Therefore, utilizing the combination of ancestry and race can be impactful to define biological determinants that drive cancer phenotypes and treatment outcomes. (**b**) In analyzing genomic sequencing data, there are structural alterations in both prostate and breast cancer tumors that are conserved in self-reported race groups, without regard to ancestry, which indicated significant genetic correlations that are relevant to cancer biology. (Adapted from [81])

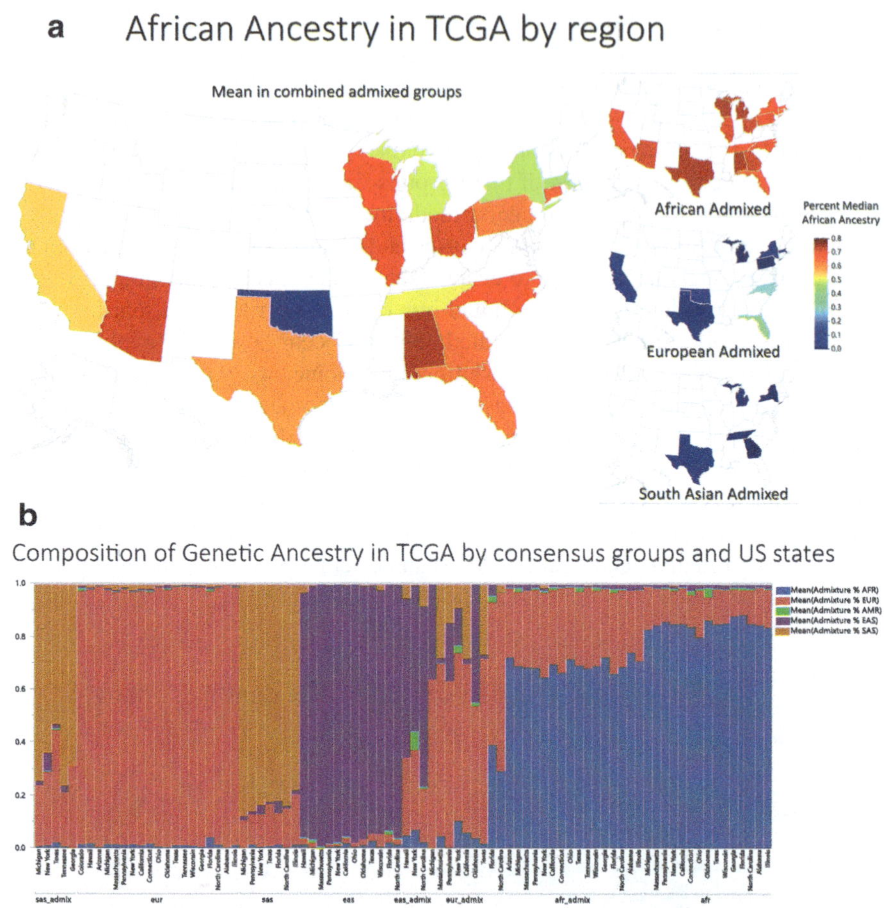

Fig. 2 The genetic composition of US patients in TCGA databases. (**a**) Regional representation of genetic ancestry of African origin indicates several states have contributed a significant proportion of samples with African ancestry. Color coding indicates the median African ancestry of all the samples donated from within the indicated states*. The highest African ancestry samples are in states in the southeast. Insets: consensus "admixed" patients as determined by Carrot-Zhang et al. African admixed patients have varying African ancestry, with the patients having highest proportions in the southeast and Texas. Some European admixed patients have nearly 40% ancestry in Florida cases. Very little African ancestry is found in South Asian admixed patients, regardless of region or state. (**b**) Average admixture composition of 1000 Genomes ancestry is shown for each state*, stratified by the consensus ancestry call groups. Of note, the highest African ancestry in the African and African-admixed groups is found in Georgia and Alabama. The largest proportion of Native American ancestry is found in the East Asian admixed population of New York. **State annotations with less than 20 samples were not included for privacy protection of patients*

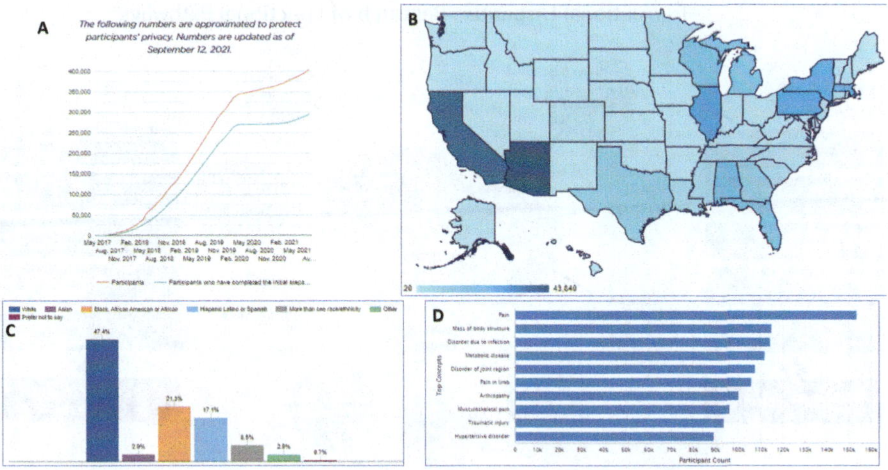

Fig. 3 Diversity in *all* of the USA. (**a**) The cumulative numbers of enrollees are upward of 400K as of September 2021. (**b**) The regional distribution of these enrollment numbers is shown as a state-centered heatmap. The most enrollments are in the west coast, with the next populous states in east and mid-west having significant enrollment. (**c**) The racial diversity of these enrollments is shown as self-reported categories, with nearly 50% representing non-European populations. (**d**) Of the top presenting medical afflictions in the cohorts, cancer/neoplasms are the second-highest reported disease

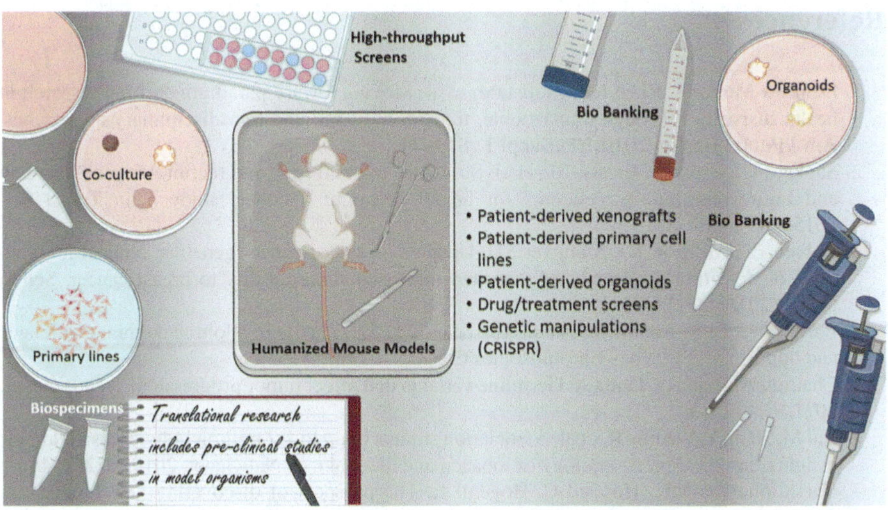

Fig. 4 Clinical and preclinical studies in disparities. Using the tools of preclinical precision medicine studies, we can leverage ex vivo and in vivo models to interrogate the findings from clinical cohorts that identify the mechanisms of varying tumor biology. Bio-banking is also a key aspect of population studies that requires the engagement and recruitment of patients from minoritized race groups. Establishing replenishable resources, such as primary 2D or 3D organoid lines, will be an instrumental step in conducting high-throughput mechanistic screens and drug screens. Preclinical studies are the bridge to translational medicine

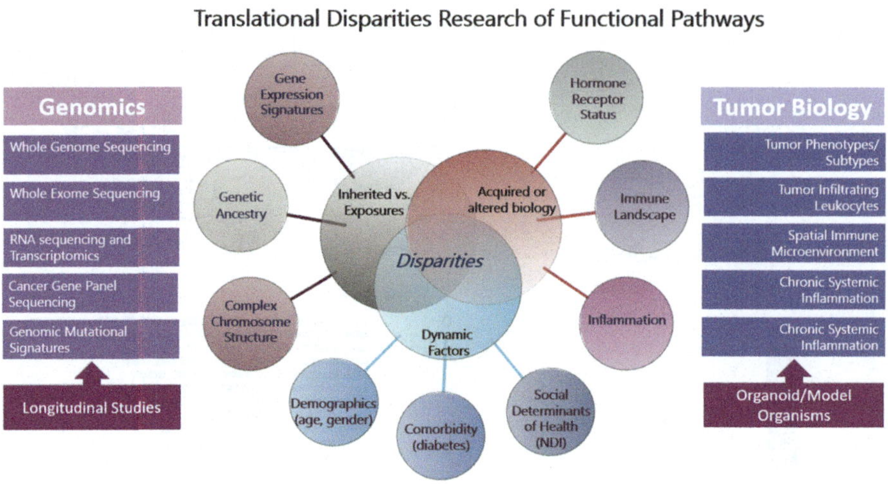

Fig. 5 The alternate lenses of research focus to employ precision medicine tools in translational cancer disparities research. The integration of multiple disciplines is required to address the multi-faceted issues that can play a role in disparate outcomes. Any given patient may have a constellation of factors that track with poor outcomes, which correlate with race. To truly identify the actionable causes for individualized treatment, translational research is required to disaggregate the mechanisms that could all link together in driving tumor biology and treatment response differences

References

1. Dankwa-Mullan I, Rhee KB, Stoff DM, et al. Moving toward paradigm-shifting research in health disparities through translational, transformational, and transdisciplinary approaches. Am J Public Health. 2010;100(Suppl 1):S19–24.
2. Sankare IC, Bross R, Brown AF, et al. Strategies to build trust and recruit African American and Latino community residents for health research: a cohort study. Clin Transl Sci. 2015;8:412–20.
3. Cobain EF, Milliron KJ, Merajver SD. Updates on breast cancer genetics: clinical implications of detecting syndromes of inherited increased susceptibility to breast cancer. Semin Oncol. 2016;43:528–35.
4. Barbosa K, Li S, Adams PD, et al. The role of TP53 in acute myeloid leukemia: challenges and opportunities. Genes Chromosomes Cancer. 2019;58:875–88.
5. Chatrath A, Ratan A, Dutta A. Germline variants that affect tumor progression. Trends Genet. 2021;37:433–43.
6. Liu M, Jiang Y, Wedow R, et al. Association studies of up to 1.2 million individuals yield new insights into the genetic etiology of tobacco and alcohol use. Nat Genet. 2019;51:237–44.
7. Christophersen MK, Hogdall C, Hogdall E. The prospect of discovering new biomarkers for ovarian cancer based on current knowledge of susceptibility loci and genetic variation (review). Int J Mol Med. 2019;44:1599–608.
8. Montazeri Z, Li X, Nyiraneza C, et al. Systematic meta-analyses, field synopsis and global assessment of the evidence of genetic association studies in colorectal cancer. Gut. 2020;69:1460–71.
9. Yin J, Liu H, Liu Z, et al. Pathway-analysis of published genome-wide association studies of lung cancer: a potential role for the CYP4F3 locus. Mol Carcinog. 2017;56:1663–72.

10. Haiman CA, Hsu C, de Bakker PI, et al. Comprehensive association testing of common genetic variation in DNA repair pathway genes in relationship with breast cancer risk in multiple populations. Hum Mol Genet. 2008;17:825–34.
11. Hamann U. Hereditary breast cancer: high risk genes, genetic testing and clinical implications. Clin Lab. 2000;46:447–61.
12. Konstantinopoulos PA, Norquist B, Lacchetti C, et al. Germline and somatic tumor testing in epithelial ovarian cancer: ASCO guideline. J Clin Oncol. 2020;38:1222–45.
13. Hereditary Cancer Syndromes and Risk Assessment: ACOG COMMITTEE OPINION, Number 793. Obstet Gynecol. 2019;134:e143–9.
14. Muller C, Lee SM, Barge W, et al. Low referral rate for genetic testing in racially and ethnically diverse patients despite universal colorectal cancer screening. Clin Gastroenterol Hepatol. 2018;16:1911–1918e2.
15. Peterson JM, Pepin A, Thomas R, et al. Racial disparities in breast cancer hereditary risk assessment referrals. J Genet Couns. 2020;29:587–93.
16. Garland V, Cioffi J, Kirelik D, et al. African-Americans are less frequently assessed for hereditary colon cancer. J Natl Med Assoc. 2021;113:336–41.
17. Ademuyiwa FO, Salyer P, Ma Y, et al. Assessing the effectiveness of the National Comprehensive Cancer Network genetic testing guidelines in identifying African American breast cancer patients with deleterious genetic mutations. Breast Cancer Res Treat. 2019;178:151–9.
18. Olopade OI, Fackenthal JD, Dunston G, et al. Breast cancer genetics in African Americans. Cancer. 2003;97:236–45.
19. Ndugga-Kabuye MK, Issaka RB. Inequities in multi-gene hereditary cancer testing: lower diagnostic yield and higher VUS rate in individuals who identify as Hispanic, African or Asian and Pacific islander as compared to European. Familial Cancer. 2019;18:465–9.
20. Bishop MR, Omeler-Fenaud SM, Huskey ALW, et al. Gene panel screening for insight towards breast cancer susceptibility in different ethnicities. PLoS One. 2020;15:e0238295.
21. Roberts ME, Susswein LR, Janice Cheng W, et al. Ancestry-specific hereditary cancer panel yields: moving toward more personalized risk assessment. J Genet Couns. 2020;29:598–606.
22. Martin AR, Kanai M, Kamatani Y, et al. Clinical use of current polygenic risk scores may exacerbate health disparities. Nat Genet. 2019;51:584–91.
23. Thomas M, Sakoda LC, Hoffmeister M, et al. Genome-wide modeling of polygenic risk score in colorectal cancer risk. Am J Hum Genet. 2020;107:432–44.
24. Dixon P, Keeney E, Taylor JC, et al. Can polygenic risk scores contribute to cost-effective cancer screening? A systematic review. Genet Med. 2022;24(8):1604–17.
25. Yanes T, Young MA, Meiser B, et al. Clinical applications of polygenic breast cancer risk: a critical review and perspectives of an emerging field. Breast Cancer Res. 2020;22:21.
26. Heckler MM. Secretary Heckler: health-care needs and political needs must mix. Hosp Manage. 1983;Q:2–4.
27. Centers for Disease Control. Report of the secretary's task force on black and minority health. MMWR Morb Mortal Wkly Rep. 1986;35:109–12.
28. Nickens H. Report of the Secretary's Task Force on Black and Minority Health: a summary and a presentation of health data with regard to blacks. J Natl Med Assoc. 1986;78:577–80.
29. DuBois WE. The health and physique of the Negro American. 1906. Am J Public Health. 2003;93:272–6.
30. Sprague Martinez L, Freeman ER, Winkfield KM. Perceptions of cancer care and clinical trials in the black community: implications for care coordination between oncology and primary care teams. Oncologist. 2017;22:1094–101.
31. Fam E, Ferrante JM. Lessons learned recruiting minority participants for research in urban community health centers. J Natl Med Assoc. 2018;110:44–52.
32. Jaiswal J. Whose responsibility is it to dismantle medical mistrust? Future directions for researchers and health care providers. Behav Med. 2019;45:188–96.

33. DeSantis CE, Ma J, Gaudet MM, et al. Breast cancer statistics, 2019. CA Cancer J Clin. 2019;69:438–51.
34. DeSantis CE, Miller KD, Goding Sauer A, et al. Cancer statistics for African Americans, 2019. CA Cancer J Clin. 2019;69:211–33.
35. Mitchell E, Alese OB, Yates C, et al. Cancer healthcare disparities among African Americans in the United States. J Natl Med Assoc. 2022;114:236.
36. Martini R, Newman L, Davis M. Breast cancer disparities in outcomes; unmasking biological determinants associated with racial and genetic diversity. Clin Exp Metastasis. 2022;39:7–14.
37. Lord BD, Martini RN, Davis MB. Understanding how genetic ancestry may influence cancer development. Trends Cancer. 2022;8:276–9.
38. Leong SP, Witz IP, Sagi-Assif O, et al. Cancer microenvironment and genomics: evolution in process. Clin Exp Metastasis. 2022;39:85–99.
39. Davis M, Martini R, Newman L, et al. Identification of distinct heterogenic subtypes and molecular signatures associated with African ancestry in triple negative breast cancer using quantified genetic ancestry models in admixed race populations. Cancers (Basel). 2020;12:1220.
40. Davis MB. Genomics and cancer disparities: the justice and power of inclusion. Cancer Discov. 2021;11:805–9.
41. Halbert CH, Allen CG. Basic behavioral science research priorities in minority health and health disparities. Transl Behav Med. 2021;11:2033–42.
42. Chen CH, Lu YS, Cheng AL, et al. Disparity in tumor immune microenvironment of breast cancer and prognostic impact: Asian versus Western populations. Oncologist. 2020;25:e16–23.
43. Curran T, Sun Z, Gerry B, et al. Differential immune signatures in the tumor microenvironment are associated with colon cancer racial disparities. Cancer Med. 2021;10:1805–14.
44. Deshmukh SK, Srivastava SK, Tyagi N, et al. Emerging evidence for the role of differential tumor microenvironment in breast cancer racial disparity: a closer look at the surroundings. Carcinogenesis. 2017;38:757–65.
45. Kim G, Pastoriza JM, Condeelis JS, et al. The contribution of race to breast tumor microenvironment composition and disease progression. Front Oncol. 2020;10:1022.
46. Mitchell KA, Zingone A, Toulabi L, et al. Comparative transcriptome profiling reveals coding and noncoding RNA differences in NSCLC from African Americans and European Americans. Clin Cancer Res. 2017;23:7412–25.
47. O'Meara T, Safonov A, Casadevall D, et al. Immune microenvironment of triple-negative breast cancer in African-American and Caucasian women. Breast Cancer Res Treat. 2019;175:247–59.
48. Powell IJ, Chinni SR, Reddy SS, et al. Pro-inflammatory cytokines and chemokines initiate multiple prostate cancer biologic pathways of cellular proliferation, heterogeneity and metastasis in a racially diverse population and underlie the genetic/biologic mechanism of racial disparity: update. Urol Oncol. 2021;39:34–40.
49. Chand GB, Dwyer DB, Erus G, et al. Two distinct neuroanatomical subtypes of schizophrenia revealed using machine learning. Brain. 2020;143:1027–38.
50. Coram MA, Fang H, Candille SI, et al. Leveraging multi-ethnic evidence for risk assessment of quantitative traits in minority populations. Am J Hum Genet. 2017;101:218–26.
51. Hobbs BD, Putman RK, Araki T, et al. Overlap of genetic risk between interstitial lung abnormalities and idiopathic pulmonary fibrosis. Am J Respir Crit Care Med. 2019;200:1402–13.
52. Kaiser P, Peralta CA, Kronmal R, et al. Racial/ethnic heterogeneity in associations of blood pressure and incident cardiovascular disease by functional status in a prospective cohort: the Multi-Ethnic Study of Atherosclerosis. BMJ Open. 2018;8:e017746.
53. Raffield LM, Iyengar AK, Wang B, et al. Allelic heterogeneity at the CRP locus identified by whole-genome sequencing in multi-ancestry cohorts. Am J Hum Genet. 2020;106:112–20.
54. van der Wouden CH, Cambon-Thomsen A, Cecchin E, et al. Implementing pharmacogenomics in Europe: design and implementation strategy of the ubiquitous pharmacogenomics consortium. Clin Pharmacol Ther. 2017;101:341–58.

55. Wojcik GL, Graff M, Nishimura KK, et al. Genetic analyses of diverse populations improves discovery for complex traits. Nature. 2019;570:514–8.
56. Zhao X, Qiao D, Yang C, et al. Whole genome sequence analysis of pulmonary function and COPD in 19,996 multi-ethnic participants. Nat Commun. 2020;11:5182.
57. Darst BF, Wan P, Sheng X, et al. A germline variant at 8q24 contributes to familial clustering of prostate cancer in men of African ancestry. Eur Urol. 2020;78:316–20.
58. Erkizan HV, Sukhadia S, Natarajan TG, et al. Exome sequencing identifies novel somatic variants in African American esophageal squamous cell carcinoma. Sci Rep. 2021;11:14814.
59. Han Y, Rand KA, Hazelett DJ, et al. Prostate cancer susceptibility in men of African ancestry at 8q24. J Natl Cancer Inst. 2016;108:djv431.
60. Chen H, Liu W, Roberts W, et al. 8q24 allelic imbalance and MYC gene copy number in primary prostate cancer. Prostate Cancer Prostatic Dis. 2010;13:238–43.
61. Hooker S, Hernandez W, Chen H, et al. Replication of prostate cancer risk loci on 8q24, 11q13, 17q12, 19q33, and Xp11 in African Americans. Prostate. 2010;70:270–5.
62. Okah E, Thomas J, Westby A, et al. Colorblind racial ideology and physician use of race in medical decision-making. J Racial Ethn Health Disparities. 2021;9:2019.
63. Hunt LM, Truesdell ND, Kreiner MJ. Genes, race, and culture in clinical care: racial profiling in the management of chronic illness. Med Anthropol Q. 2013;27:253–71.
64. Egalite N, Ozdemir V, Godard B. Pharmacogenomics research involving racial classification: qualitative research findings on researchers' views, perceptions and attitudes towards socio-ethical responsibilities. Pharmacogenomics. 2007;8:1115–26.
65. Martini R, Newman L, Davis M. Breast cancer disparities in outcomes; unmasking biological determinants associated with racial and genetic diversity. Clin Exp Metastasis. 2021;39:7.
66. Apprey V, Wang S, Tang W, et al. Association of genetic ancestry with DNA methylation changes in prostate cancer disparity. Anticancer Res. 2019;39:5861–6.
67. Yao S, Hong CC, Ruiz-Narvaez EA, et al. Genetic ancestry and population differences in levels of inflammatory cytokines in women: role for evolutionary selection and environmental factors. PLoS Genet. 2018;14:e1007368.
68. Ramakodi MP, Devarajan K, Blackman E, et al. Integrative genomic analysis identifies ancestry-related expression quantitative trait loci on DNA polymerase beta and supports the association of genetic ancestry with survival disparities in head and neck squamous cell carcinoma. Cancer. 2017;123:849–60.
69. Evans DS, Avery CL, Nalls MA, et al. Fine-mapping, novel loci identification, and SNP association transferability in a genome-wide association study of QRS duration in African Americans. Hum Mol Genet. 2016;25:4350–68.
70. Henderson BE, Lee NH, Seewaldt V, et al. The influence of race and ethnicity on the biology of cancer. Nat Rev Cancer. 2012;12:648–53.
71. Robine N, Varmus H. New York's Polyethnic-1000: a regional initiative to understand how diverse ancestries influence the risk, progression, and treatment of cancers. Trends Cancer. 2022;8(4):269–272. https://doi.org/10.1016/j.trecan.2021.11.005. Epub 2021 Dec 9. PMID: 34895873.
72. Martini R, Chen Y, Jenkins BD, Elhussin IA, Cheng E, Hoda SA, Ginter PS, Hanover J, Zeidan RB, Oppong JK, Adjei EK, Jibril A, Chitale D, Bensenhaver JM, Awuah B, Bekele M, Abebe E, Kyei I, Aitpillah FS, Adinku MO, Ankomah K, Osei-Bonsu EB, Nathansan SD, Jackson L, Jiagge E, Petersen LF, Proctor E, Nikolinakos P, Gyan KK, Yates C, Kittles R, Newman LA, Davis MB. Investigation of triple-negative breast cancer risk alleles in an International African-enriched cohort. Sci Rep. 2021;11(1):9247. https://doi.org/10.1038/s41598-021-88613-w. PMID: 33927264; PMCID: PMC8085076.
73. White JA, Kaninjing ET, Adeniji KA, Jibrin P, Obafunwa JO, Ogo CN, Mohammed F, Popoola A, Fatiregun OA, Oluwole OP, Karanam B, Elhussin I, Ambs S, Tang W, Davis M, Polak P, Campbell MJ, Brignole KR, Rotimi SO, Dean-Colomb W, Odedina FT, Martin DN, Yates C. Whole-exome sequencing of nigerian prostate tumors from the prostate cancer transatlantic consortium (CaPTC) reveals DNA repair genes associated with african

ancestry. Cancer Res Commun. 2022;2(9):1005–1016. https://doi.org/10.1158/2767-9764.CRC-22-0136. PMID: 36922933; PMCID: PMC10010347.
74. Kaur P, Porras TB, Ring A, et al. Comparison of TCGA and GENIE genomic datasets for the detection of clinically actionable alterations in breast cancer. Sci Rep. 2019;9:1482.
75. Lewis KL, Heidlebaugh AR, Epps S, et al. Knowledge, motivations, expectations, and traits of an African, African-American, and Afro-Caribbean sequencing cohort and comparisons to the original ClinSeq((R)) cohort. Genet Med. 2019;21:1355–62.
76. Spratt DE, Chan T, Waldron L, et al. Racial/ethnic disparities in genomic sequencing. JAMA Oncol. 2016;2:1070–4.
77. Fang H, Hui Q, Lynch J, et al. Harmonizing genetic ancestry and self-identified race/ethnicity in genome-wide association studies. Am J Hum Genet. 2019;105:763–72.
78. Weiss GJ, Byron SA, Aldrich J, et al. A prospective pilot study of genome-wide exome and transcriptome profiling in patients with small cell lung cancer progressing after first-line therapy. PLoS One. 2017;12:e0179170.
79. Palmer JR, Ambrosone CB, Olshan AF. A collaborative study of the etiology of breast cancer subtypes in African American women: the AMBER consortium. Cancer Causes Control. 2014;25:309–19.
80. Nichols HB, Graff M, Bensen JT, et al. Genetic variants in anti-Mullerian hormone-related genes and breast cancer risk: results from the AMBER consortium. Breast Cancer Res Treat. 2021;185:469–78.
81. Chen Y, Sadasivan SM, She R, et al. Breast and prostate cancers harbor common somatic copy number alterations that consistently differ by race and are associated with survival. BMC Med Genet. 2020;13:116. https://doi.org/10.1186/s12920-020-00765-2. PMID: 32819446; PMCID: PMC7441621.
82. Martini R, Chen Y, Jenkins BD, et al. Investigation of triple-negative breast cancer risk alleles in an International African-enriched cohort. Sci Rep. 2021;11:9247.
83. Newman LA, Jenkins B, Chen Y, et al. Hereditary susceptibility for triple negative breast cancer associated with Western Sub-Saharan African ancestry: results from an international surgical breast cancer collaborative. Ann Surg. 2019;270:484–92.
84. Jiagge E, Jibril AS, Davis M, et al. Androgen receptor and ALDH1 expression among internationally diverse patient populations. J Glob Oncol. 2018;4:1–8.
85. Freedman JA, Al Abo M, Allen TA, et al. Biological aspects of cancer health disparities. Annu Rev Med. 2021;72:229–41.
86. Halbert CH, Allen CG, Jefferson M, et al. Lessons learned from the Medical University of South Carolina Transdisciplinary Collaborative Center (TCC) in precision medicine and minority men's health. Am J Mens Health. 2020;14:1557988320979236.
87. Mancilla VJ, Peeri NC, Silzer T, et al. Understanding the interplay between health disparities and epigenomics. Front Genet. 2020;11:903.
88. Shim JK, Ackerman SL, Darling KW, et al. Race and ancestry in the age of inclusion: technique and meaning in post-genomic science. J Health Soc Behav. 2014;55:504–18.
89. Colditz GA, Wei EK. Preventability of cancer: the relative contributions of biologic and social and physical environmental determinants of cancer mortality. Annu Rev Public Health. 2012;33:137–56.
90. Gehlert S, Colditz GA. Cancer disparities: unmet challenges in the elimination of disparities. Cancer Epidemiol Biomark Prev. 2011;20:1809–14.
91. Cassel KD. Using the Social-Ecological Model as a research and intervention framework to understand and mitigate obesogenic factors in Samoan populations. Ethn Health. 2010;15:397–416.
92. Davis MB, Newman LA. Breast cancer disparities: how can we leverage genomics to improve outcomes? Surg Oncol Clin N Am. 2018;27:217–34.
93. Singla N, Singla S. Harnessing big data with machine learning in precision oncology. Kidney Cancer J. 2020;18:83–4.

94. Crichton DJ, Altinok A, Amos CI, et al. Cancer biomarkers and big data: a planetary science approach. Cancer Cell. 2020;38:757–60.
95. Jourquin J, Reffey SB, Jernigan C, et al. Susan G. Komen big data for breast cancer initiative: how patient advocacy organizations can facilitate using big data to improve patient outcomes. JCO Precis Oncol. 2019;3:1.
96. Cammarota G, Ianiro G, Ahern A, et al. Gut microbiome, big data and machine learning to promote precision medicine for cancer. Nat Rev Gastroenterol Hepatol. 2020;17:635–48.
97. Pastorino R, De Vito C, Migliara G, et al. Benefits and challenges of Big Data in healthcare: an overview of the European initiatives. Eur J Pub Health. 2019;29:23–7.
98. Jiang P, Sellers WR, Liu XS. Big data approaches for modeling response and resistance to cancer drugs. Annu Rev Biomed Data Sci. 2018;1:1–27.
99. Ow GS, Kuznetsov VA. Big genomics and clinical data analytics strategies for precision cancer prognosis. Sci Rep. 2016;6:36493.
100. Klann JG, Estiri H, Weber GM, et al. Validation of an internationally derived patient severity phenotype to support COVID-19 analytics from electronic health record data. J Am Med Inform Assoc. 2021;28:1411–20.
101. Salvatore M, Gu T, Mack JA, et al. A phenome-wide association study (PheWAS) of COVID-19 outcomes by race using the electronic health records data in Michigan medicine. J Clin Med. 2021;10:1351.
102. Guo Y, Zhang Y, Lyu T, et al. The application of artificial intelligence and data integration in COVID-19 studies: a scoping review. J Am Med Inform Assoc. 2021;28:2050–67.
103. Mysona DP, Kapp DS, Rohatgi A, et al. Applying artificial intelligence to gynecologic oncology: a review. Obstet Gynecol Surv. 2021;76:292–301.
104. Su TH, Wu CH, Kao JH. Artificial intelligence in precision medicine in hepatology. J Gastroenterol Hepatol. 2021;36:569–80.
105. Benissan-Messan DZ, Merritt RE, Bazan JG, et al. National utilization of surgery and outcomes for primary tracheal cancer in the United States. Ann Thorac Surg. 2020;110:1012–22.
106. Breen N, Berrigan D, Jackson JS, et al. Translational health disparities research in a data-rich world. Health Equity. 2019;3:588–600.
107. Chino F, Suneja G, Moss H, et al. Health care disparities in cancer patients receiving radiation: changes in insurance status after medicaid expansion under the affordable care act. Int J Radiat Oncol Biol Phys. 2018;101:9–20.
108. Karalexi MA, Baka M, Ryzhov A, et al. Survival trends in childhood chronic myeloid leukaemia in southern-Eastern Europe and The United States of America. Eur J Cancer. 2016;67:183–90.
109. Ramirez AG, Thompson IM. How will the 'cancer moonshot' impact health disparities? Cancer Causes Control. 2017;28:907–12.
110. Panel's "moonshot" goals released. Cancer Discov. 2016;6:1202–3.
111. Oh A, Vinson CA, Chambers DA. Future directions for implementation science at the National Cancer Institute: implementation science centers in cancer control. Transl Behav Med. 2021;11:669–75.
112. Jaffee EM, Dang CV, Agus DB, et al. Future cancer research priorities in the USA: a Lancet Oncology Commission. Lancet Oncol. 2017;18:e653–706.
113. Stevens KR, Masters KS, Imoukhuede PI, et al. Fund black scientists. Cell. 2021;184:561–5.
114. Kaiser J. Biomedical research funding. NIH uncovers racial disparity in grant awards. Science. 2011;333:925–6.
115. Ginther DK, Schaffer WT, Schnell J, et al. Race, ethnicity, and NIH research awards. Science. 2011;333:1015–9.
116. Woods-Burnham L, Basu A, Cajigas-Du Ross CK, et al. The 22Rv1 prostate cancer cell line carries mixed genetic ancestry: implications for prostate cancer health disparities research using pre-clinical models. Prostate. 2017;77:1601–8.

117. Myers JS, Vallega KA, White J, et al. Proteomic characterization of paired non-malignant and malignant African-American prostate epithelial cell lines distinguishes them by structural proteins. BMC Cancer. 2017;17:480.
118. Yates C, Long MD, Campbell MJ, et al. miRNAs as drivers of TMPRSS2-ERG negative prostate tumors in African American men. Front Biosci (Landmark Ed). 2017;22:212–29.
119. Sanchez TW, Zhang G, Li J, et al. Immunoseroproteomic profiling in African American men with prostate cancer: evidence for an autoantibody response to glycolysis and plasminogen-associated proteins. Mol Cell Proteomics. 2016;15:3564–80.
120. Jones J, Mukherjee A, Karanam B, et al. African Americans with pancreatic ductal adenocarcinoma exhibit gender differences in Kaiso expression. Cancer Lett. 2016;380:513–22.
121. Reams RR, Agrawal D, Davis MB, et al. Microarray comparison of prostate tumor gene expression in African-American and Caucasian American males: a pilot project study. Infect Agent Cancer. 2009;4(Suppl 1):S3.
122. Davis M, Tripathi S, Hughley R, et al. AR negative triple negative or "quadruple negative" breast cancers in African American women have an enriched basal and immune signature. PLoS One. 2018;13:e0196909.
123. Theodore SC, Davis M, Zhao F, et al. MicroRNA profiling of novel African American and Caucasian Prostate Cancer cell lines reveals a reciprocal regulatory relationship of miR-152 and DNA methyltranferase 1. Oncotarget. 2014;5:3512–25.
124. Lee CP, Irwanto A, Salim A, et al. Breast cancer risk assessment using genetic variants and risk factors in a Singapore Chinese population. Breast Cancer Res. 2014;16:R64.
125. Conti DV, Darst BF, Moss LC, et al. Trans-ancestry genome-wide association meta-analysis of prostate cancer identifies new susceptibility loci and informs genetic risk prediction. Nat Genet. 2021;53:65–75.
126. Robbins C, Torres JB, Hooker S, et al. Confirmation study of prostate cancer risk variants at 8q24 in African Americans identifies a novel risk locus. Genome Res. 2007;17:1717–22.
127. Freedman ML, Haiman CA, Patterson N, et al. Admixture mapping identifies 8q24 as a prostate cancer risk locus in African-American men. Proc Natl Acad Sci U S A. 2006;103:14068–73.
128. Li Y, Li Y, Yang T, et al. Clinical significance of EML4-ALK fusion gene and association with EGFR and KRAS gene mutations in 208 Chinese patients with non-small cell lung cancer. PLoS One. 2013;8:e52093.
129. Bai H, Mao L, Wang HS, et al. Epidermal growth factor receptor mutations in plasma DNA samples predict tumor response in Chinese patients with stages IIIB to IV non-small-cell lung cancer. J Clin Oncol. 2009;27:2653–9.
130. Guerrero-Preston R, Lawson F, Rodriguez-Torres S, et al. JAK3 variant, immune signatures, DNA methylation, and social determinants linked to survival racial disparities in head and neck cancer patients. Cancer Prev Res (Phila). 2019;12:255–70.
131. Maxwell GL, Allard J, Gadisetti CV, et al. Transcript expression in endometrial cancers from Black and White patients. Gynecol Oncol. 2013;130:169–73.
132. Krishnan B, Rose TL, Kardos J, et al. Intrinsic genomic differences between African American and White patients with clear cell renal cell carcinoma. JAMA Oncol. 2016;2:664–7.

Patient Navigation for Cancer Screening and Treatment

Evan M. Graboyes and Elizabeth A. Calhoun

Introduction

Since President Nixon declared war on cancer in 1971, there has been tremendous progress in reducing cancer incidence, mortality, and morbidity in the USA through risk-factor modification, improved screening capability and uptake, and biomedical advances resulting in novel therapeutics and treatment paradigms. Unfortunately, profound disparities in cancer incidence and outcomes based on race/ethnicity, income, health insurance coverage, and geography persist in the USA [1]. These observed disparities in cancer incidence and outcomes in the USA are predominantly driven by differences in social determinants of health [2] (i.e., the social, economic, and physical conditions in which individuals are born, live, work, and age) and subsequent social risk factors (i.e., the adverse social conditions associated with poor health such as food, housing, or transportation insecurity) [3, 4]. Differences in key social risk factors between racial, ethnic, socioeconomic, and geographic groups result in differential barriers to care; subsequent access to and utilization of timely, high-quality cancer care; and subsequently cancer outcomes [5]. This relationship was eloquently articulated in the 1989 *Report to the Nation: Cancer in the Poor* [6] and has been repeated in numerous treatises on the topic in the intervening 30 years [7, 8].

In recognition of the fact that barriers to accessing and obtaining timely, high-quality cancer care directly contribute to observed disparities in cancer outcomes,

E. M. Graboyes (✉)
Department of Otolaryngology – Head & Neck Surgery, Medical University of South Carolina, Charleston, SC, USA

Department of Public Health Sciences, Medical University of South Carolina, Charleston, SC, USA
e-mail: graboyes@musc.edu

E. A. Calhoun
Department of Population Health, University of Illinois at Chicago, Chicago, IL, USA

C. Hughes Halbert (ed.), *Cancer Health Disparities*,
https://doi.org/10.1007/978-3-031-37638-2_5

Dr. Harold P. Freeman developed patient navigation (PN) in 1990 [9]. As part of the Harlem Cancer Education and Demonstration Project, the initial PN program aimed to improve follow-up and decrease diagnostic delays for patients with suspicious findings on screening mammography in Harlem, NY [10]. In a primarily urban, low socioeconomic, uninsured Black patient population, this study demonstrated that PN resulted in higher rates of completing recommended breast biopsies and an increased proportion of patients who obtained the recommended biopsy in a timely manner [10]. Following up on the promising results of Dr. Freeman's PN project in 1995 [10], the Patient Navigator Research Program (PRNP) demonstrated, in a seminal multi-site randomized controlled trial, that PN can reduce disparities in cancer care [11].

Since these landmark studies, there has been an explosion of PN programs targeting cancer disparities across the USA [12–14]. Over time, PN programs have increased their scope to target disparities across a wide variety of types of cancers and in diverse settings. PN programs have also expanded their purview to address barriers across the cancer care continuum, enhancing timely movement of individuals from detection through diagnosis, treatment, and subsequent cancer survivorship (although PN remains understudied for treatment and survivorship) [12, 15]. Concurrent with the widescale dissemination of PN programs for cancer care, evidence has accumulated that PN is acceptable to its target population and highly efficacious at reducing disparities in access to cancer care and outcomes for specific racial and ethnic, socioeconomic, and geographic groups [12]. It is thus now well recognized that PN has, and will continue to play, a critically important role in attempts to eradicate disparities in access to cancer care and cancer outcomes for underrepresented and medically vulnerable populations [5, 13].

In this chapter, we (1) describe core principles of PN, PN services, and the rationale for PN as an appealing strategy to eliminate disparities in cancer care and outcomes; (2) evaluate the efficacy of PN at reducing racial and ethnic, socioeconomic, and geographic disparities in outcomes across the cancer care continuum; and (3) discuss practical considerations to implementing effective PN programs aimed at reducing disparities in cancer incidence and outcomes.

What Is Patient Navigation?

PN is a patient-centered, healthcare service delivery intervention that aims to eliminate barriers to cancer care in a culturally sensitive manner, thereby improving outcomes and decreasing disparities in health and healthcare [9, 16, 17]. PN addresses barriers to care across the increasingly complicated cancer care continuum to enhance timely care and for all patients, with a focus on those at risk for treatment delays and lower-quality care. Through their knowledge of the healthcare system, navigators communicate with patients and caregivers to identify, and potentially even anticipate, obstacles to timely, high-quality care and then work to address each patient's barriers using a culturally competent and patient-centered approach.

Through this patient-centered approach, the navigator acts as the constant, go-to person who guides the patient through the byzantine healthcare system to help make sure that the patient does not fall through the cracks. PN programs engage the patient in both the community and medical settings. Navigators therefore act as a bridge between two worlds, the fragmented, poorly coordinated healthcare system and the complex biopsychosocial needs of cancer patients, especially those who are underserved [18].

As the scope of PN has expanded across the cancer care continuum, its definition has evolved. For instance, in 2008, the PNRP defined PN as "support and guidance offered to vulnerable populations with abnormal cancer screening or cancer diagnosis, with the goal of overcoming barriers to timely, quality care" [19]. Now, however, comprehensive PN includes (1) cancer prevention, (2) cancer screening adherence/uptake, (3) diagnostic resolution following abnormal screening tests, (4) cancer treatment, and (5) cancer survivorship [12, 17]. The American Cancer Society National Navigation Roundtable definition of PN in the cancer care setting is "individualized assistance offered to patients, families, and caregivers to help overcome healthcare system barriers and facilitate timely access to quality health and psychosocial care from pre-diagnosis through all phases of the cancer experience." [20] As a result of navigating across the continuum, particularly in the prevention, screening, and diagnostic resolution phases of navigation, the navigator often interacts with patients who do not in fact have cancer.

What Do Patient Navigators Do?

There is a tremendous variation in the implementation of PN programs across diverse community and healthcare delivery settings [21], to the point where some wonder if there are multiple specialties of PN (of which one specialty focuses on reducing health disparities) [22]. However, across its varied forms, PN generally used a case management model [19]. In the case management model, the navigator begins with case identification, works to elicit the patient's unique barriers to cancer care, develops an individualized plan to address the barriers, and systematically tracks the case through resolution. Core principles of PN include (1) patient-centered healthcare delivery; (2) eliminating barriers to care across the healthcare continuum; (3) ensuring timely delivery of healthcare services; and (4) connecting and coordinating within and across fragmented healthcare systems [9]. Because navigators are working with racial and ethnic minorities and other medically vulnerable groups, care must be culturally competent, compassionate, and professional throughout all aspects of care.

Barriers are categorized and organized differently across studies, making comparison about the types of barriers addressed by PN across studies challenging. Nevertheless, commonly encountered barriers to cancer care that drive disparities in cancer outcomes include (1) knowledge, attitudes, and beliefs, (2) fear/distrust, (3) communication, (4) financial/employment, (5) transportation/location of healthcare facility, (6) insurance coverage, (7) housing, (8) social/practical support, (9) language/literacy, (10) cultural views, and (11) the healthcare system [5, 13, 19]. These barriers may differ by racial or ethnic group, socioeconomic status, geography, type of cancer, and timepoint along the cancer care continuum.

Table 1 lists a variety of tools that patient navigators use to address these commonly encountered barriers [5, 13, 19]. For instance, to address gaps in knowledge about guidelines for screening, a navigator could provide education about guidelines. The navigator might also offer individualized advice for screening based on

Table 1 Barriers contributing to disparities in timely access and utilization of cancer care and associated potential patient navigation-based activities and interventions [5, 13, 19]

Barrier	Examples	Potential patient navigation intervention
Knowledge, attitudes, beliefs	Lack of knowledge about indications for screening test Lack of perceived risk Lack of perceived consequences	Provide education Provide personalized advice Organize outreach
Fear/distrust	Delay or refusal of care Lack of trust in medical system	Build trust Provide education
Communication	Difficulty understanding information from healthcare team Difficulty expressing desires/needs	Assist with bidirectional communication of clinical information to/from healthcare team
Financial/employment	Inability to pay for necessary medical tests or appointments Inability to get time off of work to receive medical care	Refer to financial counselor
Transportation/location of healthcare facility	Lack of car Living far from treatment facility	Arrange for shuttle or community-provided transportation assistance Find sources of funding to help patients pay for transportation
Insurance coverage	Lack of health insurance Help filling out insurance forms	Determine eligibility for Medicaid/Medicare Provide patient with forms and assist with completion
Housing	Lack of housing	Refer to social services
Social/practical support	Lack of caregiver	Provide support
Language/literacy	Patient speaks a different language than healthcare provider	Speak the patient's language Arrange for a medical translator Assist with reading; completing paperwork
Cultural views	Fatalism regarding cancer	Bridge cultural differences
Healthcare system	Fragmented care across specialists or healthcare systems	Arrange clinic appointments Referral tracking and follow-up

family history and personal risk factors to improve knowledge and risk perception. To overcome barriers related to accessing the medical system, the navigator could connect the patient with the appropriate resources (including Federally Qualified Health Centers). For patients who do not get the necessary care because they lack health insurance, the navigator may help the patient complete a complicated insurance application to gain insurance coverage and/or stay insured. For those who cannot attend follow-up medical appointments due to lack of transportation, the navigator could help identify alternative methods of transportation or even assist with scheduling a ride. Care coordination has been identified as a particularly important task for PN to eliminate racial and ethnic disparities and can include a range of services (e.g., scheduling appointments, directly contacting the family, facilitating communication with patients, providers, and administrators) to enhance appropriate health utilization in a multidisciplinary, multisite setting [21]. In addition to resolving many barriers independently, a key role of the navigator is to refer patients to financial counselors, social workers, psychologists, or palliative care when their expertise is needed. Navigators also link patients with key follow-up and support services within the community including food prescription assistance, child-care services, local advocacy, and community outreach groups.

To provide clarity and organization to the broad array of services provided by PN, a recent taxonomy of PN services was developed. These included (1) basic navigation (e.g., identifying patient needs, developing a plan to minimize barriers to care, and providing follow-up); (2) making arrangements and referrals to services; (3) treatment support; (4) care coordination; and (5) clinical trials and peer support [22].

Why Is Patient Navigation an Appealing Strategy to Reduce Disparities in Cancer Care and Outcomes?

The underlying rationale for PN as a tool to help eliminate disparities in access to cancer care and cancer outcomes is intuitive and compelling [5, 13, 19, 23]. Patients with barriers to cancer care experience higher rates of treatment delay relative to patients without barriers [24]. Barriers to accessing and utilizing timely, high-quality cancer care disproportionately burden certain racial and ethnic, socioeconomic, or geographic groups across the continuum [5, 6, 13, 25, 26]. Therefore, an intervention delivering personalized assistance to identify, address, and overcome the barriers that disproportionately burden certain groups should eliminate observed disparities in access to cancer care and outcomes. As described in the next section, there is an abundance of data supporting the underlying premise that PN, by addressing the barriers to cancer care that disproportionately burden racial and ethnic minorities and low-income, underinsured, rural, and other medically vulnerable populations, can help eliminate observed disparities in access to care and cancer outcomes.

Efficacy of Patient Navigation at Reducing Racial and Ethnic, Socioeconomic, and Geographic Disparities in Outcomes Across the Cancer Care Continuum

In 2005, the National Cancer Institute Center to Reduce Cancer Health Disparities established the Patient Navigator Research Program (PNRP) through $25 million in grants to ten participating centers. The landmark PNRP studies evaluated (1) patient satisfaction, (2) time to diagnostic resolution, (3) time to initiation of treatment, and (4) cost-effectiveness of a generalizable PN program implemented among vulnerable populations with abnormal screening or cancer diagnosis for four common cancers (breast, cervical, colorectal, and prostate) [19]. The study was unfortunately plagued by a myriad of issues related to randomization [19]. Nevertheless, among 10,521 participants with abnormal screening tests and 2105 participants with a diagnosis of precancer/cancer (73% racial and ethnic minority, 71% with public or no insurance), PN resulted in a moderate benefit in time to diagnostic resolution between 91 and 365 days (aHR = 1.51; 95% confidence interval [CI] 1.23–1.84) and treatment initiation (aHR = 1.43; 95% CI 1.10–1.86) [11]. When PNRP data were analyzed specifically to evaluate the efficacy of the PN at reducing racial and ethnic disparities in time to diagnostic resolution following a suspicious finding on cancer screening, they discovered that the impact of PN was greatest for Black patients who had the greatest delays in care [27]. However, PN did not fully eliminate delays in diagnostic resolution among Black participants relative to other racial and ethnic groups [27].

Numerous subsequent clinical trials have demonstrated that PN is an acceptable and effective strategy to decrease disparities in care for vulnerable populations from racial and ethnic minority groups as well as patients who are low income, underinsured, or treated at safety-net hospitals [28–34]. The results of these important individual studies were confirmed in a recent systematic review, which found that PN is highly efficacious in increasing the uptake of, and adherence to, cancer screenings and timely diagnostic resolution and follow-up as well as decreasing disparities in these outcomes [12]. In addition to demonstrating efficacy, a key component of building the evidence-base supporting PN as a promising strategy to eliminate cancer health disparities involved demonstrating reach, adoption, acceptance, and utilization of PN programs, particularly for community-based programs serving medically vulnerable populations. Numerous studies have documented that acceptance and utilization of PN is high across a variety of traditionally medically underserved populations [11, 35–37]. Below we describe select studies and summarize key evidence supporting PN as an intervention to reduce cancer disparities across the continuum for three key populations who suffer cancer disparities: (1) racial and ethnic minorities; (2) patients who are low-income, underinsured, or treated at safety-net hospitals; and (3) rural patients.

Race and Ethnic Minorities

Results of numerous studies demonstrate the efficacy of PN (implemented in a variety of forms) at decreasing disparities across the cancer care continuum (screening, diagnostic resolution, treatment initiation) for numerous racial and ethnic groups (Black, Hispanic, Southeast Asian, American Indian) across different types of cancer (e.g., colorectal, breast, cervical) [12]. While there has been a dearth of research evaluating whether PN is equally effective across racial and ethnic subgroups (as well as types of cancer and points along the cancer care continuum), a recent prospective meta-analysis of data from women in the PNRP with an abnormal breast screening test demonstrated an equal benefit of navigation across all groups, regardless of race or ethnicity [38].

Multiple RCTs implemented in diverse community and clinical settings have demonstrated that PN results in improved adherence for colorectal, breast, and cervical cancer screening among Black patients. In the Mister B trial, 731 Black men aged 50 years or older not up-to-date on CRC screening were recruited from barber shops in New York City and randomized to community-based PN or control (motivational interviewing); PN increased the likelihood of CRC screening relative to motivational interviewing (17.5% vs. 8.4%) [30]. PN delivered via a primary care setting also improves CRC screening among African Americans. An RCT among 764 African American patients in primary care practices in Philadelphia comparing preference-based tailored navigation to standard (mailed stool blood test kit and reminder) showed a twofold increase in CRC screening at 6 months (OR = 2.1; 95% CI 1.5–2.9) [39]. A multisite RCT of 1905 African American females recruited from a community-based and clinical setting in Baltimore, MD, showed that PN improved the odds of adherent mammography screening relative to control (print education) (OR 2.26; 95% CI 1.59–3.22) [40].

For patients of Hispanic ethnicity, multiple RCTs have demonstrated the efficacy of PN at reducing cancer disparities in screening and treatment initiation. A tailored PN intervention delivered outside of primary care settings to Latino Medicare enrollees resulted in higher rates of CRC screening adherence relative to mailed education materials (43.7% vs. 32.1%) [41]. The Six Studies Study showed that a culturally tailored PN program reduced the time from screening to diagnosis for Latinas with suspicious findings on mammography and improved timely initiation of treatment. In this RCT of 425 Latinas recruited from San Antonio, Texas, and five regional partners in the National Latino Cancer Research Network, the time to diagnosis was shorter in the PN group relative to control (mean 32.5 days vs. 44.6 days; HR, 1.32) and the proportion of Latinas diagnoses within 30 days higher (67.3% vs. 57.7%), primarily due to decreasing missed appointments [29]. The time from cancer diagnosis to treatment was lower in the PN group relative to controls (median, 23 days vs. 33 days), and the percentage of subjects initiating treatment within 30 days of diagnosis was higher (69.0% vs. 46.3%) [28]. Although cultural tailoring is common among PN interventions targeting Latinos, it is unclear whether culturally targeted PN is superior to standard PN. In an RCT comparing culturally targeted PN to standard PN among Latinos, Braschi et al. found no difference between the trial arms in rates of screening colonoscopy [42].

PN is also effective among Southeast Asian populations, which are disproportionately burdened by hepatitis B virus (HBV)-associated liver cancer. A lay navigator intervention among 260 Hmong adults resulted in higher rates of HBV screening relative to control (24% vs. 10%) [43]. Ma et al. demonstrated that a community-based participatory research (CBPR) intervention program featuring PN improved HPV screening and vaccination among Korean Americans. In this cluster-randomized trial involving 32 Korean church-based community organizations (1834 participants), three-series HBV vaccination completion rate was higher in the PN group relative to control (84% vs. 17.6%), a 500-fold increase in adjusted odds [31]. PN is also effective at improving diagnostic resolution following suspicious findings on cancer screening tests among Asian Americans.

For American Indians, PN programs demonstrate high levels of satisfaction, utilization, and efficacy. The Native Navigators and the Cancer Continuum, a CBPR project among numerous Native American communities, demonstrated improvements in community knowledge and access to care for participants diagnosed with cancer [44]. A retrospective review comparing a culturally competent PN program (focusing on obtaining medications, insurance issues, communicating with medical providers, and travel and lodging logistics) with historical control showed a decrease in the number of treatment breaks during radiation therapy (mean 1.7 days vs. 4.9 days) [37].

Patients Who Are Low Income, Underinsured, or Treated at Safety-Net Hospitals

In addition to reducing cancer disparities for racial and ethnic minorities, PN is also highly effective at improving outcomes across the continuum for patients who are low-income, underinsured, or treated at safety-net hospitals. In an RCT of 843 racially and ethnically diverse, low-income adults aged 50–75 years referred for colonoscopy at Boston Medical Center randomized to PN or usual care, PN resulted in higher rates of colonoscopy completion within 6 months of enrollment (61.1% vs. 53.2%; OR 1.5) [32]. In an RCT of 450 patients treated at a community health center randomized to a multifaceted PN intervention or usual care, completion of fecal occult blood testing within 6 months was significantly higher in the PN group (82.2% vs. 37.3%) [45]. A study implementing a PN program among uninsured women receiving free breast or cervical cancer screening through the Illinois Breast and Cervical Cancer Program showed favorable follow-up times [46]. In addition to improving screening adherence, PN also improves guideline-adherent adjuvant therapy for low-income women with breast cancer treated at a public safety-net hospital [47].

Geography

There has been significant recent attention to studying PN as a strategy to ameliorate the significant geographic disparities in cancer access to care and outcomes, although via less rigorous study designs. A quasi-experimental study of PN among 478 women from rural Appalachian Kentucky with abnormal pap smears showed a higher level of recommended follow-up care relative to comparison (91.6% vs. 80.8%) [48]. A different quasi-experimental study evaluating the effectiveness of PN on CRC screening among low-income rural patients treated at a FQHC in Georgia found that PN improved the odds of undergoing colonoscopy screening (35% vs. 7%; OR 7.9) and CRC screening adherence (43% vs. 11%; OR 5.9) [49]. In the prospective cohort study of Friend to Friend plus Patient Navigation Program among underserved women in rural Texas, PN participants and women with more program staff contact had greater odds of receiving a mammogram and a pap compared with their reference groups [50].

Practical Considerations for the Implementation of Effective PN Programs to Eliminate Cancer Disparities

Because of its efficacy in identifying barriers to care and addressing cancer care disparities across the continuum, PN has been standard of care and required for accreditation by the American College of Surgeons Commission on Cancer since 2015 [51]. There is, however, tremendous variation in the implementation of PN programs including type of individual serving as a navigator, core intervention tasks, program structure, work setting, health conditions navigated, navigation training, and patient population [21, 52]. With an eye toward implementation of effective PN aimed at eliminating cancer disparities, this section analyzes heterogeneity of existing PN programs in terms of the type of navigator, training, certification, and evaluation. Because the cost and cost-effectiveness of PN programs represent a potential existential threat to their continued implementation and sustainability, we also discuss financial considerations of PN. Finally, we highlight the importance having a patient navigator champion to the implementation and sustainability of PN.

Types of Patient Navigators

Patient navigators can broadly be categorized as nonlicensed (i.e., without a clinical practitioner license; also referred to as lay or nonclinical) or licensed (i.e., with a clinical practitioner license in nursing or social work) [52]. Five "types" of navigator categories have been described: including (1) nurse (completion of at least a

2-year educational degree or higher in nursing), (2) social worker/counselor (at least a bachelor's degree in social work), (3) lay (no professional degree, clinical licensure or credential and education no higher than a bachelor's degree), (4) allied health (non-nurse professional with a clinical background [e.g., medical assistant] or nonclinical degree beyond a bachelor's degree), and (5) other [21]. Using this taxonomy, a recent national respondent-driven survey reported that 35% of PN were nurse navigators, 28% lay navigators, 20% social work/counselor navigators, 7% allied health resources, and 10% "other." [21]

Importantly, when considering the ability of a PN program to eliminate racial disparities, the type of PN utilized was strongly associated with substantial differences in program implementation [21]. Lay navigators were less likely to work in rural settings and assist underserved populations relative to other types of navigators. Nurse navigators were more likely to work in a hospital setting, have clinical responsibilities, and less likely to navigate racial minority patients. Social work/counselor navigators were more likely to assist with a Medicare population and less likely to serve an underserved population. Despite observed differences in types of navigators and program implementation, there is insufficient data to analyze the association between PN implementation strategies and patient outcomes [21].

Although a key principle of PN is that the role and responsibilities of the navigator should be clearly defined and the scope of practice for the navigator distinct from other providers, this has remained challenging in practice [9, 52]. The challenge defining and delimiting the scope of practice for PN is both driven (and compounded) by the varied professional backgrounds and types of individuals providing PN. In addition, the scope of PN has evolved over time. Earlier formulations of PN sought to bring case managers, patient advocates, community health works, and care coordinators under the PN umbrella [19]. However, navigators now seek to distinguish themselves from these other allied health specialties. In so doing, it has been suggested that the distinguishing characteristic of PN relative to other support personnel in healthcare delivery is that patient navigators provide flexible problem-solving to overcome perceived barriers to care rather than the providing a predefined set of services [13].

Navigator Training, Certification, and Evaluation

Since the seminal publication outlining the national patient navigator training program [53], there has been a steady growth in the number of PN training programs across the USA (Table 2) [52]. As a reflection of the ongoing challenges clearly defining the scope of practice for a patient navigator, these training programs vary widely in terms of target audience (cancer navigation vs. general navigation; licensed navigator vs. non-licensed navigator), content, components, duration (mean, 59.5 hours; range, 8–160 hours), method of delivery (online, in person, interactive online, or print manual), cost (range: free to $1500), and background/expertise of the trainer [52]. In addition to the heterogeneity in nationally available

Table 2 Patient navigation training programs reviewed by the National Navigation Roundtable Task Group [52]

Patient navigation training program	Website
GW Cancer Center's Online Academy	https://cme.smhs.gwu.edu/gw-cancer-center-/group/gw-cancer-center
Patient Navigator Training Collaborative	https://patientnavigatortraining.org
Native American Cancer Research Corporation	https://natamcancer.org
Academy of Oncology Nurse & Patient Navigators	https://aonnonline.org
Otero Junior College	https://www.ojc.edu/catalog/workforcedegrees/cathealthnavaas.aspx
National Community Health Worker Training Center	https://nchwtc.tamhsc.edu
Smith Center for Healing and the Arts	https://smithcenter.org/institute-for-integrative-oncology-navigation/
Health Navigator Certification Training Program: Pacific Clinical Training Institute in collaboration with the USC School of Social Work	http://www.healthnavigation.org/health-navigation-training

navigation training programs, another challenge to PN training is that many protocols are research-specific rather than public PN programs [54].

As a result of this heterogeneity in navigator scope of practice and training, there has been a renewed interest in standardizing training for patient navigators and developing a standardized set of core competencies for certification and evaluating ongoing performance monitoring. Key national organizations including the National Accreditation Program for Breast Centers, Academy of Oncology Nurse & Patient Navigators [AONN+], Patient Navigator Training Collaborative, and George Washington Cancer Center's Online Academy are working toward establishing standardized core PN competencies for knowledge, skill, and performance [52]. The National Navigation Roundtable Task Group has been at the forefront of developing and articulating competency-based navigation training and certification; a proposed set of competencies is shown in Table 3 [52]. This competency-based training would aim to deliver the knowledge and skills necessary to meet the level of mastery dictated by the specific position and role [52].

Having a Patient Navigator Champion

A champion who can initiate and support a new PN program as it is implemented into a healthcare setting is key to its long-term maintenance. Key functions of champions include (1) demonstrating organizational need; (2) identifying key decision-makers across relevant levels of healthcare delivery settings (clinicians, staff, and administrators) and getting "buy-in"; (3) exploring potential barriers and facilitators to implementation (including program scope, cost, and implementation strategy); (4) implementing the program, designing a reporting structure, and hiring and

Table 3 Domains for training and certification competencies proposed by the National Navigation Roundtable Task Group [52]

Competency domain	Performance of competency
Ethical, cultural, legal, and professional	Demonstrates sensitivity and responsiveness to a diverse patient population, including but not limited to respecting confidentiality, organizational rules and regulations, ethical principles, and diversity in sex, age, culture, race, ethnicity, religion, abilities, sexual orientation, and geography
Client and care team interaction	Apply insight and understanding concerning human emotional responses to create and maintain positive interpersonal actions leading to trust and collaboration between the patient/client/family and the healthcare team. Patient safety and satisfaction are a priority
Health knowledge	Demonstrate knowledge of health, the cancer continuum, psychosocial and spiritual belief systems, and types of patient attitudes and behaviors specific to patient navigators (licensed or nonmedical licensure) role
Patient care coordination	Participate in the development of an evidence-based or promising/best practice patient-centered plan of care which is inclusive of a client's personal assessment and health provider/system and community resources.
Practice-based learning	Optimize navigator practice through continual professional development and the assimilation of scientific evidence, based on individual patient navigator gaps in knowledge, skills, attitudes, and abilities, to continuously improve patient care
System-based practice	Advocate for quality patient care by acknowledging and monitoring needed (desirable) improvements in systems of care for patients along the cancer care continuum through end of life. This includes enhancing community relationships and developing skills and knowledge to monitor and evaluate patient care and the effectiveness of the program
Communication/ interpersonal skills	Promote effective communication and interactions with patients in shared decision-making based on their needs, goals, strengths, barriers, solutions, and resources. Resolution of conflict among patients, family members, community partners, and members of the oncology care team is demonstrated in professional and culturally acceptable behaviors

training a PN; and (5) assessing program efficacy and cost-effectiveness through outcome tracking and quantitative evaluation of key quality and financial metrics.

Cost and Economic Feasibility of Patient Navigation

The economic feasibility of PN remains a major hurdle to the implementation and long-term sustainability of PN programs [55]. A recent national survey of PN programs reported that 82% are funded primarily via operational/departmental budgets. From an institutional and administration perspective, some have described the requirement by the Commission on Cancer to have PN processes (with current reimbursement models) as an unfunded mandate [25]. As a result of the current operational/departmental funding stream, long-term strategies are needed to address the cost of PN programs and reimbursement of PN services.

Unfortunately, a significant obstacle to demonstrating the cost-effectiveness of PN programs for reducing cancer disparities is the lack of financial data. In a recent study of over 750 oncology PN programs, only 22% reported collecting operational or financial data. Without collecting data, analyzing the cost-effectiveness and financial return on these programs is not possible. In addition, costs of over the program life are also poorly characterized, although it is known that startup cost of a PN program requires a much more significant investment than its ongoing maintenance.

However when financial data are collected (and analyzed and reported), PN appears to be a cost-effectiveness intervention [12]. By increasing healthcare utilization (e.g., number of screening colonoscopy procedures performed), PN programs may actually generate net revenue. In a cost analysis study of an RCT examining PN to improving screening colonoscopy among patients with public health insurance, Jandorf et al. showed that their PN program generated net income of $44,956 relative to the national average after accounting for the average contribution margins of each procedure type [56]. Another study conducted at three urban public hospitals showed that PN generated net revenue, primarily due to the increase in monthly colonoscopy volume (44–67 additional procedures per month) [57]. There was, however, variability in the revenue generation between the three hospitals, primarily driven by differences in the cost of the PN program. In addition to being cost-effective by generating revenue, PN programs may also be cost-effective (for the healthcare system) by reducing the cost of medical treatment paid by the healthcare payer. Modeling from colorectal and breast cancer PN programs estimates that by decreasing the time to diagnostic resolution of screening abnormalities (without including medical treatment costs saved for avoiding stage migration), the PN program decreased costs by $511 to $2080 per patient with breast cancer and by $1192 to $9708 per patient with colorectal cancer [58]. Analysis of a lay PN program for geriatric cancer patients implemented across two academic and ten community cancer centers showed that mean total costs declined by $781 more per quarter per navigated patient relative to non-navigated patients. The authors estimated that lay PN resulted in a $19 million decline in Medicare costs per year across the network, due to decreases in both inpatient and outpatient costs [59].

Conclusions

From Dr. Freeman's initial PN demonstration program through the landmark studies of the PNRP, PN has a rich and evidence-based track record as a strategy to help eliminate cancer disparities among racial and ethnic minorities; patients who are low income, underinsured, or treated at safety-net hospitals; and patients residing in the rural USA. Because of their success, PN programs have expanded in scope to target cancer disparities across a wide variety of types of cancers and in diverse settings. PN programs have also expanded their purview to address barriers across the cancer care continuum, enhancing timely movement of individuals from detection through diagnosis, treatment, and subsequent cancer survivorship. Although practical considerations abound for the continued dissemination and implementation of PN programs in diverse settings across the cancer care continuum, PN has, and will continue to play, a critically important role in our attempts to eradicate disparities in access to cancer care and cancer outcomes for underrepresented and medically vulnerable populations.

References

1. 2018 National Healthcare Quality and Disparities Report. Rockville: Agency for Healthcare Research and Quality, 2018.
2. World Health Organization. Social determinants of health. Available at: https://www.who.int/social_determinants/sdh_definition/en/. Accessed 30 Aug 2020.
3. Social determinants of health. Available at: https://www.healthypeople.gov/2020/topics-objectives/topic/social-determinants-of-health. Accessed 30 Aug 2020.
4. Green K, Zook M. When talking about social determinants, precision matters. Health Affairs Blog 2019. https://www.healthaffairs.org/do/10.1377/forefront.20191025.776011/
5. Natale-Pereira A, Enard KR, Nevarez L, Jones LA. The role of patient navigators in eliminating health disparities. Cancer. 2011;117:3543–52.
6. A summary of the American Cancer Society Report to the Nation: cancer in the poor. CA Cancer J Clin 1989;39:263–5.
7. Smedley B, Stith A, Nielsen A. Unequal treatment: confronting racial and ethnic disparities in health care. Institute of Medicine. Washington, DC: The National Academies Press; 2003.
8. Cancer trends progress report. Available at: https://progressreport.cancer.gov. Accessed 1 Sept 2020.
9. Freeman HP, Rodriguez RL. History and principles of patient navigation. Cancer. 2011;117:3539–42.
10. Freeman HP, Muth BJ, Kerner JF. Expanding access to cancer screening and clinical follow-up among the medically underserved. Cancer Pract. 1995;3:19–30.
11. Freund KM, Battaglia TA, Calhoun E, et al. Impact of patient navigation on timely cancer care: the Patient Navigation Research Program. J Natl Cancer Inst. 2014;106:dju115.
12. Bernardo BM, Zhang X, Beverly Hery CM, Meadows RJ, Paskett ED. The efficacy and cost-effectiveness of patient navigation programs across the cancer continuum: a systematic review. Cancer. 2019;125:2747–61.
13. Dohan D, Schrag D. Using navigators to improve care of underserved patients: current practices and approaches. Cancer. 2005;104:848–55.
14. Hendren S, Griggs JJ, Epstein RM, et al. Study protocol: a randomized controlled trial of patient navigation-activation to reduce cancer health disparities. BMC Cancer. 2010;10:551.
15. Guadagnolo BA, Dohan D, Raich P. Metrics for evaluating patient navigation during cancer diagnosis and treatment: crafting a policy-relevant research agenda for patient navigation in cancer care. Cancer. 2011;117:3565–74.
16. Freeman HP. Patient navigation: a community centered approach to reducing cancer mortality. J Cancer Educ. 2006;21:S11–4.
17. Freeman HP. Harold P. Freeman Patient Navigation Institute. Available at: http://www.hpfreemanpni.org. Accessed 27 Aug 2020.
18. Carroll JK, Humiston SG, Meldrum SC, et al. Patients' experiences with navigation for cancer care. Patient Educ Couns. 2010;80:241–7.
19. Freund KM, Battaglia TA, Calhoun E, et al. National Cancer Institute Patient Navigation Research Program: methods, protocol, and measures. Cancer. 2008;113:3391–9.

20. About patient navigation. Available at: https://navigationroundtable.org/about-patient-navigation/. Accessed 1 Oct 2020.
21. Valverde PA, Calhoun E, Esparza A, Wells KJ, Risendal BC. The early dissemination of patient navigation interventions: results of a respondent-driven sample survey. Transl Behav Med. 2018;8:456–67.
22. Wells KJ, Valverde P, Ustjanauskas AE, Calhoun EA, Risendal BC. What are patient navigators doing, for whom, and where? A national survey evaluating the types of services provided by patient navigators. Patient Educ Couns. 2018;101:285–94.
23. Freund KM. Patient navigation: the promise to reduce health disparities. J Gen Intern Med. 2011;26:110–2.
24. Ramachandran A, Snyder FR, Katz ML, et al. Barriers to health care contribute to delays in follow-up among women with abnormal cancer screening: data from the Patient Navigation Research Program. Cancer. 2015;121:4016–24.
25. Krok-Schoen JL, Brewer BM, Young GS, et al. Participants' barriers to diagnostic resolution and factors associated with needing patient navigation. Cancer. 2015;121:2757–64.
26. Hendren S, Chin N, Fisher S, et al. Patients' barriers to receipt of cancer care, and factors associated with needing more assistance from a patient navigator. J Natl Med Assoc. 2011;103:701–10.
27. Ko NY, Snyder FR, Raich PC, et al. Racial and ethnic differences in patient navigation: results from the Patient Navigation Research Program. Cancer. 2016;122:2715–22.
28. Ramirez A, Perez-Stable E, Penedo F, et al. Reducing time-to-treatment in underserved Latinas with breast cancer: the Six Cities Study. Cancer. 2014;120:752–60.
29. Ramirez AG, Perez-Stable EJ, Penedo FJ, et al. Navigating Latinas with breast screen abnormalities to diagnosis: the Six Cities Study. Cancer. 2013;119:1298–305.
30. Cole H, Thompson HS, White M, et al. Community-based, preclinical patient navigation for colorectal cancer screening among older black men recruited from barbershops: the MISTER B trial. Am J Public Health. 2017;107:1433–40.
31. Ma GX, Lee MM, Tan Y, et al. Efficacy of a community-based participatory and multilevel intervention to enhance hepatitis B virus screening and vaccination in underserved Korean Americans. Cancer. 2018;124:973–82.
32. DeGroff A, Schroy PC 3rd, Morrissey KG, et al. Patient navigation for colonoscopy completion: results of an RCT. Am J Prev Med. 2017;53:363–72.
33. Rodday AM, Parsons SK, Snyder F, et al. Impact of patient navigation in eliminating economic disparities in cancer care. Cancer. 2015;121:4025–34.
34. Paskett ED, Katz ML, Post DM, et al. The Ohio Patient Navigation Research Program: does the American Cancer Society patient navigation model improve time to resolution in patients with abnormal screening tests? Cancer Epidemiol Biomark Prev. 2012;21:1620–8.
35. Halbert CH, Briggs V, Bowman M, et al. Acceptance of a community-based navigator program for cancer control among urban African Americans. Health Educ Res. 2014;29:97–108.
36. Steinberg ML, Fremont A, Khan DC, et al. Lay patient navigator program implementation for equal access to cancer care and clinical trials: essential steps and initial challenges. Cancer. 2006;107:2669–77.
37. Guadagnolo BA, Boylan A, Sargent M, et al. Patient navigation for American Indians undergoing cancer treatment: utilization and impact on care delivery in a regional healthcare center. Cancer. 2011;117:2754–61.
38. Battaglia TA, Darnell JS, Ko N, et al. The impact of patient navigation on the delivery of diagnostic breast cancer care in the National Patient Navigation Research Program: a prospective meta-analysis. Breast Cancer Res Treat. 2016;158:523–34.
39. Myers RE, Sifri R, Daskalakis C, et al. Increasing colon cancer screening in primary care among African Americans. J Natl Cancer Inst. 2014;106:dju344.
40. Marshall JK, Mbah OM, Ford JG, et al. Effect of patient navigation on breast cancer screening among African American medicare beneficiaries: a randomized controlled trial. J Gen Intern Med. 2016;31:68–76.

41. Enard KR, Nevarez L, Hernandez M, et al. Patient navigation to increase colorectal cancer screening among Latino Medicare enrollees: a randomized controlled trial. Cancer Causes Control. 2015;26:1351–9.
42. Braschi CD, Sly JR, Singh S, Villagra C, Jandorf L. Increasing colonoscopy screening for Latino Americans through a patient navigation model: a randomized clinical trial. J Immigr Minor Health. 2014;16:934–40.
43. Chen MS Jr, Fang DM, Stewart SL, et al. Increasing hepatitis B screening for hmong adults: results from a randomized controlled community-based study. Cancer Epidemiol Biomark Prev. 2013;22:782–91.
44. Burhansstipanov L, Krebs LU, Dignan MB, et al. Findings from the native navigators and the Cancer Continuum (NNACC) study. J Cancer Educ. 2014;29:420–7.
45. Castaldi M, Safadjou S, Elrafei T, McNelis J. A multidisciplinary patient navigation program improves compliance with adjuvant breast cancer therapy in a public hospital. Am J Med Qual. 2017;32:406–13.
46. Baker DW, Brown T, Buchanan DR, et al. Comparative effectiveness of a multifaceted intervention to improve adherence to annual colorectal cancer screening in community health centers: a randomized clinical trial. JAMA Intern Med. 2014;174:1235–41.
47. Simon MA, Tom LS, Nonzee NJ, et al. Evaluating a bilingual patient navigation program for uninsured women with abnormal screening tests for breast and cervical cancer: implications for future navigator research. Am J Public Health. 2015;105:e87–94.
48. Dignan M, White C, Schoenberg N, et al. Effectiveness of an intervention for adherence to follow-up recommendations for abnormal pap tests in Appalachian Kentucky. Health Behav Policy Rev. 2014;1:6–15.
49. Honeycutt S, Green R, Ballard D, et al. Evaluation of a patient navigation program to promote colorectal cancer screening in rural Georgia, USA. Cancer. 2013;119:3059–66.
50. Falk D, Cubbin C, Jones B, et al. Increasing breast and cervical cancer screening in rural and border texas with friend to friend plus patient navigation. J Cancer Educ. 2018;33:798–805.
51. Optimal resources for cancer care (2020 Standards). Available at: https://www.facs.org/2020standards. Accessed 16 Sept 2020.
52. Valverde PA, Burhansstipanov L, Patierno S, et al. Findings from the National Navigation Roundtable: a call for competency-based patient navigation training. Cancer. 2019;125:4350–9.
53. Calhoun EA, Whitley EM, Esparza A, et al. A national patient navigator training program. Health Promot Pract. 2010;11:205–15.
54. Ustjanauskas AE, Bredice M, Nuhaily S, Kath L, Wells KJ. Training in patient navigation: a review of the research literature. Health Promot Pract. 2016;17:373–81.
55. Freund KM, Haas JS, Lemon SC, et al. Standardized activities for lay patient navigators in breast cancer care: recommendations from a citywide implementation study. Cancer. 2019;125:4532–40.
56. Jandorf L, Stossel LM, Cooperman JL, et al. Cost analysis of a patient navigation system to increase screening colonoscopy adherence among urban minorities. Cancer. 2013;119:612–20.
57. Elkin EB, Shapiro E, Snow JG, Zauber AG, Krauskopf MS. The economic impact of a patient navigator program to increase screening colonoscopy. Cancer. 2012;118:5982–8.
58. Donaldson EA, Holtgrave DR, Duffin RA, et al. Patient navigation for breast and colorectal cancer in 3 community hospital settings: an economic evaluation. Cancer. 2012;118:4851–9.
59. Rocque GB, Pisu M, Jackson BE, et al. Resource use and medicare costs during lay navigation for geriatric patients with cancer. JAMA Oncol. 2017;3:817–25.

Tobacco Control and Lung Cancer Screening to Address Disparities

Chanita Hughes Halbert

Introduction

Behavioral risk factors such as cigarette smoking play an important role in cancer health disparities. In particular, cigarette smoking is a well-established behavioral risk factor for lung cancer, and this disease continues to be a leading cause of racial disparities in cancer morbidity and mortality adults in the USA [1]. National data show that many adults continue to smoke cigarettes, even in states that have made rigorous efforts to implement evidence-based strategies for tobacco control. According to 2020 data from the Behavioral Risk Factor Surveillance Survey, for instance, 8.9% of adults in California are current smokers overall and there are racial disparities in smoking status. 18.9% of African American residents in California are current smokers compared to 8.9% of white California residents. While current smoking rates are higher in states that have weaker tobacco control, smoking rates are comparable among African Americans. South Carolina, for instance, has a lower rating for statewide tobacco control relative to California and 18.1% of adults in South Carolina are current smokers. However, 15.7% of African American residents in South Carolina are current smokers (compared to 18.9% of African American residents in California) [2]. Using data from the Tobacco Use Supplement from the Current Population Survey (TUS-CPS), Leventhal and colleagues found that many adult smokers in the USA are interested in quitting and many make a quit attempt. However, less than 10% of adults in the TUS-CPS were successful at sustaining cessation overall, and there were racial disparities in cessation. African Americans had a lower likelihood of sustained cessation compared to whites from 2014 to 2019 [3]. At the same time, low-dose computed tomography (LDCT) is now available as an evidence-based approach for lung cancer early detection in clinical settings. The demonstrated ability of LDCT to reduce lung

C. Hughes Halbert (✉)
University of Southern California, California, CA, USA
e-mail: hughesha@usc.edu

C. Hughes Halbert (ed.), *Cancer Health Disparities*,
https://doi.org/10.1007/978-3-031-37638-2_6

cancer mortality is a significant clinical and public health advance because it is the only evidence-based approach for detecting lung cancer at an early stage when treatment is most likely to be curative. However, prior studies have demonstrated that patients from disparity populations have reduced access and uptake of LDCT [4, 5]. The purpose of this chapter is to identify multilevel determinants of smoking behaviors, cessation efforts, and uptake of early detection strategies.

Cigarette Smoking and Cessation Among African Americans

Despite ongoing efforts, African Americans continue to experience disproportionately high morbidity and mortality from lung cancer because of behavioral risk factors such as cigarette smoking [1]. Previous efforts to address racial disparities in lung cancer morbidity and mortality have focused on describing differences in smoking behaviors and cessation outcomes between African Americans and whites [6]. This work has been important for documenting racial disparities in exposure to menthol versus non-menthol cigarettes, characterizing differences in physiological responses to nicotine between African Americans and whites, and evaluating smoking cessation outcomes [6]. This research has shown that African Americans are more likely than whites to initiate smoking at a later age and smoke menthol cigarettes [6]. Data from randomized trials have demonstrated the efficacy of pharmacological therapy among African Americans [7, 8]; but, even with these evidence-based treatments, smoking cessation rates are low among African Americans [9]. In addition to racial background, having fewer socioeconomic resources is associated with a lower likelihood of smoking cessation [10, 11]. Perceived stress also influences cigarette smoking among African Americans [6, 12–14]; exposure to stressors contributes to a distinct pattern of smoking among African Americans that includes smoking intermittently, greater nicotine dependence despite smoking a limited number of cigarettes, and smoking with greater intensity [6]. Smoking in response to stress and smoking to obtain the physiological rewards from smoking are more common among African Americans (vs. whites) [6]. Relatedly, several observational studies have also shown that greater perceived stress is associated with smoking initiation and the likelihood of cessation among African Americans [6].

Smoking Cessation in African Americans

Smoking cessation is an important component of lung cancer prevention; there are several FDA-approved cessation pharmacotherapies. Nevertheless, African Americans are likely to attempt to quit smoking on their own [15–17] because of concerns and distrust against pharmacological strategies and do not believe in the efficacy of cessation products [18]. African Americans are also less likely than whites to receive recommended approaches for smoking cessation counseling from health-care providers (e.g., physician advice about cessation, asking about tobacco use and willingness to quit, and arranging follow-up) [19–22]. Racial disparities in the 5As of behavioral counseling and referral for smoking cessation ultimately contribute to inequities in lung cancer morbidity and mortality. For this reason, improving access utilization of evidence-based strategies for smoking cessation among disparity populations continues to be important priorities for cancer health equity. Programs such as quitlines for smoking cessation have been developed to enhance access to tobacco control among medically underserved groups. Quitlines were designed to be anonymous and easy to use, but utilization of this program is low [23]. Previous research has shown that smokers have negative attitudes about this program and only 34% of smokers contacted the state quitline after an intervention that was designed to enhance referrals to this program [24]. While utilization of cessation medications was greater among smokers who contacted the quitline (vs. non-callers), quitline callers and non-callers did not differ significantly in terms of quit attempts and abstinence rates [24].

Smoking cessation takes place within a physiological, social, and environmental context; empirical data are emerging about the physiological impact of cessation efforts among African American and white smokers. For instance, Hooper and colleagues found that African Americans (vs. whites) have lower cortisol levels at critical time points in the trajectory of a smoking cessation intervention (e.g., at the beginning and end of treatment) [25]. Cortisol slopes at baseline, end of treatment, and 1-month follow-up were also flatter among African American smokers compared to white smokers [25]. The relationship between nicotine, stress, smoking, and HPA-axis functioning is complex. Previous research has shown that (1) nicotine increases activation of the HPA-axis, (2) the HPA-axis is also activated by acute and daily stressors, (3) smoking is a response to acute and daily stressors, (4) stress and nicotine can increase cortisol concentrations, and (5) smoking in response to stress exposure can reinforce the rewarding effects of nicotine [26–28]. Research has been conducted to disentangle these effects [28]; following exposure to a laboratory-based stressor, smokers were most likely to have a blunted cortisol response compared to non-smokers and occasional smokers [29]. Cigarette craving also increased among daily smokers, and cortisol responses were positively associated with these cravings [29]. Smokers also demonstrate a blunted cortisol response to stress and nicotine during abstinence; blunted stress responses were associated with reduced control over smoking behavior, an increased craving for tobacco, and greater withdrawal [30, 31]. McKee and colleagues found that following stress induction, activity in the HPA-axis system increased as cigarettes were smoked [30]. Additionally, smoking intensity increased, smokers perceived greater reward and satisfaction from smoking, and they also had greater difficulty resisting the urge to smoke [30].

Improving the Precision of Smoking Cessation Interventions

Current smoking cessation interventions focus on increasing the precision of pharmacological treatment for cigarette smoking by identifying the most effective configuration of intervention components [32, 33], using biomarkers such as nicotine metabolism rates (NMR) [34, 35] and genetic variants that are associated with risk for treatment failure [36]. These efforts are important but may not consider the biological underpinning and mechanisms involved risk factors (e.g., perceived stress and stress responses) for smoking initiation, maintenance, and cessation relapse. That is to say, several studies have demonstrated a positive association between self-reported perceived stress and smoking, initiation, and relapse. At the same time, previous research has shown that nicotine activates the HPA-axis and smoking can dysregulate cortisol responses [29]. Other work has shown that African Americans may be likely to smoke following stress exposure because the positive physiological effects of nicotine reduce the adverse effects of stress by activating the HPA-axis system [6]. Thus, cortisol responses following stress exposure may be important to consider as biological mediators between racial background and smoking behaviors, but these responses are expressed in a social, psychological, and structural context. For instance, African American and other groups with greater exposure to discrimination experience more severe smoking urge and anxiety and risk of smoking relapse when abstaining from tobacco [37, 38]. However, few efforts have been made to translate cross-sectional data on the association between perceived stress, physiological stress responses, and smoking behaviors into evidence-based interventions for smoking cessation and tobacco control in African Americans and other disparity populations. Empirical data on racial disparities in HPA-axis functioning within the context of social, psychological, and structural variables is needed among smokers to enhance the precision of pharmacological treatment for smoking cessation for African Americans and other disparity populations.

Early Detection for Lung Cancer

In addition to the observational research and randomized trials that have been conducted to identify risk factors for cigarette smoking and evaluate the effects of pharmacological treatments for cessation [6, 15], substantial investments have been made to develop novel clinical approaches for detecting lung cancer early and therapeutic strategies for treating this disease. The National Lung Cancer Screening Trial (NLST) demonstrated the efficacy of low-dose computed tomography (LDCT) screening in terms of reducing lung cancer-specific and overall mortality [39], and LDCT is now offered in many academic medical centers [40]. Lung cancer screening with LDCT has a Grade B recommendation from the US Preventive Services Task Force [40], and screening guidelines have been revised recently to be better aligned with the smoking behaviors and disease risk profiles of smokers from disparity populations to increase access among these groups [41]. These efforts are important but may not be sufficient for improving access and utilization of lung cancer screening among disparity populations [42]. Further, disparity populations have reduced access to high-end diagnostic tests (e.g., tumor sequencing), definitive treatment for lung cancer (e.g., lung resection), and emerging treatment approaches [43]. Recent studies have shown that African Americans and individuals from medically underserved ethnic groups are less likely to be treated with immunotherapies [44] and continue to be underrepresented in immunotherapy trials and precision oncology studies [45, 46] even though considerable efforts have been made to expand the infrastructure for minority accrual to clinical trials through initiatives such as the NCI Community Oncology Research Program (NCORP) [47].

Patient navigation is emerging as an efficacious strategy for improving access to and utilization of health-care services, especially among racial minorities. Navigation is an approach that provides targeted support to address individual-level barriers to health-care services [48]; it is a strategy that is being used to address racial disparities in access to cancer care services [49, 50]. For the most part, studies have shown that patient navigation is effective at improving utilization of cancer screening tests and research is now being conducted to evaluate the efficacy of patient navigation on diagnostic and treatment outcomes following cancer diagnosis [51]. Navigation can be applied to other health services; recently, Halbert and colleagues developed a community-based navigator program for cancer control among African Americans and found high acceptance and satisfaction rates [52]. Other research has shown that primary care providers are receptive to smoking cessation navigation, believe that it is an effective strategy for addressing patient barriers that are beyond the scope of practice, and are interested in implementing this approach into primary care [53]. This may be because providers have a limited amount of time to address smoking cessation among patients and also have limited knowledge and expertise on how to address cessation needs adequately, particularly among African American smokers. Findings from previous research also demonstrate the beneficial effects of patient navigation for smoking cessation. For instance, Lasser et al. [54] used navigation to promote smoking cessation among low-income primary care patients and found that it was associated with greater engagement in smoking cessation compared to usual care. Compared to low-income patients in usual care, those who received navigation were more likely to use smoking cessation treatment (e.g., used quitline, discussed treatment for tobacco use with a health-care provider). Similarly, smokers who received a navigation plus financial incentive intervention had significantly greater cessation rates compared to those in the control condition [54].

Empirical evidence is also emerging about patient navigation for lung cancer screening. Reports have described the rationale for using patient navigation to address barriers to LDCT [55], defined intervention protocols [55], and recommended metrics for evaluating outcomes of navigation interventions [56]. Percac-Lima et al. [57], for instance, compared the effects of patient navigation for lung cancer screening versus usual care on the proportion of primary care patients who were screened, the reach of the intervention, and the number and proportion of screened patients who needed follow-up care. As navigation programs for lung cancer screening continue to be developed as a solution for addressing disparities in lung cancer risk and outcomes in medically underserved groups, it is important that these interventions address the fundamental causes of reduced access to care in addition to addressing knowledge about LCDT and ensuring that patients understand the risks and benefits of screening as part of shared decision-making. For instance, in the research conducted by Cappelletti and colleagues, participants who had unmet basic needs related to social determinants (e.g., financial hardship, food insecurity, housing) had greater psychosocial stress, were unlikely to complete personalized referrals for preventive health care services, and did not recall the information that was provided as part of the tailored intervention [58]. Accordingly, navigation interventions are now being developed to address SDOH; in pediatric settings, SDOH screening and navigation for caregivers were associated with a significant reduction in the number of unmet social needs and a significant improvement in the child's health [59]. Findings from prior studies have demonstrated that patients and providers are likely to be receptive to SDOH screening and navigation [60, 61], but this approach has not yet been widely integrated into lung cancer screening navigation interventions, and empirical data on the effects of navigation for lung cancer screening is emerging. The time is ripe to translate the promise of patient navigation to address underutilization of cessation support and lung cancer screening among African American smokers and those at increased risk for developing this disease. Navigation can be particularly effective in enhancing access to early detection and tobacco control strategies in primary care because it is a strategy that addresses individual barriers and needs for cessation using a culturally appropriate delivery strategy.

Conclusions and Future Directions

Now more than ever, health-care systems and providers are expected to identify patients who have unmet social needs and address social risk factors among patients as part of efforts to improve access to care, enhance the efficiency and quality of health-care delivery, and enhance the public's health. In particular, SDOH have emerged as important determinants of cancer health disparities in lung cancer risk behaviors and outcomes because these factors intersect with biological mechanisms and pathways, geographic factors, and clinical variables to contribute to poorer outcomes in disparity populations. For instance, previous research has shown that African Americans metabolize nicotine more slowly than whites and several other racial groups [62, 63]. This is important because faster nicotine metabolism is a biomarker that provides an indication of the extent to which smokers may have an urge to smoke and have increased vulnerability to relapse [62, 63]. Despite overrepresentation of this putatively protective biological factor and evidence that US African Americans (vs. whites) smoke fewer cigarettes per day, and are more likely to report an interest in quitting and make quit attempts, a smaller percentage of

African Americans than other racial/ethnic groups successfully quit smoking each year [64]. At the same time, findings from observational studies have shown that greater perceived stress, stress relief, and the avoidance of adverse psychological and physiological reactions are among the primary reasons for smoking initiation, maintenance of smoking behaviors, and relapse in all populations [6]. While stress is a universal mechanism underlying smoking and other cancer control behaviors, the quantity and quality of stress experienced by groups subject to health disparities is unique due to SDOH. For instance, African American and other groups with greater exposure to discrimination experience more severe smoking urge and anxiety and risk of smoking relapse when abstaining from tobacco [37, 38]. Stress exposure has both psychological and physiological consequences that are important to nicotine addiction and cessation behaviors and outcomes. That is to say, individuals can perceive that they are unable to cope with or manage challenging situations, but there are also physiological reactions that include activation of the sympathetic nervous system (SNS) and HPA-axis. However, disparities in physiological stress responses have not been examined within the context of multilevel determinants that include clinical factors, geographic variables, and tobacco control behaviors in diverse racial and ethnic groups who are at increased risk for developing lung cancer because diverse cohorts have not been established to support this research. Recent studies have shown that disparity populations (e.g., African Americans, Hispanics) continue to be underrepresented in precision oncology studies [45, 46], the cohorts that are used to conduct fundamental oncological discovery science, and randomized trials that compare early detection strategies. For instance, only 4% of participants in the NLST were African Americans [46]. Multilevel data on SDOH (e.g., race/ethnicity, social deprivation) are also not included in most registries and national cohorts. Without annotation and documentation of these variables in cohorts and registries, it is not possible to examine the effects of multilevel determinants on disparities in lung cancer risk factors, access to early detection and tobacco control interventions, or treatment.

Lung cancer prevention and early detection are at a critical juncture where it is essential to move beyond descriptive studies that compare racial/ethnic groups in tobacco control and cessation behaviors to solutions that address the primary drivers of inequity in lung cancer outcomes. Reduced access to evidence-based strategies for lung cancer prevention and early detection through smoking cessation interventions and lung cancer screening continues to be a primary driver of lung cancer disparities that sets the stage for delays in obtaining appropriate follow-up of abnormal results, access to molecular diagnosis that drive care decisions and definitive treatment, and equitable access to precision oncology trials and therapies. Progress on each step in this continuum will ultimately reduce disparities in lung cancer morbidity and mortality, especially if strategies leverage current investments in population-based research, clinical care, and discovery science and include efforts to establish diverse cohorts that will enable transdisciplinary translational studies to be conducted in disparity populations.

References

1. American Cancer Society. Cancer facts and figures, 2022. Atlanta: American Cancer Society; 2022.
2. Behavioral risk factor surveillance survey data. 2020. Available at: https://www.cdc.gov/brfss/data_tools.htm
3. Leventhal AM, Dai H, Higgins ST. Smoking cessation prevalence and inequalities in the United States: 2014–2019. J Natl Cancer Inst. 2022;114(3):381–90.
4. Watson KS, Blok AC, Buscemi J, Molina Y, Fitzgibbon M, Simon MA, Williams L, Matthews K, Studts JL, Lillie SE, Ostroff JS, Carter-Harris L, Winn RA. Society of Behavioral Medicine supports implementation of high quality lung cancer screening in high-risk populations. Transl Behav Med. 2016 Dec;6(4):669–71.
5. Zeliadt SB, Hoffman RM, Birkby G, Eberth JM, Brenner AT, Reuland DS, Flocke SA. Challenges implementing lung cancer screening in federally qualified health centers. Am J Prev Med. 2018 Apr;54(4):568–75.
6. National Cancer Institute. A socioecological approach to addressing tobacco-related health disparities, National Cancer Institute Tobacco Control monograph 22. Bethesda: U.S. Department of Health and Human Services, National Institutes of Health, National Cancer Institute; 2017.
7. Ahluwalia JS, Harris KJ, Catley D, Okuyemi KS, Mayo MS. Sustained-release bupropion for smoking cessation in African Americans: a randomized controlled trial. JAMA. 2002;288:468–74.
8. Cox LS, Nollen NL, Mayo MS, et al. Bupropion for smoking cessation in African American light smokers: a randomized controlled trial. J Natl Cancer Inst. 2012;104:290–8.
9. Centers for Disease Control and Prevention. African Americans and tobacco use. Available at: https://www.cdc.gov/tobacco/disparities/african-americans/
10. Barbeau EM, Krieger N, Soobader MJ. Working class matters: socioeconomic disadvantage, race/ethnicity, gender, and smoking in NHIS 2000. Am J Public Health. 2004;94:269–78.
11. Winkleby MA, Cubbin C, Ahn DK, Kraemer HC. Pathways by which SES and ethnicity influence cardiovascular disease risk factors. Ann N Y Acad Sci. 1999;896:191–209.
12. Kendzor DE, Cofta-Woerpel LM, Mazas CA, et al. Socioeconomic status, negative affect, and modifiable cancer risk factors in African-American smokers. Cancer Epidemiol Biomarker Prev. 2008;17:2546–54.
13. Kendzor DE, Costello TJ, Li Y, et al. Race/ethnicity and multiple cancer risk factors among individuals seeking smoking cessation treatment. Cancer Epidemiol Biomarker Prev. 2008;17:2937–45.
14. Williams DR, Yan Y, Jackson JS, Anderson NB. Racial differences in physical and mental health: socio-economic status, stress and discrimination. J Health Psychol. 1997;2:335–51.
15. Ahluwalia JS, Resnicow K, Clark WS. Knowledge about smoking, reasons for smoking, and reasons for wishing to quit in inner-city African Americans. Ethn Dis. 1998;8:385–93.
16. Royce JM, Hymowitz N, Corbett K, Hartwell TD, Orlandi MA. Smoking cessation factors among African Americans and whites. COMMIT Research Group. Am J Public Health. 1993;83:220–6.
17. Ryan KK, Garrett-Mayer E, Alberg AJ, Cartmell KB, Carpenter MJ. Predictors of cessation pharmacotherapy use among black and non-Hispanic white smokers. Nicotine Tob Res. 2011;13:646–52.
18. Carpenter MJ, Ford ME, Cartmell K, Alberg AJ. Misperceptions of nicotine replacement therapy within racially and ethnically diverse smokers. J Natl Med Assoc. 2011;103:885–94.
19. Chase EC, McMenamin SB, Halpin HA. Medicaid provider delivery of the 5A's for smoking cessation counseling. Nicotine Tob Res. 2007;9:1095–101.
20. Cokkinides VE, Halpern MT, Barbeau EM, Ward E, Thun MJ. Racial and ethnic disparities in smoking-cessation interventions: analysis of the 2005 National Health Interview Survey. Am J Prev Med. 2008;34:404–12.

21. Agency for Healthcare Research and Quality. Treating tobacco use and dependence. Available at: http://www.ahrq.gov/professionals/clinicians-providers/guidelines-recommendations/tobacco/clinicians/update/index.htmlQuality
22. U.S. Preventive Services Task Force. Final update summary: Tobacco smoking cessation in adults, including pregnant women: Behavioral and pharmacotherapy interventions. September 2015. Available at: https://www.uspreventiveservicestaskforce.org/Page/Document/UpdateSummaryFinal/tobacco-use-in-adults-and-pregnant-women-counseling-and-interventions1
23. Solomon LJ, Hughes JR, Livingston A, et al. Cognitive barriers to calling a smoking quitline. Nicotine Tob Res. 2009;11:1339–46.
24. Mathew AR, Burris JL, Alberg AJ, Cummings KM, Carpenter MJ. Impact of a brief telephone referral on quitline use, quit attempts and abstinence. Health Educ Res. 2015;30:134–9.
25. Webb Hooper M. Racial/ethnic differences in physiological stress and relapse among treatment seeking tobacco smokers. Int J Environ Res Public Health. 2019;16(17):3090.
26. Jensen KP, Sofuoglu M. Stress response genes and the severity of nicotine withdrawal. Pharmacogenomics. 2016;17(1):1–3.
27. Wong JA, Pickworth WB, Waters AJ, al'Absi M, Leventhal AM. Cortisol levels decrease after acute tobacco abstinence in regular smokers. Hum Psychopharm Clin. 2014;29(2):152–62.
28. Richards JM, Stipelman BA, Bornovalova MA, Daughters SB, Sinha R, Lejuez CW. Biological mechanisms underlying the relationship between stress and smoking: state of the science and directions for future work. Biol Psychol. 2011;88(1):1–12.
29. Buchmann AF, Laucht M, Schmid B, Wiedemann K, Mann K, Zimmermann US. Cigarette craving increases after a psychosocial stress test and is related to cortisol stress response but not to dependence scores in daily smokers. J Psychopharmacol. 2010;24(2):247–55.
30. McKee SA, Sinha R, Weinberger AH, Sofuoglu M, Harrison EL, Lavery M, Wanzer J. Stress decreases the ability to resist smoking and potentiates smoking intensity and reward. J Psychopharmacol. 2011;25(4):490–502.
31. Childs E, de Wit H. Effects of acute psychosocial stress on cigarette craving and smoking. Nicotine Tob Res. 2010;12(4):449–53.
32. Piper ME, Cook JW, Schlam TR, Smith SS, Bolt DM, Collins LM, Mermelstein R, Fiore MC, Baker TB. Toward precision smoking cessation treatment II: proximal effects of smoking cessation intervention components on putative mechanisms of action. Drug Alcohol Depend. 2017;171:50–8.
33. Piper ME, Schlam TR, Cook JW, Smith SS, Bolt DM, Loh WY, Mermelstein R, Collins LM, Fiore MC, Baker TB. Toward precision smoking cessation treatment I: moderator results from a factorial experiment. Drug Alcohol Depend. 2017;171:59–65.
34. Lerman C, Schnoll RA, Hawk LW Jr, Cinciripini P, George TP, Wileyto EP, Swan GE, Benowitz NL, Heitjan DF, Tyndale RF, Group P-PR. Use of the nicotine metabolite ratio as a genetically informed biomarker of response to nicotine patch or varenicline for smoking cessation: a randomised, double-blind placebo controlled trial. Lancet. Respir Med. 2015;3(2):131–8.
35. Allenby CE, Boylan KA, Lerman C, Falcone M. Precision medicine for tobacco dependence: development and validation of the nicotine metabolite ratio. J Neuroimmune Pharmacol. 2016;11(3):471–83.
36. Chen LS, Horton A, Bierut L. Pathways to precision medicine in smoking cessation treatments. Neurosci Lett. 2018;669:83–92.
37. Bello MS, Liautaud MM, De La Cerda JT, Pang RD, Ray LA, Ahluwalia JA, Leventhal AM. Association of frequency of perceived exposure to discrimination with tobacco withdrawal symptoms and smoking lapse behavior in African Americans. Addiction. 2021;116(4):914–25.
38. Kendzor DE, Businelle MS, Reitzel LR, Rios DM, Scheuermann TS, Pulvers K, Ahluwalia JS. Everyday discrimination is associated with nicotine dependence among African American, Latino, and White smokers. Nicotine Tob Res. 2014;16(6):633–40.
39. National Lung Screening Trial Research Team, Aberle DR, Adams AM, Berg CD, Black WC, Clapp JD, Fagerstrom RM, Gareen IF, Gatsonis C, Marcus PM, Sicks JD. Reduced

lung-cancer mortality with low-dose computed tomographic screening. N Engl J Med. 2011;365(5):395–409.
40. US Preventive Services Task Force, Krist AH, Davidson KW, Mangione CM, Barry MJ, Cabana M, Caughey AB, Davis EM, Donahue KE, Doubeni CA, Kubik M, Landefeld CS, Li L, Ogedegbe G, Owens DK, Pbert L, Silverstein M, Stevermer J, Tseng CW, Wong JB. Screening for lung cancer: US preventive services task force recommendation statement. JAMA. 2021 Mar 9;325(10):962–70.
41. Rivera MP, Katki HA, Tanner NT, Triplette M, Sakoda LC, Wiener RS, Cardarelli R, Carter-Harris L, Crothers K, Fathi JT, Ford ME, Smith R, Winn RA, Wisnivesky JP, Henderson LM, Aldrich MC. Addressing disparities in lung cancer screening eligibility and healthcare access. An official American Thoracic Society statement. Am J Respir Crit Care Med. 2020 Oct 1;202(7):e95–112.
42. Landy R, Young CD, Skarzynski M, Cheung LC, Berg CD, Rivera MP, Robbins HA, Chaturvedi AK, Katki HA. Using prediction models to reduce persistent racial and ethnic disparities in the draft 2020 USPSTF lung cancer screening guidelines. J Natl Cancer Inst. 2021;113(11):1590–4.
43. Gross CP, Meyer CS, Ogale S, Kent M, Wong WB. Associations between medicaid insurance, biomarker testing, and outcomes in patients with advanced NSCLC. J Natl Compr Cancer Netw. 2022;20(5):479–87.
44. Verma V, Haque W, Cushman TR, Lin C, Simone CB 2nd, Chang JY, McClelland S 3rd, Welsh JW. Racial and insurance-related disparities in delivery of immunotherapy-type compounds in the United States. J Immunother. 2019;42(2):55–64.
45. Aldrighetti CM, Niemierko A, Van Allen E, Willers H, Kamran SC. Racial and ethnic disparities among participants in precision oncology clinical studies. JAMA Netw Open. 2021;4(11):e2133205.
46. Tanner NT, Gebregziabher M, Hughes Halbert C, Payne E, Egede LE, Silvestri GA. Racial differences in outcomes within the National Lung Screening Trial. Implications for widespread implementation. Am J Respir Crit Care Med. 2015;192(2):200–8.
47. St Germain D, Denicoff AM, Dimond EP, Carrigan A, Enos RA, Gonzalez MM, Wilkinson K, Mathiason MA, Duggan B, Einolf S, McCaskill-Stevens W, Bryant DM, Thompson MA, Grubbs SS, Go RS. Use of the National Cancer Institute community cancer centers program screening and accrual log to address cancer clinical trial accrual. J Oncol Pract. 2014;10(2):e73–80.
48. Parker VA, Clark JA, Leyson J, et al. Patient navigation: development of a protocol for describing what navigators do. Health Serv Res. 2010;45:514–31.
49. Paskett ED, Harrop JP, Wells KJ. Patient navigation: an update on the state of the science. CA Cancer J Clin. 2011;61:237–49.
50. Paskett ED, Katz ML, Post DM, et al. The Ohio Patient Navigation Research Program: does the American Cancer Society patient navigation model improve time to resolution in patients with abnormal screening tests? Cancer Epidemiol Biomarker Prev. 2012;21:1620–8.
51. Graboyes EM, Sterba KR, Li H, Warren GW, Alberg AJ, Calhoun EA, Nussenbaum B, McCay J, Marsh CH, Osazuwa-Peters N, Neskey DM, Kaczmar JM, Sharma AK, Harper J, Day TA, Hughes-Halbert C. Development and evaluation of a navigation-based, multilevel intervention to improve the delivery of timely, guideline-adherent adjuvant therapy for patients with head and neck cancer. JCO Oncol Pract. 2021;17(10):e1512–23.
52. Halbert CH, Briggs V, Bowman M, et al. Acceptance of a community-based navigator program for cancer control among urban African Americans. Health Educ Res. 2014;29:97–108.
53. Lubetkin EI, Lu WH, Krebs P, Yeung H, Ostroff JS. Exploring primary care providers' interest in using patient navigators to assist in the delivery of tobacco cessation treatment to low income, ethnic/racial minority patients. J Community Health. 2010;35:618–24.
54. Lasser KE, Kenst KS, Quintiliani LM, et al. Patient navigation to promote smoking cessation among low-income primary care patients: a pilot randomized controlled trial. J Ethn Subst Abus. 2013;12:374–90.

55. Ruane B, Giamboy TE, Sundaram B, Evans NR, Myers RE, Kane GC. The case for patient navigation in lung cancer screening in vulnerable populations: a systematic review. Popul Health Manag. 2019;22(4):347–61.
56. Gerber DE, Hamann HA, Santini NO, Abbara S, Chiu H, McGuire M, Quirk L, Zhu H, Lee SJC. Patient navigation for lung cancer screening in an urban safety-net system: protocol for a pragmatic randomized clinical trial. Contemp Clin Trials. 2017;60:78–85.
57. Percac-Lima S, Ashburner JM, Rigotti NA, Park ER, Chang Y, Kuchukhidze S, Atlas SJ. Patient navigation for lung cancer screening among current smokers in community health centers a randomized controlled trial. Cancer Med. 2018;7(3):894–902.
58. Cappelletti ER, Kreuter MW, Boyum S, Thompson T. Basic needs, stress and the effects of tailored health communication in vulnerable populations. Health Educ Res. 2015;30(4):591–8.
59. Gottlieb LM, Hessler D, Long D, Laves E, Burns AR, Amaya A, Sweeney P, Schudel C, Adler NE. Effects of social needs screening and in-person service navigation on child health: a randomized clinical trial. JAMA Pediatr. 2016;170(11):e162521.
60. Hamity C, Jackson A, Peralta L, Bellows J. Perceptions and experience of patients, staff, and clinicians with social needs assessment. Perm J. 2018;22:18–105.
61. Schickedanz A, Hamity C, Rogers A, Sharp AL, Jackson A. Clinician experiences and attitudes regarding screening for social determinants of health in a large integrated health system. Med Care. 2019;57:S197–201.
62. Perez-Stable EJ, Herrera B, Jacob P 3rd, Benowitz NL. Nicotine metabolism and intake in black and white smokers. JAMA. 1998;280(2):152–6.
63. Ross KC, Gubner NR, Tyndale RF, Hawk LW Jr, Lerman C, George TP, Cinciripini P, Schnoll RA, Benowitz NL. Racial differences in the relationship between rate of nicotine metabolism and nicotine intake from cigarette smoking. Pharmacol Biochem Behav. 2016;148:1–7.
64. Babb S, Malarcher A, Schauer G, Asman K, Jamal A. Quitting smoking among adults – United States, 2000–2015. MMWR Morb Mortal Wkly Rep. 2017 Jan 6;65(52):1457–64.

Evidence-Based Interventions for Cancer Equity, Clinic-Based Interventions to Promote Patient-Centered Care, and Weight Loss and Management

Marian L. Fitzgibbon, Jennifer Sanchez-Flack, Mirjana Antonic, and Mackenzie Ferguson

Introduction

There is an urgent need for evidence-based obesity prevention and weight management strategies to address the public health problem of overweight/obesity in the USA. Recent epidemiological data reflect that approximately 37.9% of adults and 17% of children and adolescents in the USA are obese [1]. Additionally, there are striking racial/ethnic disparities in obesity, as 48.5% of African Americans and 42.7% of Latinos in the USA are obese compared to 37.1% percent of non-Latino whites [1]. Addressing obesity among historically underrepresented groups is significant to the prevention of cancer health inequities and control given the association between excess body weight and a number of cancers, including colorectal cancer, postmenopausal breast cancer, endometrial cancer, and cancers of the kidney and pancreas [2]. The link between obesity and increased cancer incidence and mortality is well-established, and it is estimated that 14% of cancer deaths in men and 20% in women can be linked to obesity [3]. With current trends toward increases in overweight/obesity, the global burden of cancer is expected to rise, and overweight/obesity is likely to overtake smoking as a primary risk factor for cancer [4].

In the USA, the risk of developing cancer has increased in younger generations for 6 of 12 obesity-related cancers: multiple myeloma, colorectal, uterine corpus, gallbladder, kidney, and pancreatic cancer [5]. Fortunately, many modifiable lifestyle and environmental factors strongly influence cancer risk, indicating that many cancers are preventable [4]. It is estimated that between 30% and 50% of cancer cases are preventable via healthy lifestyles, specifically healthy dietary habits and physical activity, among other factors [4]. Therefore, maintaining a healthy body weight is a critical strategy to protect against cancer [4]. Efforts to reduce and

M. L. Fitzgibbon (✉) · J. Sanchez-Flack · M. Antonic · M. Ferguson
University of Illinois at Chicago, Chicago, IL, USA
e-mail: mlf@uic.edu

C. Hughes Halbert (ed.), *Cancer Health Disparities*,
https://doi.org/10.1007/978-3-031-37638-2_7

prevent obesity should be targeted to both adults and children, and additional research is needed on early-life exposures in relation to carcinogenesis, such as colorectal carcinogenesis, given that the incidence for such cancers has increased exclusively in younger adults in higher-income countries [6].

Strategies to maintain a healthy weight includes a healthy diet and regular physical activity. Unfortunately, for many Americans, dietary quality has worsened in recent decades, with more than half of adults reporting a low consumption of fruit and vegetables, whole grains, and fish and high consumption of sodium and sugar-sweetened beverages [7]. Fruit and vegetables are a rich source of micronutrients and phytochemicals, which show anticancer effects in cell and rodent studies [4]. These foods also contain various nutrients that impact cancer risk, such as vitamins C and E, selenium, and folate [4]. Longitudinal human clinical trial research shows that low intake of fruits or vegetables and high intake of red meat and processed meat are associated with increased risk of colorectal cancer [5]. However, underrepresented populations, including African Americans and Latinos, do not currently meet the recommended dietary guidelines for these foods [8]. The current USDA dietary guidelines recommend US adults consume 1.5–2 cup equivalents of fruits and 2–3 cup equivalents of vegetables daily and that children, depending on age, gender, and level of physical activity, consume 1–2 cup equivalents of fruits and 1–3 cup equivalents of vegetable daily [9, 10]. Recent estimates from the National Health and Nutrition Examination Survey (NHANES) indicate that the median cup equivalent intakes for African Americans are 0.62 for fruits and 0.90 for vegetables. For Latinos, intakes are 0.78 for fruits and 1.33 for vegetables [8].

Physical activity also has a beneficial effect on cancer risk via multiple mechanisms, including reductions in insulin resistance, inflammation, and visceral fat, all of which are linked to cancer development at various sites [4]. Additionally, physical activity is an important lifestyle behavior that can prevent the onset of overweight/obesity and facilitate weight loss. For preschool-aged children, the recommendations are that they should be physically active throughout the day for growth and development [11]. For older children, ages 6–17 years, it is recommended they participate in 60 minutes or more of moderate-to-vigorous physical activity each day and participate in muscle- and bone-strengthening activities 3 days a week [11]. For adults, 150 minutes of moderate to vigorous activity are recommended each week, in addition to 2 or more days of muscle-strengthening activities [12]. However, African American and Latino adults and children do not currently meet recommended physical activity guidelines [13]. According to the American Heart Association, African Americans and Latinos are more likely to be physically inactive, 41.1% and 42.2% respectively, than their non-Latino white counterparts (27.7%) [13]. Given this evidence, there is a pressing need to address obesity disparities in the USA. Preventing overweight/obesity early in life and promoting weight management among adults by improving healthier obesogenic behaviors, including diet and physical activity, could reduce the lifetime risk of obesity-related cancers [14].

The US Preventive Services Task Force recommends behavioral-based interventions for obesity prevention and treatment, given the evidence that multicomponent behavioral-based interventions in obese adults and children can lead to clinically significant improvements in weight status [15]. Lifestyle interventions promoting healthy dietary habits and increased physical activity show moderate, short-term weight loss that are associated with fewer adverse events than more aggressive pharmacological or surgical interventions [16]. For lifestyle interventions to be effective, they need to be multifactorial and consider the social determinants of health, which are "conditions in which people are born, grow, work, line and age, and the wider set of forces and systems shaping the conditions of daily life" [17]. These conditions influence many health behaviors, including diet and physical activity, which contribute to obesity risk (e.g., access to healthy foods, safe communities to exercise) [18]. Multifactorial lifestyle interventions could be integrated into healthcare and clinic settings via primary care providers (PCPs) [19, 20]. Clinics can be an initial avenue for intervention by screening patients at risk for obesity, providing brief advice and referral to services that can assist patients with long-term maintenance of healthier dietary habits and physical activity [21]. A meta-analysis conducted by Rose and colleagues (2013) reported that advice can have a positive impact on patient weight management [22]. However, PCPs within clinic settings face challenges in providing weight management counseling, such as a lack of skills and training, self-efficacy, sufficient reimbursement, staff support, and time constraints [21, 23–25]. Therefore, to reduce obesity-related cancer disparities, multifactorial approaches that utilize clinics as one area of intervention must be used.

Theoretical Foundations and Conceptual Frameworks

The Chronic Care Model

The Chronic Care Model (Fig. 1) is designed to help healthcare systems and clinics improve patient health outcomes by improving care delivery [26]. This model proposes that health care delivery can be enhanced through six interrelated system shifts meant to make patient-centered, evidence-based care easier. The Chronic Care Model aims to transform care for patients with chronic illnesses from acute and reactive to proactive, planned, and population-based [26, 27]. The model posits that healthcare and clinic settings can accomplish these goals via a combination of effective team-based care, self-management support bolstered by more effective use of community resources, integrated decision support, and patient registries, and other supportive information technology [26, 27]. Improved patient outcomes are a result of an improved and committed patient interacting with a prepared care team [26, 27]. To meet these goals, it is necessary for PCPS in healthcare systems and clinics to be connected with resources in the broader community [26, 27]. However, such resources, in addition to policies, primarily operate in the background versus critical component of the model [26, 27].

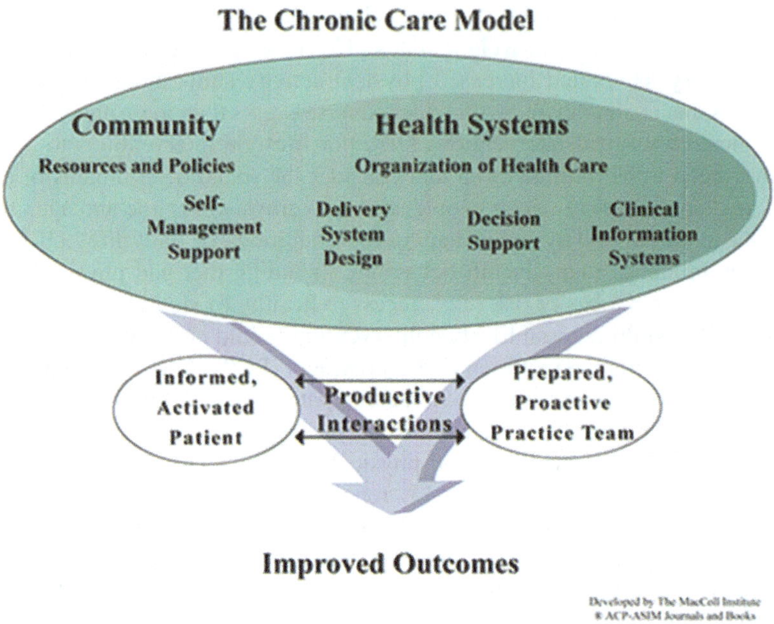

Fig. 1 The Chronic Care Model. (Developed by The MacColl Institute® ACP-ASIM Journals and Books)

Framework for Integrated Clinical and Community Systems of Care

An iteration of the Chronic Care Model, the Framework for Integrated Clinical and Community Systems of Care (Fig. 2), focuses on obesity and its related diseases [28]. This framework illustrates that improved patient experience, population health, and reduced cost of care for obese patients cannot be achieved by PCP-delivered interventions alone [28]. This framework integrates both clinical and community systems to address obesity and its related chronic diseases. This framework reflects an integrated healthcare system centered on patient and family engagement and empowerment and restructured clinical services by PCPs sensitive to the stigmatization of obesity and who use behavior change strategies to encourage healthier lifestyle behaviors [28]. In addition to complementary community systems that make healthier options, including healthy eating and physical activity, the default or easier option (e.g., increased access to healthy foods and/or safe spaces to exercise) [28]. From the clinical side, patient behavior change is a result of the PCP-patient interaction. From the community side, behavior change results from population-level policies, initiatives, and interventions that change social norms and the built environment [28].

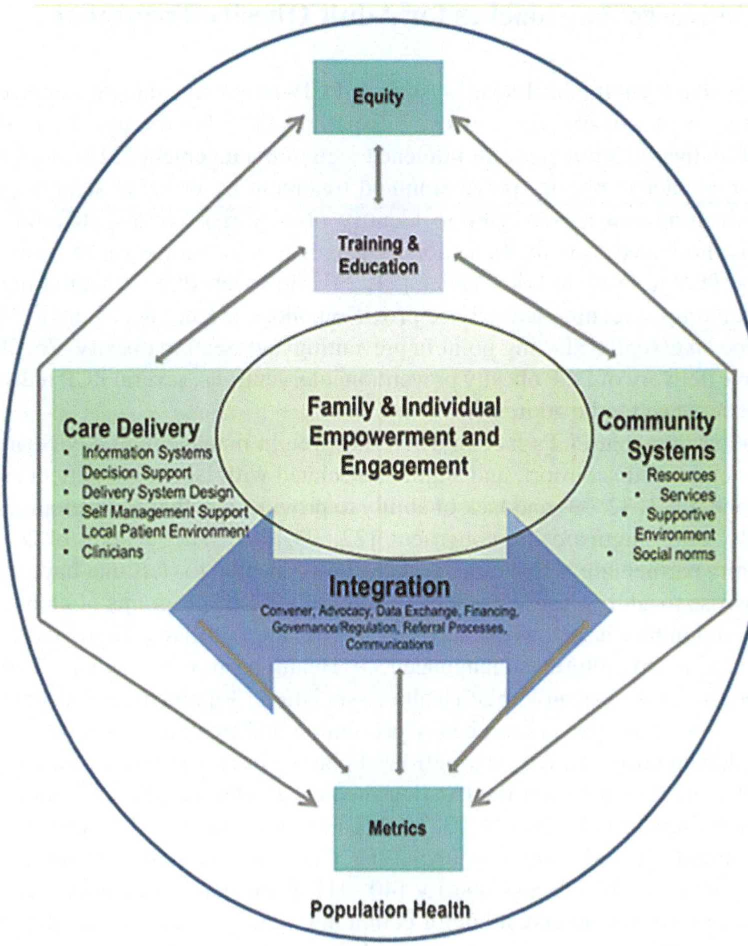

Fig. 2 Framework for integrated clinical and community systems of care

As indicated in both models, PCP-delivered intervention strategies to reduce obesity among diverse populations could be utilized in conjunction with other community-level strategies. Such multicomponent, or multilevel, interventions can be implemented with the development and adoption of clinical-community partnerships [28]. However, to effectively design and implement these multilevel interventions and effectively foster clinical-community partnerships, an understanding of the strengths and limitations of PCP-delivered intervention strategies needs to be understood and appropriately addressed [28].

PCP-Delivered Approaches for Adult Obesity Treatment

It is recognized that the healthcare system or PCP-delivered strategies alone cannot reduce the impact of obesity or obesity disparities [19], but the healthcare system and PCP-delivered strategies can influence weight management [21]. PCPs can be an initial contact in obesity prevention and treatment by utilizing screening practices. Screening can allow PCPs to identify obesity risk factors, determine if a patient is motivated to make behavioral changes to address their risk factors, and allow the PCP to provide brief advice [21, 29]. However, PCP-delivered interventions, including screening and advice provision, alone are not necessarily effective but can be an essential starting point in preventing and treating obesity [25, 29–31]. Before the delivery of PCP obesity prevention interventions, several PCP individual-level barriers need to be addressed.

Some barriers that PCPs face in delivering weight management advice are their own perceptions, discomfort, and stigma associated with labeling a patient as overweight/obese [21, 32, 33] and lack of ability to provide care that is developmentally, culturally, and linguistically congruent [22, 24, 34]. The benefit of a clinic-community partnership is that clinicians can be connected to staff that have the time and expertise to address these barriers. Community-based programs often hire staff, such as community health workers (CHWs), who are familiar with the target community in terms of culture and language [35]. Health promoters, such as CHWs, are endorsed by the American Public Health Association [36] and are consistently recognized as essential players in obesity prevention and treatment interventions [37, 38]. Implementation of PCP-only delivered obesity interventions is often hindered by the discordance between the existing medical model and the upstream, multi-level determinants of obesity [21, 23, 34, 39]. Fostering partnerships between clinic- and community-based programs, including CHW referrals, is recognized as an effective approach to address obesity [40, 41] given that community-based programs have a strong understanding of community contexts and needs. Not only do these partnerships improve an intervention's credibility, but they may also prove to be beneficial to PCPs. These partnerships can address barriers faced by PCPs in addressing obesity, including lack of time, training, and resources [23, 24, 42, 43], in addition to time and space constraints, associated with conducting obesity prevention interventions in clinic-based settings (e.g., space availability) [23]. Moreover, additional trips to clinics may be burdensome to patients, creating adherence issues [23]. Referring patients to resources in their communities would eliminate the need to additional trips to see a PCP.

Such community-based approaches can be utilized to target obesity prevention and control with a strategy such as clinic-community partnerships. In community-based care, PCPs, other healthcare personnel (e.g., registered dieticians, nurses, pharmacists), CHWs, and community organizations, can work together to support patients in implementing and supporting diet and physical activity behaviors by utilizing resources within their communities [44]. With a clinical-community partnership, high-risk groups, such as African Americans and Latinos, can be better reached through education and research and allow community involvement to reduce obesity disparities [45]. CHWs and others at community organizations can reinforce clinicians' recommendations and have an intensive role in delivering behavioral-based interventions, supplemented by regular monitoring from PCPs [23, 30, 46]. Clinic-community partnerships are in line with the American Academy of Pediatrics recommendations, highlighting the importance of clinician-community connectedness in the prevention and treatment of public health issues, such as obesity [25]. Therefore, developing a clinic-community partnership may be an effective way to address this barrier, given that community programs are typically well versed in these complex upstream factors [47].

Additional noted barriers are time constraints [23, 24, 39], unfamiliarity with billing codes, and lack of reimbursement by third-party payers [33]. To address such barriers, PCPs can engage with other nonphysician personnel in their clinics, such as registered dieticians. PCPs often provide obese patients with referrals to registered dieticians to support obese patients in setting and implementing diet-related behavioral goals [43]. Nonphysician personnel may have more time to work with obese patients and can be trained to become versed in billing codes and reimbursement policies [43]. Prior research demonstrates that intensive interventions delivered by nonphysician personnel effectively achieve clinically significant weight loss outcomes in the primary-care setting [30]. Additionally, the involvement of PCPs appears to increase retention rates and uptake of interventions delivered by nonphysician personnel [30].

Despite the barriers mentioned above, PCP-delivered interventions are worthwhile, given that PCPs are consistently recognized as trusted sources of information [23–25, 30, 39]. Patients with obesity may be more apt to listen to PCPs regarding their risk factors and the need to engage in obesity prevention efforts. Obesity prevention or treatment interventions can build off this provider-patient relationship and encourage PCPs to refer patients to community-based interventions and programs that provide ongoing support for building and maintaining healthy dietary and physical activity behaviors [21, 23, 43, 48]. Additionally, such community-based interventions can utilize PCPs to bolster their program's credibility to patients [23–25, 30, 39].

PCP-Delivered Approaches for Pediatric Obesity Treatment

Preventative approaches should be utilized to address pediatric obesity. For instance, PCPs can begin obesity prevention counseling during preconception, given that maternal BMI and gestational weight gain are associated with childhood obesity [49]. Therefore, women should follow recommendations for weight gain throughout pregnancy to help prevent obesity in their children [50]. Additionally, during the postpartum period, women should be encouraged to breastfeed as breastfeeding is a protective factor against childhood obesity [51]. Like adult obesity prevention and treatment methodologies, PCPs can act as a first point of contact by screening children for obesity or obesity risk and by offering advice and/or referrals for obesity prevention or treatment [33]. In addition to offering advice during preconception, pregnancy, and postpartum phases, PCPs can also provide advice and encourage parents to partake in obesity prevention efforts at home. This can include health behaviors such as increasing the number of meals consumed at home or limiting the number of meals consumed from restaurants, reducing portion sizes, limiting the consumption of sugar-sweetened beverages, increasing the number of meals eaten together as a family without distractions (e.g., not eating in front of the television), increasing the number of fruit and vegetables consumed, and increasing physical activity while reducing screen time [52]. Overall, the basis of pediatric obesity prevention and treatment should be that energy expenditure surpasses energy consumption [49].

Data suggest that 26 or more hours of contact between a patient, family, and treatment program, with a focus on family-based approaches, are needed to improve a child's weight status [49, 53]. In family-based approaches, the parent's body mass index (BMI) is considered a risk factor for pediatric obesity, and in these approaches, strategies are targeted to motivate behavior changes in both parents and children [49]. As a result, parents lose weight and act as role models for the behavior in their children [54]. Such family-based approaches could be complemented with motivational interviewing (MI), a technique where PCPs become a facilitator in the health behavior change process and display acceptance of the patient no matter their motivation, attitudes, barriers, or beliefs [55]. MI is an approach that is customized to the patient and their specific barriers and helps set specific, attainable goals (e.g., taking family walks after school three time per week or adding a vegetable side at dinner time) [49, 55]. PCPs can be trained in MI and utilize such approaches during child well visits.

However, similar to adult approaches, PCPs need to evaluate the feasibility of parents' ability to change obesity-related health behaviors given contextual factors. For instance, when recommending structured (e.g., games and exercise training sessions) and unstructured (e.g., free play) physical activity and healthier dietary behaviors (e.g., increased consumption of fruit and vegetables with meals) among families, it is important to consider social and environmental factors that may pose barriers [44, 56]. This could include a parent's perceived level of safety to participate in physical activity in their neighborhood or access to food outlets that stock healthy foods [44]. To address such barriers, PCPs can connect with local community organizations to address barriers cited by parents that limit their ability to engage in healthier obesity-related behavior change [44]. For instance, in the Families in Training program in Winston-Salem, North Carolina, a pediatric obesity treatment, prevention, research, and education program, clinical-community partnerships were developed to help patients meet their obesity-related health behavior change goals [44]. PCPs provided referrals to local community-based obesity efforts so that parents and children could engage in hands-on opportunities to prevent and treat obesity. Such hands-on opportunities included cooking classes, physical activity programming, and parenting classes. This program is innovative for extending clinical treatment and prevention programs to community settings, which addressed the contextual factors that limited the ability of parents and children to make positive health behavior changes.

Conclusion

The rate of adult and pediatric obesity has declined slightly, yet stark racial/ethnic disparities still exist. Many multilevel factors (e.g., individual-, interpersonal-, environmental-, and policy-level) influence obesity risk and outcomes, and the root causes are not as simple as energy intake and expenditure. Although clinic-based approaches represent one potential avenue to reduce obesity and obesity disparities, clinic-based approaches should be used in conjunction with other intervention approaches. As discussed, PCP-delivered obesity prevention strategies are not effective in isolation but are effective when integrated within clinic-community partnerships and approaches. Clinic-community partnerships can assist in addressing PCP barriers (e.g., time, ability to provide culturally competent care) to obesity prevention and treatment delivery while simultaneously providing a more holistic approach to obesity prevention and treatment by addressing the contextual barriers of adults, parents, and children in reducing their own obesity risk and weight status. PCPs can provide individual-level obesity prevention and treatment in the form of screening and advice and refer their patients to other healthcare personnel (e.g., registered dieticians) and to local community resources that can support a patient's ability to change their obesity-related behavior, specifically dietary and physical activity and support, and to support maintenance of these behavior changes.

References

1. Flegal KM, Kruszon-Moran D, Carroll MD, Fryar CD, Ogden CL. Trends in obesity among adults in the United States, 2005 to 2014. JAMA. 2016;315:2284.
2. Hruby A, et al. Determinants and consequences of obesity. Am J Public Health. 2016;106:1656–62.
3. Gregor MF, Hotamisligil GS. Inflammatory mechanisms in obesity. Annu Rev Immunol. 2011;29:415–45.
4. WCRF. Diet, nutrition, physical activity and cancer: a global perspective. Continuous update project expert report 2018. 2018.
5. Sung H, Siegel RL, Rosenberg PS, Jemal A. Emerging cancer trends among young adults in the USA: analysis of a population-based cancer registry. Lancet Public Health. 2019;4:e137–47.
6. Siegel RL, et al. Global patterns and trends in colorectal cancer incidence in young adults. Gut. 2019;68:2179–85.
7. Rehm C, Peñalvo J, Afshin A, Mozaffarian D. Dietary intake among US adults, 1999–2012. JAMA. 2016;315(23):2542–53.
8. Moore L, et al. Using behavioral risk factor surveillance system data to estimate the percentage of the population meeting US Department of Agriculture Food Patterns fruit and. Am J Epidemiol. 2015;181:979–88.

9. USDA. USDA MyPlate all about the vegetable group. 2015. Available at: http://www.choosemyplate.gov/vegetables. Accessed: 1 Sept 2015.
10. USDA. USDA MyPlate, fruits gallery. 2015. Available at: http://www.choosemyplate.gov/foodgallery-fruits. Accessed: 1 Sept 2015.
11. Centers for Disease Prevention and Control. How much physical activity do children need? | Physical activity | CDC. Available at: https://www.cdc.gov/physicalactivity/basics/children/index.htm. Accessed: 27 Jan 2021.
12. Centers for Disease Prevention and Control. How much physical activity do adults need? | Physical activity | CDC. Available at: https://www.cdc.gov/physicalactivity/basics/adults/index.htm. Accessed: 27 Jan 2021.
13. Go AS, et al. Heart disease and stroke statistics-2013 update: a report from the American Heart Association. Circulation. 2013;127:42–3.
14. Dev DA, et al. Risk factors for overweight/obesity in preschool children: an ecological approach. Child Obes. 2013;9:399–408.
15. Curry SJ, et al. Behavioral weight loss interventions to prevent obesity-related morbidity and mortality in adults US preventive services task force recommendation statement. JAMA J Am Med Assoc. 2018;320:1163–71.
16. Norris SL et al. Long-term non-pharmacological weight loss interventions for adults with prediabetes. Cochrane Database Syst Rev. 2005. https://doi.org/10.1002/14651858.cd005270.
17. The World Health Organization. Social determinants of health. Available at: https://www.who.int/health-topics/social-determinants-of-health#tab=tab_1. Accessed: 27 Jan 2021.
18. Esther KC, Martha CR. Social determinants of childhood obesity: beyond individual choices. Curr Pediatr Rev. 2012;8:237–52.
19. Epping-Jordan JE, Pruitt SD, Bengoa R, Wagner EH. Innovative care for chronic conditions: building blocks for action: global report. World Health Organ. 2002;2002:112.
20. Daniel H, Bornstein SS, Kane GC. Addressing social determinants to improve patient care and promote health equity: an American college of physicians position paper. Ann Intern Med. 2018;168:577–8.
21. Pearce C, Rychetnik L, Wutzke S, Wilson A. Obesity prevention and the role of hospital and community-based health services: a scoping review. BMC Health Serv Res. 2019;19:453.
22. Rose SA, Poynter PS, Anderson JW, Noar SM, Conigliaro J. Physician weight loss advice and patient weight loss behavior change: a literature review and meta-analysis of survey data. Int J Obes. 2013;37:118–28.
23. Seburg EM, Olson-Bullis BA, Bredeson DM, Hayes MG, Sherwood NE. A review of primary care-based childhood obesity prevention and treatment interventions. Curr Obes Rep. 2015;4:157–73.
24. Tripicchio GL, et al. Clinical-community collaboration: a strategy to improve retention and outcomes in low-income minority youth in family-based obesity treatment. Child Obes. 2018;14:141–8.
25. Vine M, Hargreaves MB, Briefel RR, Orfield C. Expanding the role of primary care in the prevention and treatment of childhood obesity: a review of clinic- and community-based recommendations and interventions. J Obes. 2013. https://doi.org/10.1155/2013/172035.
26. Wagner EH. Chronic disease management: what will it take to improve care for chronic illness? Eff Clin Pract. 1998;1:2–4.
27. Coleman K, Austin BT, Brach C, Wagner EH. Evidence on the chronic care model in the new millennium: thus far, the evidence on the chronic care model is encouraging, but we need better tools to help practices improve their systems. Health Aff. 2009;28:75–85.
28. Dietz WH et al. An integrated framework for the prevention and treatment of obesity and its related chronic diseases. Health Aff. 2015;34(9):1456–63.
29. Tsai AG, Wadden TA. Treatment of obesity in primary care practice in the United States: a systematic review. J Gen Intern Med. 2009;24:1073–9.

30. Yoong SL, Carey M, Sanson-Fisher R, Grady A. A systematic review of behavioural weight-loss interventions involving primary-care physicians in overweight and obese primary-care patients (1999–2011). Public Health Nutr. 2013;16:2083–99.
31. MacDonell K, Brogan K, Naar-King S, Ellis D, Marshall S. A pilot study of motivational interviewing targeting weight-related behaviors in overweight or obese African American adolescents. J Adolesc Health. 2012;50:201–3.
32. Villablanca AC, Slee C, Lianov L, Tancredi D. Outcomes of a clinic-based educational intervention for cardiovascular disease prevention by race, ethnicity, and urban/rural status. J Women's Health. 2016;25:1174–86.
33. Gibson JS. Translation of clinical practice guidelines for childhood obesity prevention in primary care mobilizes a rural Midwest community. J Am Assoc Nurse Pract. 2016;28:130–7.
34. Tolliver SO, Hefner JL, Tolliver SD, McDougle L. Primary care provider understanding of hair care maintenance as a barrier to physical activity in African American women. J Am Board Fam Med. 2019;32:944–7.
35. Balcazar H, et al. Community health workers can be a public health force for change in the United States: three actions for a new paradigm. Am J Public Health. 2011;101:2199–203.
36. American Public Health Association. Support for community health workers to increase health access and to reduce health inequities. Available at: https://www.apha.org/policies-and-advocacy/public-health-policy-statements/policy-database/2014/07/09/14/19/support-for-community-health-workers-to-increase-health-access-and-to-reduce-health-inequities. Accessed: 27 Jan 2021.
37. Schroeder K, McCormick R, Perez A, Lipman TH. The role and impact of community health workers in childhood obesity interventions: a systematic review and meta-analysis. Obes Rev. 2018;19:1371–84.
38. Perez LG, et al. Evidence-based obesity treatment interventions for Latino adults in the U.S.: a systematic review. Am J Prev Med. 2013;44:550–60.
39. Semlitsch T, Stigler FL, Jeitler K, Horvath K, Siebenhofer A. Management of overweight and obesity in primary care—a systematic overview of international evidence-based guidelines. Obes Rev. 2019;20:1218–30.
40. Taveras EM, et al. Comparative effectiveness of clinical-community childhood obesity interventions a randomized clinical trial. JAMA Pediatr. 2017;171:1–8.
41. Boudreau ADA, Kurowski DS, Gonzalez WI, Dimond MA, Oreskovic NM. Latino families, primary care, and childhood obesity: a randomized controlled trial. Am J Prev Med. 2013;44:S247–57.
42. Story MT, et al. Management of child and adolescent obesity: attitudes, barriers, skills, and training needs among health care professionals. Pediatrics. 2002;110:210–4.
43. Wadden TA, Butryn ML, Hong PS, Tsai AG. Behavioral treatment of obesity in patients encountered in primary care settings: a systematic review. JAMA J Am Med Assoc. 2014;312:1779–91.
44. Skelton JA, et al. Community engagement and pediatric obesity: incorporating social determinants of health into treatment. J Clin Transl Sci. 2020;4:279–85.
45. Pratt CA, et al. A systematic review of obesity disparities research. Am J Prev Med. 2017;53:113–22.
46. Gerber BS, et al. Design of a trial to evaluate the impact of clinical pharmacists and community health promoters working with African-Americans and Latinos with diabetes. BMC Public Health. 2012;12:891.
47. Dietz WH, et al. An integrated framework for the prevention and treatment of obesity and its related chronic diseases. Health Aff. 2015;34:1456–63.
48. LeBlanc E, O'Connor E, Whitlock E, Patnode C, Kapka T. Review annals of internal medicine effectiveness of primary care – relevant treatments for obesity in. Ann Intern Med. 2011;155:434–47.
49. Pujalte GGA, Ahanogbe I, Thurston MJ, White RO, Roche-Green A. Addressing pediatric obesity in clinic. Glob Pediatr Health. 2017;4:1–7.

50. Fraser A, et al. Association of maternal weight gain in pregnancy with offspring obesity and metabolic and vascular traits in childhood. Circulation. 2010;121:2557–64.
51. Ip S, Chung M, Raman G, Trikalinos TA, Lau J. A summary of the agency for healthcare research and quality's evidence report on breastfeeding in developed countries. Breastfeed Med. 2009;4:S17–30.
52. American Academy of Pediatrics Committee on Nutrition. Feeding the child. In: Kleinman RE, editor. Pediatric nutrition handbook, vol. 146. Elk Grove Village: American Academy of Pediatrics; 2009.
53. Whitlock EP, O'Connor EA, Williams SB, Beil TL, Lutz KW. Effectiveness of weight management interventions in children: a targeted systematic review for the USPSTF. Pediatrics. 2010;125:e396–418.
54. Wrotniak BH, Epstein LH, Paluch RA, Roemmich JN. Parent weight change as a predictor of child weight change in family-based behavioral obesity treatment. Arch Pediatr Adolesc Med. 2004;158:342–7.
55. Saelens BE, Lozano P, Scholz K. A randomized clinical trial comparing delivery of behavioral pediatric obesity treatment using standard and enhanced motivational approaches. J Pediatr Psychol. 2013;38:954–64.
56. O'Malley G, et al. Physical activity and physical fitness in pediatric obesity: what are the first steps for clinicians? Expert conclusion from the 2016 ECOG workshop. Int J Exerc Sci. 2017;10:487–96.

Integrating Social Determinants into Health Care

Courtnee Hamity, Tamara Cadet, Artair Rogers, and Ana Jackson

Introduction

In many ways, the health of communities and individuals is shaped by factors other than the clinical care available to them. Given the definition of cancer health disparities, which are "adverse differences in cancer incidence (new cases), cancer prevalence (all existing cases), cancer death (mortality), cancer survivorship, and burden of cancer or related health conditions that exist among specific population groups in the United States" [1], understanding the social influences that affect cancer health disparities is complex. Cancer health disparities highlight population differences by race, ethnicity, gender, sexual orientation, disability, education, income, or geographic location. Because individuals and populations can identify with more than one group, it becomes difficult to pinpoint one factor that contributes to cancer health disparities. Thus, it is important to acknowledge and recognize that disparities are the result of factors at the policy, community/neighborhood, and individual levels. Typically, there is a focus on individual behaviors as it relates to disparities [2, 3]. However, this narrow perspective on improving disparities ignores powerful factors that impact patients' health. According to Marmot (2018), cancer prevention will not happen by simply urging people to behave better but will require action on the social determinants of health [4].

C. Hamity (✉) · A. Jackson
Blue Shield of California Foundation, San Francisco, CA, USA
e-mail: Courtnee.Hamity@Blueshieldcafoundation.org;
ana.jackson@blueshieldcafoundation.org

T. Cadet
University of Pennsylvania, Philadelphia, PA, USA
e-mail: cadet@upenn.edu

A. Rogers
Harvard Graduate School of Arts and Sciences, Boston, MA, USA
e-mail: arogers@g.harvard.edu

C. Hughes Halbert (ed.), *Cancer Health Disparities*,
https://doi.org/10.1007/978-3-031-37638-2_8

Health disparities are indicative of underlying societal, economic, geographic, and political disadvantages that impact access to opportunities, support networks, and resources. Inequities in access to support and resources affect many populations and demographics, and reflect structural and systemic barriers and biases across a broad swath of sectors. Federal and state policies have begun to respond to evidence of these underlying causes of health disparities by incentivizing health-care systems and providers to comprehensively improve health outcomes and health equity by identifying and addressing patients' social needs through interventions that account for factors beyond biology and care quality.

Many health-care organizations have taken on the challenge of starting to systematically screen patients for social needs and building new infrastructure and relationships, often with community-based organizations, to help address identified needs. This chapter summarizes the ways in which health-care organizations have integrated social interventions into care and highlights early evidence of these interventions' acceptability and effectiveness in cancer care, as well as outlining key considerations in designing new social interventions to improve cancer inequities.

The Intersection of Social Influence and Health

Understanding disparities of any kind requires consideration of both population-level and individual-level factors that impact outcomes of interest. Often, to understand the influencers that affect public health outcomes at the individual levels, an ecological framework is utilized [5]. The ecological framework [6] suggests that there is a dynamic, ongoing, interactive relationship between individuals, their relationships (with family, friends), their communities (workplace, school, neighborhoods), and society. The Centers for Disease Control uses this four-level social-ecological model to better understand the effect of potential prevention strategies because it allows for the understanding of the various factors that put individuals at risk for poor health and mortality [7]. The overlapping rings in the figure below illustrate how levels are interrelated with factors at all other levels.

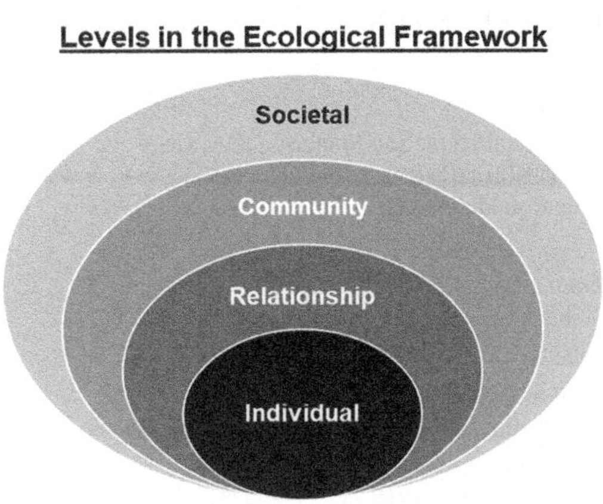

The individual level encompasses those factors that are personal or biologically related to an individual's likelihood of being affected by a particular risk. Some of those factors, regardless of the risk, are age, education, and income. Strategies to minimize risk at this level often target attitudes, beliefs, and behaviors that support or hinder a positive outcome. The relationship level includes the individuals' social circle (friends, family members) who can influence their behaviors. Risk mitigation strategies at this level, like caregiver education or social media campaigns, often target members of the social circle along with the individual. At the community level, strategies are often focused on settings such as schools, workplaces, and neighborhoods in which the individual's broader social relationships may occur. Thus, strategies at this level often aim to impact the social and physical environment including improving economic and housing opportunities in neighborhoods or changing policies within school and workplace settings. The fourth and final societal level includes intervening on those factors that help create the climate for an issue to occur and be sustained, including health, economic, educational, and social policies that create or help to maintain inequalities between groups. Acknowledging the complex and interconnected relationship between individual, relationship, community, and societal risk paves the way for breaking down silos in efforts to impact individual-level outcomes and any effective strategy must be responsive to the broader factors that influence individual risk.

A Framework for the Relationship Between Social Factors and Cancer Disparities

In cancer care, there is an increased recognition of the multitude of factors that contribute to individual risk and the likelihood of survival after a cancer diagnosis. These include a multitude of influences, like biological/genetic, environmental, behavioral, health-care, and social determinants [6]. Similar to the ecological framework, this comprehensive view incorporates the multilevel, complex, and interacting influences on cancer risk and expands perspectives for more comprehensive strategies to improve cancer outcomes [8, 9].

There are multiple frameworks that can be utilized to understand the dynamic, interactive, and ongoing relationship between social influencers and cancer care. While each framework is presented slightly differently, they each essentially highlight that social and economic conditions, such as structural inequities and social justice, shape population health and that the following constructs are associated with health outcomes: (1) economic stability, (2) educational level, (3) neighborhood and built environment, (4) health and health care, and (5) social and community context [9–11].

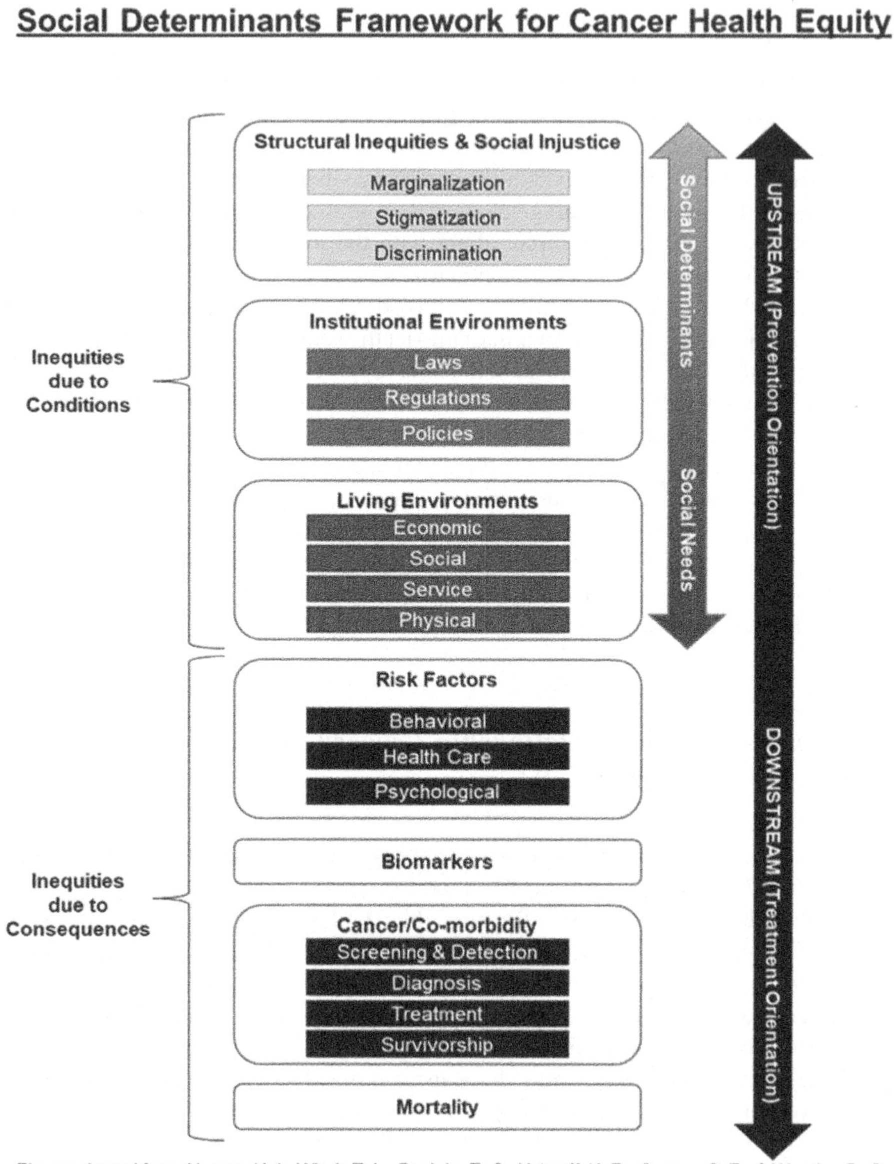

Figure adapted from Alcaraz, K. I., Wiedt, T. L., Daniels, E. C., Yabroff, K. R., Guerra, C. E., & Wender, R. C. (2020). Understanding and addressing social determinants to advance cancer health equity in the United States: A blueprint for practice, research, and policy. *CA: A Cancer Journal for Clinicians*, *70*(1), 31-46.

Alcarez et al. (2019) note in their framework, which integrates and expands other frameworks including the Bay Area Regional Health Inequities (2018) [12] and the NASEM report (2018) [13], that health-related disparities stem from conditions where social-structural factors resulted in excluding certain populations from access to resources in society and has consequently produced social stratification and social inequities. Individual behavioral or biological factors may play a role, but the systematic deprivation of resources for certain groups has exacerbated, if not been a primary contributor to, disparities in many health outcomes, including cancer [14].

Economic, physical, social, and service conditions each impact disparities in cancer pre-disease, preclinical, incidence, morbidity and mortality [15, 16]. Specifically, social circumstances such as housing status, environmental exposures, educational attainment, employment opportunities, and access to high-quality health care not only increase the likelihood of cancer but also dictate the quality and length of survival following a cancer diagnosis. The lack of access to advances in cancer prevention, early detection, treatment, and survivorship care in low socio-economic communities is a substantial barrier to improving the number of cancer survivors.

Targeting the upstream factors recognized as influencers of cancer health, such as financial security, housing stability and quality, education, health food access, and access to transportation, begins to reduce downstream factors of cancer survivorship. Health-care organizations can play a key role in more holistically accounting for the factors that contribute to cancer disparities by examining beyond an individual's behavior, for example, ensuring that care facilities are located in places with ample public transportation or offering after business-hour care options for patients that cannot be absent during a typical workday. Findings from Peipins et al. (2013) indicate that women who lived in predominantly African American neighborhoods had far longer travel times to reach radiation therapy facilities than women who lived in predominantly white neighborhoods [17, 18]. This lack of access is influenced by factors such as employment type and an individual's proximity to physicians and health-care facilities. However, access is also shaped by health insurance status, which is considered both a living and institutional issue. Evidence suggests that Americans generally have easier access to recommended health screenings and improved access to earlier diagnoses due to the Affordable Care Act [19], financial barriers to cancer care and overall racial disparities in access to cancer care persist [20–23]. While broader helath insurance access effectively addressed an institutional issue in access to care, it did not account for living environmental issues in care access that remain today.

Discussion

In a 2011 study that attempted to understand why a particular Baltimore community had abnormally high rates of comorbidities, Laveist et al. did not find racial differences in rates of diabetes and hypertension in a racially integrated, low-income neighborhood. The health status of both White and Black residents was the same.

What other factors, beyond individual-level characteristics, could have contributed to the higher rates of comorbid conditions across races in this study? What strategies may help to improve this community's health and what strategies could prevent future incidence of comorbidities in this community?

LaVeist, T., Pollack, K., Thorpe, R., Jr, Fesahazion, R., & Gaskin, D. (2011). Place, not race: disparities dissipate in southwest Baltimore when blacks and whites live under similar conditions. Health affairs (Project Hope), 30 (10), *1880–1887. https://doi.org/10.1377/hlthaff.2011.0640*

Social Determinants and Social Needs

To improve health equity, it is critical to identify and address both upstream and downstream opportunities to reduce disparities. The ineffectiveness of siloed upstream social determinant-informed policies and downstream interventions highlights an important distinction between social determinants of health and social needs. The World Health Organization defines social determinants of health as "the circumstances in which people are born, grow up, live, work and age, and the systems put in place to deal with illness. These circumstances are in turn shaped by a wider set of forces: economics, social policies, and politics" [24]. Social determinants of health are factors that fundamentally influence everyone's health and well-being both positively and negatively. Ultimately reducing health inequities resulting from social determinants of health requires the political will to promote policies that invest in equitable access to resources and opportunities, and minimize discriminatory practices and policies. The health-care sector can advocate for policies that impact social determinants of health, but the behavioral, social, economic, political, and environmental factors that are powerful *contributors* to health inequities do not *determine* individuals' health and well-being.

The term "determinants" suggests that factors contributing to inequities and health disparities are decidedly fixed. However, individuals may have negative circumstances influencing their health that may not be associated with their immediate unmet social needs, such as access to healthy food, safe and reliable housing, transportation, or financial stability, that more directly impact their access to care, as well as their health and well-being. Acknowledging that individuals' circumstances does not exactly or independently correlate with their health outcomes and that immediate social needs more directly impact health outcomes offers the opportunity to intervene on those needs and potentially improve the health of disproportionately disadvantaged individuals.

Interventions to Address Individual-Level Social Needs

Historically, health-care organizations have focused solely on addressing individual-level clinical needs. Of late, however, many organizations and providers have begun to address community and societal contributors to health, in part due to the health-care sector's shift toward value-based payments that incentivize prevention, as well as improved health and health-care outcomes for individuals and populations, rather than service delivery alone [25]. For instance, the Henry Ford Health System (HFHS) partnered with Uber, Lyft, and Ford Motor Company to provide transportation to its patient population, with a particular focus on those in underserved communities [26, 27]. At the same time, HFHS is campaigning to modify existing transportation infrastructure in the city of Detroit in order to facilitate greater care access in vulnerable communities [25–27]. Multipronged social interventions in health care have great promise in comprehensively improving the health of whole communities and reducing health disparities.

Consistent with the National Academies of Sciences, Engineering, and Medicine (NASEM) report, *Integrating Social Care into the Delivery of Health* Care*: Moving Upstream to Improve the Nation's Health* (2019), interventions that address social needs related to health must be integrated into clinical care and a structure should to be in place to coordinate efforts to minimize inequities. The NASEM report (2019) recommends five key activities for clinical integration, and these areas can be applied to cancer care [25]. They are awareness, adjustment, assistance, alignment, and advocacy.

- *Awareness* activities identify the social circumstances of defined patients and populations.
- *Adjustment* activities alter clinical care to accommodate identified social barriers.
- *Assistance* activities reduce social needs by connecting patients with social care resources.
- *Alignment* activities enable health-care systems to understand their communities' existing social care assets, facilitate synergies, and invest in and deploy them to positively affect health outcomes.
- *Advocacy* activities bring together as partners health care and social care organizations to promote policies that facilitate the creation and redeployment of resources to address health and social needs.

While activities outlined above will ultimately benefit all patients, *adjustment* and *assistance* focus on improving care provided specifically to individual patients based on information about their social needs. *Alignment* and *advocacy* relate to roles that the health-care sector can play in influencing and investing in social care resources at the community level. All of these care delivery and community-level activities are informed by efforts that increase *awareness* of individual or community-level social needs in a health-care system's geographic region or for its served population. Further, some of the specific steps that health-care organizations can take include:

- *Recognizing* that comprehensive health care should include understanding an individual's social context. Evidence is rapidly accumulating about the most effective strategies for screening and assessing for social circumstances and social needs. Such strategies should include standardized and validated questions, as available, and should use interoperable data systems to document results, with the ability to share results across care settings and health systems.
- *Using* patient-centered care models to more routinely incorporate social needs data into care decisions.

- *Designing* and implementing integrated care systems using approaches that engage patients, community partners, frontline staff, social workers, and clinicians in care planning and patient needs assessments while incorporating the preferences of patients and communities.
- *Including* social care workers, specifically social workers as integral to a team-based approach to designing and delivering health care.
- *Establishing* linkages and communication pathways between health-care and social service providers. This is important for personal care aides, home care aides, and others who provide care and support for seriously ill and disabled patients and who have extensive knowledge of patients' social needs.
- *Developing and financing* referral relationships with selected social care providers when feasible, supported by operational integration such as co-location or patient information systems. Social care and health-care providers should establish a formal understanding and accountability within their contracting and referral relationships.

These recommendations and key messages of this report highlight the complex nature of health disparities and cancer disparities specifically. They also highlight the substantial changes needed to better integrate of social care needs into the cancer care delivery system.

To that end, many organizations have developed reports with recommendations for health organizations to effectively incorporate social needs into care [8, 28, 29] and outline the need to start by screening patients for their immediate resource needs like healthy food, safe housing, transportation, or financial resources. Once needs are identified, this context may assist in offering more patient-centered care planning and provide care team members with a more complete understanding of the circumstances that may affect patients' behavior and impact their health and well-being. Although it is not always the case, social needs intervention may also include referring patients to resources like community-based organizations to help with addressing identified needs or connections to community health workers, care navigators, or social workers for care or resource coordination. Some health systems have found ways to integrate resources directly through interventions to provide transportation services to and from appointments or onsite farmers markets with subsidized fresh produce for patients. Regardless of how social needs information from screening is used, social needs interventions within health care settings should be designed to improve effectiveness in care coordination, care quality, risk adjustment, and minimizing disparities [30]. Key considerations within each component of a social needs intervention will impact a program's ability to achieve these objectives and ultimately promote equity in cancer care outcomes.

Social Needs Screening in Health Care

At a patient level, social needs screening data can guide health-care intervention efforts to address needs and adjust clinical care based on patients' identified social needs and preferences [31]. Collectively, this type of data at a population level assists in understanding and documenting the prevalence of an issue, the distribution of needs, and the most common needs. Population-level information also allows health-care providers to see the relationship between social needs, comorbidities, and health-care utilization [32]. Additionally, social needs screening data can also inform where additional funding within communities may be needed to minimize social needs through policy changes and investment in local resources [33].

Currently Available Screening Tools

There are numerous screening instruments to assess social needs. Some health systems have created their own screening tools internally, like Kaiser Permanente's Your Current Life Situation (YCLS) tool, which is a compliation of validated questions about a number of social needs, ranging from housing insecurity and social isolation to financial strain [34]. Multiple health systems have used the Protocol for Responding to and Assessing Patients' Assets, Risks, and Experiences (PRAPARE) tool to evaluate patients' social circumstances as it has been integrated into several electronic health records, including EPIC, GE Centricity, and NextGen. The PRAPARE tool places an emphasis on collecting data that is actionable and aligns with national efforts to reduce health disparities, like Healthy People 2020 [35]. The tool's developers partnered with multiple networks, like the National Association of Community Health Centers (NACHC), to obtain patient feedback to evaluate the adoptability and validity of the tool [36]. As a result of the prominence of integrating social care into clinical care, the Center for Medicare and Medicaid Services (CMS) created a questionnaire to accompany its rollout of the Accountable Health Communities (AHC) program, which focuses on addressing social needs and risks [35]. Like the PRAPARE tool, a national panel of experts also shaped the AHC's questionnaire design. The tool focuses on connecting Medicare, Medicaid, and Dual Eligible enrollees to community-based organizations and social service providers who can provide services and resources to address housing instability, food insecurity, transportation difficulties, utility assistance needs, and interpersonal safety [35].

No-Cost Social Needs Screening Tools for Adult Populations

Screening Tool Name	AHC-Tool	HealthBegins	Health Leads	MLP IHELLP	Medicare Total Health Assessment	NAM domains	PRAPARE	WellRx	Your Current Life Situation
Patient or Clinic Population	Medicare & Medicaid	NS	NS	NS	Medicare	NS	CHCs	PC	NS
# Social Needs Questions	19	24	10	10	7	12	17	10	19
# Non-Social Needs Questions	8	4	0	0	30	12	4	1	10
Reading Level*	7th grade	6th grade	7th grade	6th grade	5th grade	5th grade	7th grade	2nd grade	10th grade
Domains: Interpersonal Violence	✓	✓		✓		✓	✓	✓	✓
Social Support	✓	✓	✓		✓	✓	✓		✓
Housing Instability/Homelessness	✓	✓	✓	✓	✓		✓	✓	✓
Food Insecurity	✓	✓	✓		✓		✓	✓	✓
Education	✓	✓		✓		✓	✓	✓	✓
Stress	✓	✓			✓	✓	✓		✓
Transportation	✓	✓	✓				✓	✓	✓
Employment	✓	✓		✓			✓	✓	
Utilities	✓		✓				✓	✓	✓
Financial Strain	✓	✓				✓			✓
Care/Treatment Access & Affordability			✓				✓		✓
Housing Quality	✓	✓		✓	✓				✓
Immigration/Migrant/Refugee Status		✓		✓			✓		

Adapted from the Social Interventions Research & Evaluation Network, Social Need Screening Tools Comparison Table Available at: https://sirenetwork.ucsf.edu/tools-resources/mmi/screening-tools-comparison/adult-nonspecific (Last Accessed September 2020).

While the above screening tools are not disease-specific, they may be useful in cancer care. In a survey of oncologists in a health system, more than 90% said that social determinants of health such as financial security, access to food, and social isolation impact outcomes for cancer patients [37]. Specifically, oncologists noted that the top social determinants of health are financial security/lack of health insurance, lack of transportation, health literacy, and social isolation—nonmedical issues that affect cancer outcomes. Evidence suggests that access to health care, health literacy, economic and employment factors, and barriers to transportation impact screening access, early detection, treatment options following a cancer diagnosis, adherence to the treatment regimen, access to clinical trials, and outcomes following treatment completion [22]. Findings from Beavis et al. [38] indicated that in a gynecologic oncology outpatient clinic, patients reported financial strain, transportation, and difficulty reading hospital materials as their top social determinants of health. Findings from Neuss et al. (2017) supported similar social determinants of health [39].

There are also several cancer-specific tools used to assess social risks for distress, including the Social Difficulties Inventory and the National Comprehensive Cancer Network's (NCCN) Distress Thermometer and Problem List. Both tools use a scoring scale that helps inform clinical staff and practitioners' care planning, which includes referral to appropriate services to meet essential resource needs [40, 41]. In 2015, the American College of Surgeons Commission on Cancer also mandated routine distress screening at cancer centers in 2015 as the Commission acknowledged the value of understanding cancer patients' social circumstances in cancer care delivery. Although not widely implemented, this distress screening assesses difficulty addressing essential resource needs or social risks [42].

Screening Tool Accessibility, Acceptability, and Adoptability

Any screening intervention is only as effective as the tool used to identify and understand patient-reported information. That is to say, ensuring that social needs screening tools yield meaningful information and align with patient and clinician preferences and expectations is foundational to any successful social intervention. Tools should provide information that is simple for clinicians and care teams to meaningfully use and that closely aligns with the intervention's intended outcomes. To date, there is growing availability of standardized screening tools; however, evidence of the accessibility, acceptability, and adoptability of the screening tools are major outstanding considerations in the implementation of a social needs intervention. To truly examine these esigners, implementers, and evaluators of social interventions must partner with patients, communities, and health-care providers to truly examine these three factors.

Often, when analyzing the accessibility of a screening tool, health literacy becomes a focus. Health literacy is the ability to understand and interpret health information to make health decisions. Health literacy can be affected whether information is received verbally or in written form [43]. Therefore, it is important to have multiple modalities for patients [44]; some patients may comprehend the screening assessment better with a member of the care team reading the information to them while others may process information better reading the screening tool individually. Either approach calls for all items within the screening tool to be written at a grade level to accommodate those who may read at a low literacy level. It is also encouraged for the assessment to be brief and translated into the languages that are most prevalent within the health system's ambulatory and inpatient settings [45]. Services should also be provided to assist patients who may experience a physical or mental disability in completing the screening instrument.

Acceptability of screening tools is often driven by rigorous psychometric testing to establish their validity and reliability. Validity refers to the exactness or accuracy of the measure, which helps implementers and evaluators ensure that those who screen for social risks have a social risk. Reliability looks at the screening tool's ability to assess patients correctly consistently [46]. It is also important to keep in mind that acceptability of screening may differ across communities and may change over time. For all screening tools implemented within a care delivery setting, particularly newly established assessment instruments, it is beneficial to regularly collect feedback on whether the tool is easy for patients with diverse backgrounds to understand and complete and easy for providers to use.

There is also a need to understand the sustained adoptability of a social needs assessment tool within a care delivery setting. While many available tools have undergone extensive evaluation in a research setting and have been tested in specific clinics or health-care systems, each care setting serves a unique population and has its own systems and culture. Even tools with high validity and reliability may yield different results in different settings among different populations. Lastly, patients' social circumstances are not static. Their social needs can shift frequently, suddenly, and potentially as a result of their health condition. Therefore, social needs screening ideally would occur regularly and could even be considered part of annual screening along with other behavioral and health screening protocols [47]. It is also prudent to have social needs screening along with the occurrence of major life events like the loss of a spouse or unanticipated hospitalization. For cancer care, assessment of social needs should occur at multiple stages throughout the clinical care plan. Still the exact timing of social needs screening and the overall adoptability of an assessment instrument into specific care settings is unknown until it is tested or implemented.

User Testing

User testing, unlike psychometric analyses, does not need to be resource- or time-intensive but can be an effective means of collecting information about a screening tool's accessibility, acceptability, and adoptability. When done thoughtfully, initial (and repeated) testing of a social needs questionnaire can result in a better understanding of the burden on patients to complete (e.g., if the tool is difficult for patients to understand or whether it triggers patient discomfort or anxiety), the length of time to takes to complete, the modes of administration that patients prefer (e.g., self-administered on paper or orally administered by a care team member), and the actionability of the information elicited from the tool. Information gleaned from user testing can help to inform decisions about:

- Whether to use a different questionnaire.
- Whether to add, remove, or modify questions.
- How to revise instructions and scripting to best set patient expectations and ease concerns.
- How to minimize any risks to patients.
- How often to administer the tool in alignment with change social or care needs.

The developers of the PRAPARE tool engaged in user testing to refine the instrument, listening to reactions and responses from multiple stakeholder groups. Insights from patients and the care team, specifically, helped discern if the screening assessment was relevant to the served or affected patient population [36]. Gleaning those perspectives through direct patient and provider feedback early in an intervention and regularly once an intervention is implemented into care can also help identify questions that are too general and yield false positives or are too focused and result in false negatives. It is this type of inclusive stakeholder participatory process that allows a social needs screening tool to be successfully piloted and scaled.

Interventions to Address Social Needs

After patients' needs have been identified, it is the health system's responsibility to use the information from the screening in a meaningful way. This could include sharing responses with clinicians to provide a more holistic understanding of their patients' circumstances, to inform care planning, or to refer patients to resources that assist in addressing identified needs. Some organizations have designed interventions that address general social risk or needs by connecting patients with health workers, promotoras, and patient navigators, who help patients prioritize the social risks they want to minimize, assist in connecting them to resources, and advocate on their behalf. Other approaches include referring patients to community-based organizations to address specific identified needs like food insecurity or lack of transportation. In any attempt to address social risk and needs, health systems likely have to form new relationships with entities more traditionally relegated to the social sphere. Ideally, these partner organizations within patients' communities to ensure they can be responsive to the unique needs of patients.

Partnering to Address Patients' Social Needs

Health systems, particularly nonprofit ones, have traditionally used community benefit dollars to invest in local social service providers that address community or public health needs. The types of organizations and level of investment is often determined by community health needs assessments that survey community members to understand local needs [48]. The level of partnership between health systems and community-based organizations using the health system's community benefit dollars varies substantially. With new investments made by payers, like Medicaid, for efforts to tackle social determinants of health, a new level of partnership is required between health care and community-based organizations [49].

Many health-care organizations are partnering with local community-based organizations to address essential resource needs [50]. For instance, Kaiser Permanente Colorado (KPCO), a large integrated health system, and Hunger Free Colorado, a nonprofit organization that leads efforts throughout the state to connect people to food resources and restructure systems within the state to reduce food insecurity, collaborated to develop a social needs intervention focused on addressing food insecurity for patients within the KPCO system. The pilot, which started at two pediatric clinics, used a screening tool to delineate whether patients are eligible for the Supplemental Nutrition Assistance Program (SNAP) or Women, Infants, and Children (WIC) program. Additionally, KPCO would refer patients to Hunger Free Colorado for information regarding food banks and pantries. As KPCO and Hunger Free Colorado worked in partnership with a shared vision for the program, the collaboration expanded to include ten departments within over ten medical offices [51].

While the KPCO and Hunger Free Colorado partnership has been a successful one, their work, like other new relationships between health-care systems and community-based organizations, necessitated alignment and shared decision-making between the two entities. Community-based organizations often see advantages in partnering with health-care organizations: in a Massachusetts study, community-based organizations noted that, together, partnerships with health organizations could result in greater combined expertise and experience in helping individuals connect to resources. However, some local nonprofits felt that partnerships with hospitals and clinics were the only way to keep large health systems from duplicating social services that already existed in the community. Given their often large size and market power, health-care organizations should be aware of dynamics that result in misalignment of goals [51]. To circumvent some of these issues, it is essential to include community-based partners throughout the decision-making process as the social needs interventions are developed, designed, implemented, improved, and evaluated [52].

Furthermore, true community partnership moves beyond health-care systems' collaboration with local community-based organizations and social service providers to also center the perspectives of the patients. Community-based participatory research (CBPR) principles provide framing that promotes shared power between large anchor institutions, like hospitals and clinics, community-based organizations, and community members [53]. CBPR elevates the voice of the community as this research approach anchors on the strengths and resources within the community; focuses on capacity-building for all entities involved in the partnership; addresses issues of systemic oppression; and prioritizes evaluation and sustainability that aligns with all partners' interests [54]. These principles can be applied to how health systems can facilitate true partnership with community-based organizations and community members.

Patient-Centeredness As with community partnerships, attempts to meaningfully use social information in health care should also be done in partnership with patients. There should be transparency about how social needs information will be used and who it will be shared with, especially if referrals will be made on the patient's behalf. Providers must also be accepting of patients' preferences. Patients can screen positive for several social needs; however, a positive screen does not equate to a patient's desire for help addressing that need [45, 55, 56]. Programs that solely attempt to address social risks or needs may neglect to assess what the patient wants, may result in blaming the patient for not being adherent to protocols, and may miss an opportunity to have a meaningful conversation. Best practices to promote patient engagement and trust should first acknowledge patient responses, especially if they screen positive for a need, to ensure they feel heard and that they know their information is being used to better understand their circumstances. Secondly, if available, providers should offerpatients referrals for social resources, without assuming that they want help for a need and giving them the opportunity to refuse. Social interventions not only have the promise of fulfilling unmet social needs and improving health outcomes; they are also likely to improve the care experience and care quality when social information serves as a catalyst for more open and inclusive communication.

Evidence from Integrating Social Interventions into Care

The body of literature on the effectiveness of social needs interventions, particularly in cancer care, is limited but emerging. To date, research has commonly, and potentially erroneously, attempted to link social needs interventions to health outcomes before first understanding interventions' ability to meet patients' social needs. Still, there is growing evidence of the acceptance and understanding of the need for social needs interventions from patients, providers, and staff. There is also early evidence of the outcomes of patient navigator and care coordination interventions, as well as of the benefits of social needs interventions in cancer care improving appointment show rates as well as treatment adherence. As more social needs interventions are embedded in the health-care setting and become more established with time, there will be considerable opportunity to more fully study interventions for effectiveness.

Overall Acceptance of Social Interventions in Health Care

Multiple studies have documented patient and clinician understanding and acceptance of social needs interventions in care. While some researchers have questioned whether it is unethical to ask questions about social risks without having the resources to address needs as they're identified [57], there is considerable evidence that patients appreciate being asked about their social needs and are generally comfortable having their social needs information documented in their medical records [58–60]. In fact, patients recognize the benefits of clinicians having information about their patients' social circumstances. In fact there is evidence that patients value social needs screening and that, even a simple acknowledgement of their responses was associated with an improved the care experience, with patients feeling cared for [61] and treated as a whole person. Best practices in setting patient expectations include explaining how social needs information will be used. This can be accomplished by including introductions to screening tools and equipping clinicians and staff with scripting that clearly explains the purpose of screening tools and how the information will be used to improve patient care (all of which can be co-designed with patients and clinicians to ensure that they are clear, accurate, and culturally sensitive). Patients also welcome health systems asking them if they would like assistance addressing their social needs. Of note, while patients are open to their care team understanding their social circumstances and offering assistance to address identified needs, many do not accept offers from their care team to help in addressing those needs [59, 61–65]. More research is needed to understand differences in willingness to accept help in addressing social needs, and, thus, close monitoring of social needs interventions in health care is also needed to ensure that disproportionate patient engagement in the interventions is not, in fact, exacerbating disparities and access to resources.

As with patients, there is also evidence that providers support incorporating social needs into care and that social needs interventions also help to reduce burnout [66]. In various surveys, clinicians reported that providing care with an organization that screens for and offers resources to intervene on social needs gives clinicians actionable options to minimize underlying factors contributing to their patients' negative behaviors and poor health, provides a more holistic understanding of their patients, and impacts medical decisions and care planning [59, 67]. Care providers appreciated interventions that offered options to meet patients' social needs, but they also highlighted the need for seamless workflows that make social needs information easy to access and act on, and clear feedback on whether patients' needs are being met reliably [29, 60, 62]. Accordingly, the most successful social needs interventions will be true partnerships with community organizations and health systems with open communication between entities to ensure that, when referrals are made, information on patients' social needs status is shared back with the care team.

The Success of Social Interventions in Cancer

To eliminate cancer disparities, there is still a need for effective interventions that account for the social and environmental contexts in which patients with cancer live and are treated. Some studies have considered the impact of social interventions on cancer care outcomes. These studies have commonly focused on the effectiveness of assistance with the cost of medicine, transportation, and understanding treatments and therapies. This could take the form of co-pay assistance programs, free drug programs, medication adherence, transportation support, and patient navigation.

Evidence indicates that social interventions that include patient navigation have improved the timeliness and appropriateness of preventive, diagnostic, and treatment services for breast, cervical, and colorectal cancer by setting patient expectations, addressing transportation and arranging financial support [68–70]. Given the top concern of financial instability among patients with high-cost medical conditions, including cancer, hospital-based financial navigation programs 1 have been instituted for cancer patients and patients with other high-cost treatment plans. These programs were able to provide cancer care that previously would have been unaffordable to many patients. Financial counselors were able to assist patients by procuring free medication and helping to cover the high co-pays that insurance companies often charge for expensive cancer medications [71].

To help patients with cancer minimize barriers to care during cancer treatment, the American Cancer Society (ACS) has partnered with a variety of private transportation vendors, including Lyft, Ride Health, and UZURV, to pay for patients' transportation services. They also have partnered with lodging companies across the country, including Extended Stay America to provide free and/or deeply discounted hotel stays away from home. To help improve extensive and equitable access for disadvantaged patients with cancer, increasing the reach of these types of transportation and lodging programs should be a high priority. Insurance companies like Humana also partners with

Lyft to help address missed appointment because of transportation barriers [72]. While there are few studies currently available about the long-term health benefits of social interventions in cancer care, it is clear that cancer patients that are unable to afford their treatment, do not have rides to their appointments, or no place to stay when seeking treatment away from home have substantial barriers to care. Interventions that address social needs are sorely needed to remove care (and health) barriers for patients along the cancer continuum, and more practice and policy initiatives at all levels are needed to yield the best health outcomes for patients.

Considerations for Social Interventions to Further Promote Equity

Despite the well-intentioned efforts of social interventions to directly tackle the social needs and risks of affected populations, there must be an awareness that these interventions implemented within a health-care system are susceptible to implicit and explicit bias and systemic racism [73]. Racism was embedded in America's health-care system's foundation and continues to influence health disparities today [74]. Therefore, intervention designers, implementers, and evaluators of social interventions in health care cannot conflate efforts to address social needs with advancing equity [73, 74] and must confront and challenge the structural barriers created by historical, institutional racism. Social needs interventions must stretch beyond individual-level, transactional resource connection approaches and work to remedy the root causes behind patients needing referrals to social service resources [75, 76].

Social interventions' ability to identify community priorities and collaboratively develop approaches to address inequities within communities dictates how these efforts help promote opportunities and restructure systems to more effectively meet the needs of marginalized individuals. Ultimately, an equity-empowered approach provides the highest likelihood of eliminating disparities and liberating patients who suffer the most health disparities. This approach not only focuses on the individual resource connection but also aims to enable needed advocacy for underrepresented groups to tackle restructuring and reforming systems, policies, and practices that are harmful to the most oppressed patient populations. Additionally, the equity-empowered social needs intervention shifts power to those with the least amount of traditional power or those who experience the most disparities. This shift in power should leverage protective factors like resiliency, and advocacy to change oppressive structures [77].

In practice, stakeholders responsible for the development of social interventions can advance equity and an antiracism agenda by having the most affected patient populations represented within the intervention's governance structure [78]. Beyond representation, these groups must have power in all aspects of the intervention, including decision-making, process or performance improvement, evaluation, and sustainability [78]. Health institutions interested in launching these programs should also prioritize partnering with community-based organizations and social service providers that have an expertise and focus with reaching the most disadvantaged communities. Collectively, patients experiencing the most inequities and community-based organizations that actively reach the most marginalized should interpret how individual resource needs highlighted through screening data and patient stories connect to larger community inequities. This community-focused governance structure and true community partnership model can facilitate opportunities to meet individual needs while uplifting a community agenda [79].

Utilizing culturally responsive and equitable evaluation (CREE) principles is also critical when considering previously developed interventions or the development of new interventions. Briefly, CREE is a lens which requires the integration of diversity, inclusion, and equity in all phases of intervention modification and development. CREE incorporates cultural, structural, and contextual factors that include historical, social, economic, racial, ethnic, and gender using a participatory process that shifts power and ownership to individuals who are most impacted by a particular issue or will be affected by an intervention. CREE informs strategy, program intervention development, decision-making, and change [80]. Thus, to successfully develop interventions, a CREE lens must be incorporated that intentionally and authentically engage community members (those impacted by cancer disparities across the cancer continuum) in discussions and decisions about interventions that work or modifications that need to be made to current interventions. This could include understanding what types of questions should be included in data collection about a possible intervention along with participation in data collection.

Summary

Despite the growing interest and spread of social needs intervention in care settings, a considerable challenge remains: social needs interventions are limited by the availability of resources to successfully address social needs. Health systems have begun to engage and advocate for community resources and resources embedded in clinical setting, but without greater government and community funding for social resources, interventions are constrained in their potential effectiveness.

References

1. National Cancer Institute. Cancer disparities. 2019. Retrieved from https://www.cancer.gov/about-cancer/understanding/disparities
2. Langston ME, Fuzzell L, Lewis-Thames MW, Khan S, Moore JX. Disparities in health information-seeking behaviors and fatalistic views of cancer by sexual orientation identity: a nationally representative study of adults in the United States. LGBT Health. 2019;6(4):192–201.
3. Rawl SM, Dickinson S, Lee JL, Roberts JL, Teal E, Baker LB, Kianersi S, Haggstrom DA. Racial and Socioeconomic Disparities in Cancer-Related Knowledge, Beliefs, and Behaviors in Indiana. Cancer Epidemiol Biomarkers Prev. 2019 Mar;28(3):462-470. doi: 10.1158/1055-9965.EPI-18-0795

4. Marmot M. Health equity, cancer, and social determinants of health. Lancet Glob Health. 2018;6:S29.
5. National Quality Forum. A roadmap for promoting health equity and eliminating disparities: the four I's for health equity. 2017. Retrieved from https://www.qualityforum.org/Publications/2017/09/A_Roadmap_for_Promoting_Health_Equity_and_Eliminating_Disparities__The_Four_I_s_for_Health_Equity.aspx
6. Bronfenbrenner U. Toward an experimental ecology of human development. Am Psychol. 1977;32:513–31.
7. Centers for Disease Control. The social-ecological model: a framework for prevention. 2020. Retrieved from https://www.cdc.gov/violenceprevention/publichealthissue/social-ecologicalmodel.html
8. Alcaraz KI, Wiedt TL, Daniels EC, Yabroff KR, Guerra CE, Wender RC. Understanding and addressing social determinants to advance cancer health equity in the United States: a blueprint for practice, research, and policy. CA Cancer J Clin. 2020;70(1):31–46.
9. Asare M, Flannery M, Kamen C. Social determinants of health: a framework for studying cancer health disparities and minority participation in research. Oncol Nurs Forum. 2017 Jan;44(1):20.
10. Purnell TS, Calhoun EA, Golden SH, Halladay JR, Krok-Schoen JL, Appelhans BM, Cooper LA. Achieving health equity: closing the gaps in health care disparities, interventions, and research. Health Aff. 2016;35(8):1410–5.
11. NEJM Catalyst, Social Determinants of Health (SDOH). Retrieved from https://catalyst.nejm.org/doi/full/10.1056/CAT.17.0312
12. Bay Area Regional Health Inequities Initiative. A public health framework for reducing health inequities. (2015). Retrieved from barhii.org/framework/
13. National Academies of Sciences, Engineering, and Medicine. (2018). Exploring equity in multisector community health partnerships: proceedings of a workshop. National Academies Press Washington, DC.
14. Pallok K, De Maio F, Ansell DA. Structural racism-a 60-year-old black woman with breast cancer. N Engl J Med. 2019;380(16):1489–93.
15. Caldwell JT, Ford CL, Wallace SP, Wang MC, Takahashi LM. Intersection of living in a rural versus urban area and race/ethnicity in explaining access to health care in the United States. Am J Public Health. 2016;106(8):1463–9.
16. Kurani SS, McCoy RG, Lampman MA, Doubeni CA, Rutten LJF, Inselman JW, et al. Association of neighborhood measures of social determinants of health with breast, cervical, and colorectal cancer screening rates in the US Midwest. JAMA Netw Open. 2020;3(3):–e200618.
17. Peipins LA, Graham S, Young R, Lewis B, Flanagan B. Racial disparities in travel time to radiotherapy facilities in the Atlanta metropolitan area. Soc Sci Med. 2013;89:32–8.
18. National Cancer Institute. Tackling cancer health disparities: small steps, big hopes. 2017. Retrieved from https://www.cancer.gov/research/areas/disparities/health-disparity-studies
19. Adamson BJ, Cohen AB, Estevez M, Magee K, Williams E, Gross CP, Meropol NJ, Davidoff AJ. Affordable Care Act (ACA) Medicaid expansion impact on racial disparities in time to cancer treatment. 2019 ASCO Annual Meeting. Abstract LBA1. Presented June 2, 2019 (2019).
20. Jemal A, Lin CC, Davidoff AJ, Han X. Changes in insurance coverage and stage at diagnosis among nonelderly patients with cancer after the Affordable Care Act. J Clin Oncol. 2017;35(35):3906–15.
21. Soni A, Sabik LM, Simon K, Sommers BD. Changes in insurance coverage among cancer patients under the Affordable Care Act. JAMA Oncol. 2018;4(1):122–4.
22. Han X, Yabroff KR, Ward E, Brawley OW, Jemal A. Comparison of insurance status and diagnosis stage among patients with newly diagnosed cancer before vs after implementation of the Patient Protection and Affordable Care Act. JAMA Oncol. 2018;4(12):1713–20.
23. Sabik LM, Adunlin G. The ACA and cancer screening and diagnosis. Cancer J. 2017;23(3):151.
24. World Health Organization. Report from the Commission on Social Determinants of Health. Geneva: WHO; 2008. Closing the gap in a generation: health equity through action on the

social determinants of health. Also available from: URL: http://www.who.int/social_determinants/thecommission/finalreport/en/index.html
25. National Academies of Sciences, Engineering, and Medicine. Integrating social care into the delivery of health care: moving upstream to improve the nation's health. Washington, DC: National Academies Press; 2019.
26. Knowles M. Henry Ford health partners with SPLT, Lyft to get patients to appointment. 2018. https://www.beckershospitalreview.com/patient-flow/henry-ford-health-partnerswith-splt-lyft-to-get-patients-to-appointments.html
27. Martinez M. Ford partners with Beaumont Health on medical transport service. 2018. https://www.crainsdetroit.com/article/20180418/news/658481/ford-partners-withbeaumont-health-on-medical-transport-service
28. Kenney GM, Waidmann TA, Skopec L, Allen EH. What would it take to reduce inequities in healthy life expectancy? Urban Institute report. Washington, DC: Urban Institute; 2019.
29. Root Cause Coalition. 2020 status of health equity report. 2020. Available at https://www.rootcausecoalition.org/sherreport/
30. Steiner JF, Bellows J, Banegas MP, Gottlieb LM. Interventions to address basic resource needs in Kaiser Permanente: a care continuum and an outcomes wheel. Perm J. 2018;22:18–130.
31. Fraze TK, Brewster AL, Lewis VA, Beidler LB, Murray GF, Colla CH. Prevalence of screening for food insecurity, housing instability, utility needs, transportation needs, and interpersonal violence by US physician practices and hospitals. JAMA Netw Open. 2019;2(9):e1911514. https://doi.org/10.1001/jamanetworkopen.2019.11514.
32. Rogers A, Hu YR, Schickedanz A, et al. Understanding high-utilizing patients based on social risk profiles: a latent class analysis within an integrated health system. J Gen Intern Med. 2020;35:2214–6. https://doi.org/10.1007/s11606-019-05510-9.
33. Green K, Zook M. When talking about social determinants, precision matters. Health Affairs. 2019 Oct 29. www.healthaffairs.org/do/10.1377/hblog20191025.776011/full/
34. Sundar KR. Universal screening for social needs in a primary care clinic: a quality improvement approach using the Your Current Life Situation survey. Perm J. 2018;22:18–089. https://doi.org/10.7812/TPP:18-089.
35. Laforge K, et al. How 6 organizations developed tools and processes for social determinants of health screening in primary care. J Ambul Care Manage. 2018;41(1):2–14. https://doi.org/10.1097/jac.0000000000000221.
36. About the PRAPARE Assessment Tool. NACHC. 2020 Aug 24. www.nachc.org/research-and-data/prapare/about-the-prapare-assessment-tool/
37. Cardinal Health. How social determinants impact cancer care. 2020. Retrieved from https://www.cardinalhealth.com/en/cmp/ext/ma/oncology-insights.html?cid=VURL-TRD-PHR-SS-HA-OncologyInsights-060117
38. Beavis AL, Sanneh A, Stone RL, Vitale M, Levinson K, Rositch AF, et al. Basic social resource needs screening in the gynecologic oncology clinic: a quality improvement initiative. Am J Obstet Gynecol. 2020;223:735.e1.
39. Neuss MN, Shyr Y, Washburn A, Elliott SL, Carson K, Carson K, Friedman DL. Determining needs for nonmedical support during cancer care. J Clin Oncol. 2017;35(8):82.
40. Klingenstein A, Samel C, Garip-Kuebler A, Miller C, Liegel RG, Priglinger SG, Foerster PI. The national comprehensive cancer network distress thermometer as a screening tool for the evaluation of quality of life in uveal melanoma patients. Acta Ophthalmol. 2020;98:e381–7. https://doi.org/10.1111/aos.14277.
41. Wright P, Smith A, Roberts K, et al. Screening for social difficulties in cancer patients: clinical utility of the social difficulties inventory. Br J Cancer. 2007;97:1063–70. https://doi.org/10.1038/sj.bjc.6604006.
42. Lazenby M, Ercolano E, Grant M, Holland JC, Jacobsen PB, McCorkle R. Supporting commission on cancer-mandated psychosocial distress screening with implementation strategies. J Oncol Pract. 2015;11(3):e413–20. https://doi.org/10.1200/JOP.2014.002816.

43. Nutbeam D. The evolving concept of health literacy. Soc Sci Med. 2008;67(12):2072–8. https://doi.org/10.1016/j.socscimed.2008.09.050.
44. Gottlieb L, et al. A randomized trial on screening for social determinants of health: the IScreen Study. Pediatrics. 2014;134(6) https://doi.org/10.1542/peds.2014-1439.
45. The Health Leads Screening Toolkit. Health Leads. www.healthleadsusa.org/resources/the-health-leads-screening-toolkit/
46. Kimberlin CL, Winterstein AG. Validity and reliability of measurement instruments used in research. Am J Health Syst Pharm. 2008;65(23):2276–84.
47. O'Gurek DT, Henke C. A practical approach to screening for social determinants of health. Fam Pract Manag. 2018;25(3):7–12.
48. Pennel CL, McLeroy KR, Burdine JN, Matarrita-Cascante D. Nonprofit hospitals' approach to community health needs assessment. Am J Public Health. 2015;105:e103–13. https://doi.org/10.2105/AJPH.2014.302286.
49. Byhoff E, Taylor LA. Massachusetts community-based organization perspectives on Medicaid redesign. Am J Prev Med. 2019;57(6S1):S74–81.
50. Baker EL, Melton RJ, Stange PV, et al. Health reform and the health of the public: forging community health partnerships. JAMA. 1994;272(16):1276–82. https://doi.org/10.1001/jama.1994.03520160060044.
51. Stenmark SH, Steiner JF, Marpadga S, Debor M, Underhill K, Seligman H. Lessons learned from implementation of the food insecurity screening and referral program at Kaiser Permanente Colorado. Perm J. 2018;22:18–093. https://doi.org/10.7812/TPP/18-093.
52. Bazzoli GJ, Stein R, Alexander JA, Conrad DA, Sofaer S, Shortell SM. Public–private collaboration in health and human service delivery: evidence from community partnerships. Milbank Q. 1997;75:533–61. https://doi.org/10.1111/1468-0009.00068.
53. Israel B, et al. Community-based participatory research: policy recommendations for promoting a partnership approach in health research. Educ Health. 2001;14(2):182–97. ProQuest, https://search.proquest.com/docview/2258169865?accountid=6724
54. Wallerstein NB, Duran B. Using community-based participatory research to address health disparities. Health Promot Pract. 2006;7(3):312–23. https://doi.org/10.1177/1524839906289376.
55. Steele R, Fitch MI. Why patients with lung cancer do not want help with some needs. Support Care Cancer. 2008;16(3):251–9.
56. Langbecker D, Ekberg S, Yates P. Don't need help, don't want help, can't get help: how patients with brain tumors account for not using rehabilitation, psychosocial and community services. Patient Educ Couns. 2017;100(9):1744–50.
57. Garg A, Boynton-Jarret R, Dworkin PH. Avoiding the unintended consequences of screening for social determinants of health. JAMA. 2016;316(8):813–4.
58. Rogers AJ, Hamity C, Sharp AL, Jackson AH, Schickedanz AB. Patients' attitudes and perceptions regarding social needs screening and navigation: multi-site survey in a large integrated health system. J Gen Intern Med. 2020;35:1–7.
59. De Marchis EH, Hessler D, Fichtenberg C, Adler N, Byhoff E, Cohen AJ, et al. Part I: a quantitative study of social risk screening acceptability in patients and caregivers. Am J Prev Med. 2019;57(6):S25–37.
60. Hamity C, Jackson A, Peralta L, Bellows J. Perceptions and experience of patients, staff, and clinicians with social needs assessment. Perm J. 2018;22:18.
61. Byhoff E, De Marchis EH, Hessler D, Fichtenberg C, Adler N, Cohen AJ, et al. Part II: a qualitative study of social risk screening acceptability in patients and caregivers. Am J Prev Med. 2019;57(6):S38–46.
62. Schickedanz A, Sharp A, Hu YR, Shah NR, Adams JL, Francis D, Rogers A. Impact of social needs navigation on utilization among high utilizers in a large integrated health system: a quasi-experimental study. J Gen Intern Med. 2019;34(11):2382–9.
63. Swavely D, Whyte V, Steiner JF, Freeman SL. Complexities of addressing food insecurity in an urban population. Popul Health Manag. 2019;22(4):300–7.

64. Gold R, Bunce A, Cowburn S, Dambrun K, Dearing M, Middendorf M, et al. Adoption of social determinants of health EHR tools by community health centers. Ann Fam Med. 2018;16(5):399–407.
65. Uwemedimo OT, May H. Disparities in utilization of social determinants of health referrals among children in immigrant families. Front Pediatr. 2018;6:207.
66. Olayiwola JN, Willard-Grace R, Dubé K, Hessler D, Shunk R, Grumbach K, Gottlieb L. Higher perceived clinic capacity to address patients' social needs associated with lower burnout in primary care providers. J Health Care Poor Underserved. 2018;29(1):415–29.
67. Tong ST, Liaw WR, Kashiri PL, Pecsok J, Rozman J, Bazemore AW, Krist AH. Clinician experiences with screening for social needs in primary care. J Am Board Fam Med. 2018;31(3):351–63.
68. Paskett ED, Katz ML, Post DM, Pennell ML, Young GS, Seiber EE, et al. The Ohio Patient Navigation Research Program: does the American Cancer Society patient navigation model improve time to resolution in patients with abnormal screening tests? Cancer Epidemiol Biomarkers Prev. 2012;21(10):1620–8.
69. Lee JH, Fulp W, Wells KJ, Meade CD, Calcano E, Roetzheim R. Patient navigation and time to diagnostic resolution: results for a cluster randomized trial evaluating the efficacy of patient navigation among patients with breast cancer screening abnormalities, Tampa, FL. PloS One. 2013;8(9):e74542.
70. Freund KM, Battaglia TA, Calhoun E, Darnell JS, Dudley DJ, Fiscella K, et al. Impact of patient navigation on timely cancer care: the Patient Navigation Research Program. J Natl Cancer Inst. 2014;106(6):dju115.
71. Yezefski T, Steelquist J, Watabayashi K, Sherman D, Shankaran V. Impact of trained oncology financial navigators on patient out-of-pocket spending. Am J Manag Care. 2018;24(5 Suppl):S74–9.
72. Bresnick J. Lyft expands work with BCBS, humana medicare advantage plans. Xtelligent Healthcare Media LLC; 2019. Retrieved from https://healthpayerintelligence.com/news/lyft-expands-work-with-bcbs-humana-medicare-advantage-plans
73. Rogers A. Warning: we're integrating social care into a racially-biased health system. Health Leads. 2019 Apr. Healthleadsusa.org/communications-center/blog/were-integrating-social-care-into-a-racially-biased-health-system/
74. Feagin J, Bennefield Z. Systemic racism and U.S. health care. Soc Sci Med. 2014;103:7–14. https://doi.org/10.1016/j.socscimed.2013.09.006.
75. Baum F, et al. Changes not for the fainthearted: reorienting health care systems toward health equity through action on the social determinants of health. Am J Public Health. 99:1967–74. https://doi.org/10.2105/AJPH.2008.154856.
76. Marmot M, Allen J. Social determinants of health equity. Am J Public Health. 2014;104:S517–9. https://doi.org/10.2105/AJPH.2014.302200.
77. Garg A, Boynton-Jarrett R, Dworkin PH. Avoiding the unintended consequences of screening for social determinants of health. JAMA. 2016;316(8):813–4. https://doi.org/10.1001/jama.2016.9282.
78. Mason C, Barraket J, Friel S, O'Rourke K, Stenta C-P. Social innovation for the promotion of health equity. Health Promot Int. 2015 Sept 1;30(suppl_2):ii116–25. https://doi.org/10.1093/heapro/dav076.
79. Mitchell SM, Shortell SM. The governance and management of effective community health partnerships: a typology for research, policy, and practice. Milbank Q. 2000;78:241–89. https://doi.org/10.1111/1468-0009.00170.
80. Expanding the Bench. Understanding the terms we use. 2020. Available at https://expandingthebench.org/about-etb/understanding-terms-we-use/

Community-Based Interventions to Address Obesity in the Context of Health Equity

Bettina Drake, Sarah Chavez, Kia Davis, Ross Brownson, and Graham Colditz

Introduction

Obesity is a significant public health challenge, affecting 42.2% of adults and 20% of children in the United States [1]. Between 1999 and 2018, the age-adjusted prevalence of obesity has increased 11.9% (30.5–42.2%), and the prevalence of severe obesity has nearly doubled (4.7–9.2%) [1]. Given the Healthy People 2020 goal of 30.5% [2], the United States is clearly trending in the wrong direction.

While obesity rates are similar across age groups, there are significantly disparities along racial and ethnic lines [3]. The prevalence is highest in non-Hispanic Black adults (49.6%), followed by Hispanic (44.8%), White (42.2%), and Asian (17.4%) adults [1]. The highest prevalence of obesity is observed in Black women (56.9%), which is over triple the lowest rate observed in Asian women (17.2%) [1]. Differences in the prevalence of obesity are also observed on the basis of socioeconomic status and geography, although these effects are complex and differ by race and ethnicity [4].

B. Drake (✉) · K. Davis · G. Colditz
Division of Public Health Sciences, Washington University in St. Louis School of Medicine, St. Louis, MO, USA

Alvin J. Siteman Cancer Center, St. Louis, MO, USA
e-mail: drakeb@wustl.edu

S. Chavez
Division of Public Health Sciences, Washington University in St. Louis School of Medicine, St. Louis, MO, USA

R. Brownson
Alvin J. Siteman Cancer Center, St. Louis, MO, USA

Brown School of Social Work, Washington University in St. Louis, St. Louis, MO, USA

C. Hughes Halbert (ed.), *Cancer Health Disparities*,
https://doi.org/10.1007/978-3-031-37638-2_9

Age-adjusted prevalence of obesity among adults in the United States, 2017–2018

	Total	Men	Women
Age 20 and over	42.4 (1.8)	43.0 (2.7)	41.9 (2.0)
Age 20–39	40.0 (2.6)	40.3 (3.8)	39.7 (2.7)
Age 40–59	44.8 (1.9)	46.4 (3.2)	43.3 (2.7)
Age 60 and over	42.8 (2.5)	42.2 (3.3)	43.3 (3.0)
Non-Hispanic White	42.2 (2.5)	44.7 (3.7)	39.8 (2.9)
Non-Hispanic Black	49.6 (1.5)	41.1 (2.2)	56.9 (1.9)
Non-Hispanic Asian	17.4 (1.3)	17.5 (2.1)	17.2 (1.3)
Hispanic (any race)	44.8 (1.6)	45.7 (1.8)	43.7 (2.0)

Adapted from Data Brief 360 [1]. (Percent and standard error) estimates for adults aged 20 and over were age adjusted by the direct method to the 2000 US Census population. Source: NCHS, National Health and Nutrition Examination Survey, 2017–2018

Obesity rates also vary along socioeconomic lines, although patterns are not consistent across all sexes, races, and ethnicity [5]. As expected, the prevalence of obesity in adults is higher in households with lower income levels in the overall population (31.2% households with >350% federal poverty level (FPL), compared to 39.0% in households with ≤130% FPL and 40.8% for households >130% to ≤350% FPL) [5]. Similar patterns are observed for non-Hispanic White and Asian households, but there is a much less significant difference by household income observed for non-Hispanic Black and Hispanic households [5]. Healthy People 2020 placed the overall target for childhood obesity at <14.5% [2], but the prevalence of obesity is significantly higher in lower-income households and in non-Hispanic Black and Hispanic households regardless of income levels [4]. Of note, the differences in childhood obesity levels are disproportionately affecting females, with prevalence rising in females while remaining consistent in males [4].

Age-adjusted prevalence of obesity by age and household income in the United States, 2011–2014

	Total	White, non-Hispanic	Black, non-Hispanic	Asian, non-Hispanic	Hispanic (any Race)
All adults	36.3 (34.7–38.0)	34.5 (32.4–36.7)	48.1 (45.5–50.7)	11.7 (9.8–13.7)	42.5 (39.8–45.3)
Adult females	38.3 (36.1–40.5)	35.5 (32.4–38.6)	56.9 (54.2–59.7)	11.9 (8.8–15.1)	45.7 (42.2–49.2)
Adult males	34.3 (32.6–36.1)	33.6 (31.4–35.7)	37.5 (34.3–40.8)	11.2 (8.8–13.6)	39.0 (35.4–42.5)
Adults ≤ 130% FPL	39.0 (36.9–41.0)	35.8 (32.8–38.7)	46.6 (43.2–50.0)	15.0 (9.7–20.3)	42.6 (38.1–47.1)
Adults > 130 to ≤ 350% FPL	40.8 (38.2–43.4)	40.2 (36.5–43.9)	48.8 (44.6–52.9)	11.2 (6.6–15.8)	45.0 (40.7–49.2)

	Total	White, non-Hispanic	Black, non-Hispanic	Asian, non-Hispanic	Hispanic (any Race)
Adults > 350% FPL	31.2 (28.3–34.2)	30.6 (27.3–34.0)	49.3 (43.4–55.1)	10.7 (8.3–13.1)	39.1 (33.9–44.3)
All youth	17.0 (15.5–18.6)	14.7 (12.3–17.3)	19.5 (17.1–22.2)	8.6 (6.4–11.2)	21.9 (20.0–23.9)
Youth females	17.1 (15.1–19.3)	15.1 (11.7–19.1)	20.7 (17.1–24.6)	5.3 (2.9–8.6)	21.4 (18.8–24.1)
Youth males	16.9 (15.1–19.0)	14.3 (11.2–17.9)	18.4 (16.1–21.0)	11.8 (8.3–16.1)	22.4 (19.9–24.9)
Youth ≤ 130% FPL	18.9 (17.3–20.6)	15.5 (12.8–18.5)	19.4 (17.0–22.0)	13.2 (8.2–19.7)	22.8 (19.4–26.5)
Youth > 130 to ≤ 350% FPL	19.9 (16.8–23.3)	18.0 (12.6–24.6)	19.9 (15.5–25.0)	8.9 (4.9–14.6)	23.7 (19.4–28.5)
Youth > 350% FPL	10.9 (8.0–14.4)	11.0 (7.3–15.7)	19.8 (12.2–29.4)	4.4 (1.9–8.4)	11.8 (7.5–17.4)

Adapted from Ogden 2018 [4]. Estimates for adults aged 20 and over were age adjusted by the direct method to the 2000 US Census population. Source: NCHS, National Health and Nutrition Examination Survey, 2011–2014

So, is there a single underlying cause of these observed disparities? Unfortunately, this is a multifactorial problem, meaning it is unlikely that public health strategies can design a one-size-fits-all approach to the problem. At the population level, it is widely accepted that different components of the environment in communities can influence behaviors that promote obesity, undermining individual efforts to control weight [3]. Obesity prevention strategies often employ the analysis grid for environments linked to obesity (ANGELO) model proposed by Swinburn et al. [6] The Institute of Medicine relied on the ANGELO model to describe strategies for obesity prevention in relation to five environments: (1) physical activity environments; (2) food and beverage environments; (3) information environments; (4) healthcare and work environments; and (5) school environments [7]. However, the APOP logic model also states that obesity prevention strategies differ significantly on the basis of race, ethnicity, socioeconomic status, and geography [7].

While obesity prevention strategies acknowledge that significant disparities exist, designing prevention strategies to effectively target disproportionately affected populations remains a significant public health challenge [3]. The equitable distribution of effective obesity prevention strategies is an even greater challenge. Kumanyika developed a "Getting to Equity" (GTE) framework designed to approach obesity prevention strategies through the lens of health equity [8].

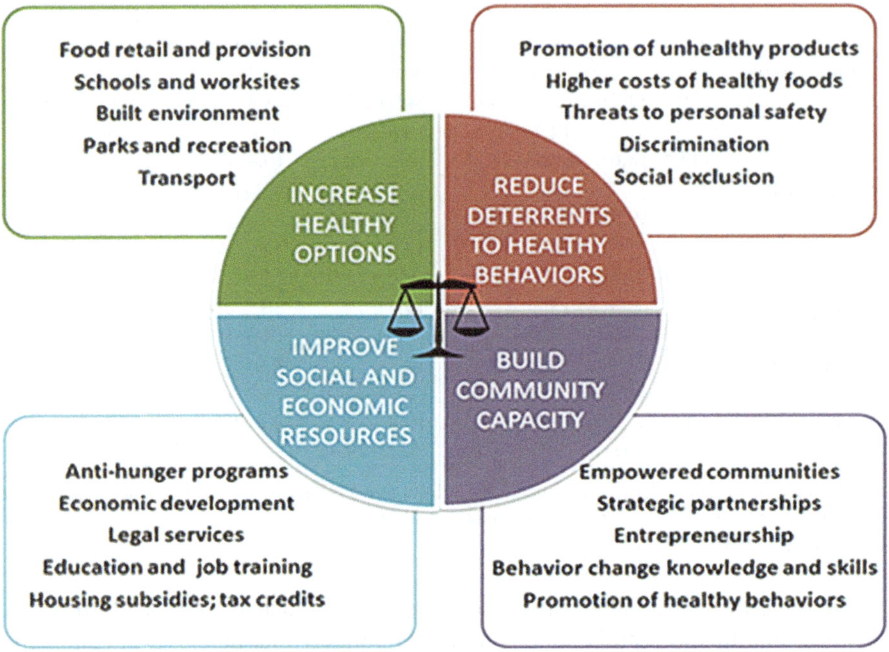

In this model, interventions include policy and systems changes to increase healthy options and reduce deterrents such as the high cost of healthy foods or the promotion of unhealthy products, as well as individual and community-based resources to build on community capacity and improve social and economic resources. The individual and community level interventions may include nutrition assistance programs, economic development, and tax credits, in addition to strategic partnerships and dissemination of educational materials designed to promote behavior change knowledge and skills [3]. This framing of obesity prevention as a health equity issue moves away from the deficit mindset of what society is doing poorly (disparities) to one that is positive about what can be achieved [9].

There are several approaches to obesity prevention, but this chapter focuses on the role of community resources to build capacity by examining community-based interventions to address obesity in the context of health equity. The two most established approaches to community-based obesity prevention, namely, diet and physical activity, are examined in the sections below.

Community-Based Interventions: Obesity Prevention Focused on Diet and Nutrition

Race and Ethnicity

Racial and ethnic minorities experience disproportionately higher rates of obesity, as well as obesity-related diseases such as cardiovascular disease, diabetes, and cancer. Previous studies have found that weight loss can significantly impact health problems and reduce the burden of comorbidities in racial and ethnic minorities.

In studies of childhood diet, relative energy and nutrient contributions vary significantly across racial and ethnic groups [10]. Because nutrients are often lost during processing of foods, it also stands to reason that energy and nutrient levels are directly impacted by the amount of processed foods ingested [10]. The International Food Information Council (IFIC) Foundation classifies foods into several categories: (1) minimally processed foods; (2) foods processed for preservation, nutrient enhancement, and freshness; (3) mixtures of combined ingredients; (4) ready-to-eat processed foods; and (5) prepared foods and meals [11]. A recent study found that among American children, regardless of race or ethnicity, 66–84% of the total energy (calories), vitamins, and nutrients are obtained from processed foods [10]. While many of these processed foods are fortified with the vitamins and nutrients that children need, they also tend to be very high in calories. Thus, dietary recommendations should focus on both the nutritional content and caloric intake, the frequency of eating, and serving sizes to be most effective [10]. While this study focused on children specifically, the same principle can be applied to adults as well.

A 2018 study by Trofholz et al. compared the home food environment and the diet of children from racially diverse households, including Black, Hmong, Latino, Native American, Somali, and White. Several distinct patterns were observed [12]. Black children had low Healthy Eating Index 2010 (HEI-2010) scores due to diets low in healthy food and high in unhealthy foods [12]. Somali children had high HEI-2010 scores, but low intake of fruits and vegetables [12]. White and Latino children also had high HEI-2010 scores, with high intake levels of both healthy and unhealthy foods [12]. Asian, Latino, and White children had higher intakes of fruit and fast food, while Hmong children had diets lower in sugar-sweetened drinks [13]. Collectively, this data suggests that interventions designed to improve home food environment should take into account race and ethnicity as a key part of strategic planning for community-based diet interventions [12].

A 2018 study by Arcan et al. used a community-based participatory approach to look at how racial/ethnic disparities may be associated with differences in perception of childhood body weight and healthy diet among Hmong, Latino, and Somali parents in Twin Cities, Minnesota [14]. This study found that parents did not associate health with weight. Instead, they sought to feed children food that they perceived to be healthy with the goal of making the children happy. The parents were interested in helping children be more active and were concerned with unhealthy food choices and lack of physical activity. The parents indicated their desire for more community-based interventions that could provide education about healthy foods and portion sizes, but the strategy should be tailored to meet their cultural norms and incorporate traditional foods to preserve their cultural identities [14].

Obesity prevalence is 20% higher in Native Hawaiian and Pacific Islanders (NH/PI) compared to non-Hispanic Whites, and the prevalence of diabetes and heart disease is also significantly higher [15]. Two long-standing studies, the PILI Ohana Project [16] and the KaHOLO Project [17], have used cultural adaptation and cultural grounded approaches to health intervention in the context of community-based participatory research [15]. The study points out that while NH/PI share similar cultures, there are many differences in terms of language, sociopolitical structures, and cultural goals and aspirations; these differences must be taken into account when designing culturally responsive health interventions. Cultural adaptations may include naming the programs in the native language, or using foods that are culturally unique and specific as examples for healthy eating [15]. The PILI Ohana studies have resulted in modest yet significant weight loss and improvement in body weight measurements, particularly with regard to long-term weight loss [16].

Income

The diet of most Americans does not meet current nutritional recommendations; however, adherence to food recommendations is significantly lower for the lowest- and middle-income groups compared to high-income populations [18]. Improving the diet and nutrition of a population requires an understanding of social context as well as the food-related knowledge and abilities of members of the population [19]. Nutrition education has been shown to improve food behaviors of adults in lower socioeconomic status (SES) who are enrolled in the Supplemental Nutrition Assistance Program (SNAP) [20]. In this sense, "nutrition literacy" can be broadly divided into two categories – functional literacy and interactive literacy [21]. Functional literacy is focused on declarative knowledge and information about factors that can affect health, while interactive literacy is focused on implementing positive dietary changes based on that functional knowledge [22]. The term "food literacy" implies the ability to apply this information about food choice to promote healthy choices by reflecting on the effect of foods on personal health and the health of society as a whole [19].

The RE-AIM framework (*reach, effectiveness, adoption, implementation*, and *maintenance*) was recently applied to address health inequities in the context of a low-income weight-loss program [23]. Be Fit, Be Well (BFBW) was a 24-month self-management trial designed to address weight loss and hypertension in low-income, predominantly African American populations [23]. As part of the ultimate goal to promote weight loss, BFBW sought to reduce common barriers to successful weight loss, including transportation, time, and access to services [24]. RE-AIM analysis of the results of this study suggested that BFBW may be expanded to additional community health centers, although it was not successful for all populations [24].

A systematic review and meta-analysis of randomized control trials examined the effects of behavioral interventions promoting healthy diet in low-income populations in the United States [25]. Previous studies have found that low-income populations may be more difficult to recruit to behavioral intervention trials [26] and may also be less successful in achieving long-term behavioral changes compared to more affluent participants [27, 28]. Thus, the concern was whether the interventions themselves could further exacerbate income-based equalities [29]. However, one study targeting the whole population argued that socioeconomic groups may experience differences in outcomes as a result of different baselines for healthy behaviors, which suggests these interventions may be successful in lower-income populations [30]. A meta-analysis was conducted in 2014 to expand on this study, and 16 studies focused on dietary interventions were included in the analysis [25]. The combined analysis found a standard mean difference (SMD) of 0.22 (95% CI 0.06 to 0.3, $I^2 = 0\%$) for all 16 studies, and SMD of 0.16 (95% CI 0.08 to 0.25, $I^2 = 41\%$) in the 8 studies that presented long-term follow-up data (6–12 months) [25]. This study concluded that interventions resulted in modest but positive influences on diet (equivalent to approximately half a portion of fruits and vegetables more than controls per day), and positive effects were maintained long term [25].

Rural vs Urban

Rural areas face barriers to obesity prevention and reducing through physical activity and health eating. Key barriers to these behaviors include limited access to healthy food retailers, as well as lack of resources to implement policy and environmental changes necessary to promote healthy diet [31]. In addition, much of the policy and environmental strategies are based on urban and suburban strategies, so these studies may have limited relevance to the unique cultures and infrastructures in rural communities [32, 33]. A recent systematic review identified 29 studies focused on nutrition-related policy and environmental strategies to prevent obesity in rural communities published between 2002 and 2013 [31]. Of note, 10 of these studies were conducted in American Indian tribes or First Nations of Canada, and only 14 provided outcome evaluations [31]. While data is limited, some trends emerged from these data.

Rural children have higher prevalence of obesity compared to urban children, independent of age, ethnicity, or socioeconomic class [34, 35]. Previous studies have proposed that school-based community health promotion programs are well-positioned to support obesity intervention efforts in rural communities [15]. The prevalence of obesity is higher amongst rural Hispanics compared to urban Hispanics [36]. Building on this work, Muzaffar et al. used a community-based participatory approach to study the burden and causes of obesity in a largely Hispanic cohort of children of migrant and seasonal farmworkers in rural Midwest communities [37].

Rates of overweight and obese adolescents were 55%, but none of the 38 participants met the recommended dietary guidelines that would achieve the HEI-2015 "good" range (score $\geq$ 80) [37]. Fat intake was higher than recommended, fiber indicate was lower, and 12% of participants did not meet daily requirements for most food groups, leading to nutrient and vitamin deficiencies [37]. The study concluded that successful community-based interventions should include physical activity, demonstrations, diet and nutrition resources, and gardening for a more complete, integrated approach [37].

Overall, three main strategies have been suggested to implement obesity prevention strategies in rural communities [31]. First, the design of these interventions must address the need to accommodate long distances to food sources [31]. Long distances can increase the cost of food, and fresh produce is often limited due to long transit times [38, 39]. Thus, stores often faced challenges providing low-cost, healthy food options to rural consumers [40, 41]. Adaptations must address the networks between food producers, retailers, and consumers. The second strategy is to tailor rural interventions to specific rural cultures and food preferences [31]. Several studies noted the importance of culture and food preparation, such as the uniquely Southern approaches to cooking and diet [42], or incorporating traditional foods unique to American Indian tribes [43]. And finally, successful strategies should build on existing local partnerships such as federal food and nutritional assistance programs, parks, healthcare providers, and health departments [31, 44, 45].

While these studies have focused on one particular socioeconomic or demographic factor, obesity prevention strategies must often address multilevel influences. The Tribal Resilience in Vulnerable Environments (THRIVE) study employed a community-based participatory research partnership between the University of Oklahoma and the Chickasaw and Choctaw Nations to study the food environment within the communities [46]. Only 57% of American Indian participants had easy access to purchase fruits and vegetables, but only 35% considered the produce to be good quality [46]. Thus, very few participants met the recommendations for daily intake of fruit or vegetables (44% and 25%, respectively) [46]. As part of the THRIVE study in American Indian communities, the prevalence of obesity was significantly higher in participants who stated that the price of fresh produce was cost-prohibitive (Prevalence Proportion Ratio (PPR) 1.24; 95% CI: 1.02–1.50) [46]. The study concluded that participants who used nontraditional food retailers had an increased prevalence of obesity (PPR 1.38; 95% CI: 1.02–1.86) [46]. The study suggested that introducing healthy options in nontraditional retail settings could significantly reduce health disparities in American Indian tribal communities by improving access to healthy food options [46].

Community-Based Interventions: Obesity Prevention Focused on Physical Activity

Physical activity has been shown to have significant improvement on mental and physical health [47]. At the population level, physical activity is influenced by many factors, with significant social and environmental influences [47,48]. Communication of physical activity guidelines is part of any comprehensive strategy, but community-based approaches offer significant benefits in terms of implementing systematic, sustainable changes to increase physical activity within a community [48, 49]. A recent meta-analysis of 123 studies concluded that physical activity messaging should focus on short-term benefits to social and mental health, but the message should be tailored to the specific needs of the target community in order to be the most impactful [49]. Thus, community-based physical activity interventions should focus on customized strategies that draw from psychology and social marketing principles to target different population subgroups [49].

One key take-away of recent studies is the need for messaging to clearly define what "counts" as physical activity. In order to assess perceptions of physical activity, work groups were asked to provide examples of what constitutes physical activity. Most individuals cited intentional, high-intensity activities such as sports or exercise, while fewer participants mentioned incidental physical activities such as gardening, housework, or active travel [48]. Younger participants were more likely to attribute social and mental health benefits to physical activities, while older participants focused on the potential to improve health and mobility [48]. Interestingly, while social connections were considered to be an important benefit of physical activity in multiple groups, mothers in the Somali Women's group saw the primary benefit as having time to themselves [48].

The content of the messaging is also crucial. Multiple groups agreed that physical activity messages should emphasize mental health, physical health, and improved social connections. The participants also recommended that the messaging provide guidance that is realistic and achievable, with more emphasis on incremental progress than the achievement of a specified goal or a precise number. However, Nobles et al. concluded that the images used in these messages should be relatable, with appearances and experiences that resonate with the message recipients, and should demonstrate cultural sensitivities [48]. Several recent studies have shown the benefit of culturally sensitive, targeted messaging in community-based physical activity interventions [50].

Race and Ethnicity

Public parks represent a widely available, free, or low-cost resource for physical activity. The System for Observing Play and Recreation in Communities (SOPARC) is a methodology for observing how people use permanent settings such as parks to engage in physical activity [51]. SOPARC data can be used to identify the demographics of park users to better inform targeted marketing efforts within specific communities. However, a recent study found that the reliability of SOPARC may be impacted when attempting to observe physical activity in specific racial and ethnic groups, contextual conditions, or physical settings [52]. Comparing the numbers reported by multiple observers, Marquet et al. found low reliability in data, possibly due to misclassification of individuals on the basis of race and ethnicity [52]. Skin color is typically the basis for identification, but this leads to inherent discrepancies in racial and ethnic groups with large phenotypic variations, including Hispanic, Latino, and American Indian populations [52]. Given that the SOPARC method is one of the most common protocols for assessing park usage, it highlights the need for more a more precise, community-based approach to target messaging to a specific population [52].

One of these community-based approaches specifically targeted American Indian youth. American Indian children are two to three times more likely to develop type II diabetes compared to non-Hispanic White children [53]. A collaboration between the University of Oklahoma and the Choctaw Nation of Oklahoma was established to study whether community-based exercise intervention with a financial incentive could increase physical activity om American Indian youth [53]. This approach had been successful with an adult cohort, so the MOVE study sought to expand its reach to the youth in the community [53]. A crucial difference between this study and previous clinical trials was that all text, exercise activities, and data collection took place within the Choctaw Nation community rather than at the city campus. Pre-implementation planning with tribal leaders was crucial to the success of the community buy-in for the study. By asking the tribal communities to identify which communities within the Choctaw Nation would be best suited to the study, that ensured the study was designed with the community needs in mind. In addition, the study identified clear strategies to promote standardization and maintain study integrity. While significant barriers exist (limited nutrition education resources, transportation barriers, and personal challenges), open and frequent communication between researchers and community partners was crucial to success [53]. Enhanced financial incentives have been shown to motivate previously sedentary, overweight, and obese adolescents to exercise longer; however, sustaining the exercise program remains a challenge [54].

In Native Hawaiian and Pacific Islander (NH/PI) communities, culturally grounded approaches have been implemented to encourage physical activity as part of obesity intervention programs [15]. These culturally grounded approaches are recommended when there is a significant need for intervention, limited data to inform adaptation strategies, and a large potential for improved health impact [55]. These approaches have been particularly successful for indigenous communities as they reflect a return to tradition, such as using traditional dance to increase physical activities [56] or adjusting dietary patterns to traditional foods to treat obesity [57]. The KaHOLO Project found that participants in hula dancing physical activity interventions successfully reduced blood pressure and improved social interactions, and hula may also potentially promote weight loss in NH/PI participants [17].

Income

While low-income communities often contained significantly more parks, these communities lack playgrounds, and the parks themselves are less likely to be well-maintained [58]. In many low-income communities, temporary spaces can provide additional spaces for physical activity [59]. Play Streets are temporary spaces created by closing streets, parking lots, or open fields to create safe play spaces during specified periods of time.

A recent study of low-income Latino families with preschool-age children found that parents recognize and appreciate the importance of physical activity for both themselves and their children [60]. Not surprisingly, daily demands for work, financial constraints, and neighborhood safety concerns acted as significant barriers to creating an environment that supports physical activity [60]. The study suggested that interventions in low-income Latino populations should take into account these barriers, using pediatricians to provide educational materials and guidance to promote the development of healthy physical activity behaviors [60].

A recent meta-analysis found that interventions targeting physical activity only were more effective than interventions targeting multiple behaviors including physical activity [25]. Interventions that targeted multiple behaviors showed a small positive effect on physical activity, but follow-up data showed that these positive effects were not maintained for physical activity [25]. This systematic review suggested that although current physical activity interventions in low-income groups are overall positive, there is a small risk of intervention-generated inequalities if the resources provided during the trial are not available post-intervention [25, 29].

Rural vs Urban

While rural areas did not experience the rapid increase in obesity initially observed in suburban areas, trends over the last decade reflect that rural populations are more likely to be overweight or obese [32, 61]. The Muzaffar et al. study of rural children of migrant and seasonal farmworkers in the Midwest found low levels of physical activity, with only 34% scoring adequate levels of physical activity [37]. However, while the physical activity score did not significantly correlate with BMI percentile or obesity, it did place these children at a higher risk of becoming obese in the future [37]. In fact, failure to meet physical activity recommendations plays a primary role in the greater risk of obesity for rural residents [32]. Rural communities often have limited access to walkable communities, recreational facilities, and parks [32, 62, 63]. However, in studies of obesity prevention efforts in diverse rural communities, strategies that increase opportunities for physical activity are deemed to be the most likely to succeed [33].

The Play Streets concept has been implemented in diverse rural communities across the United States [64]. Adapting Play Streets from an urban setting to rural communities presented unique challenges, including using locations other than streets, varying the locations to account for the more geographically disperse populations, and maximizing participation in Play Streets by coupling these times with community events [65]. Play Streets can be successfully implemented in rural areas [65]. However, other studies have suggested that children were more likely to show improvements in physical activity levels at Play Streets, while most adults remained sedentary [64].

Physical activity is also critically important to cancer survivors, but the barriers to physical activity that exist in rural areas may account for some of the health disparities observed in rural cancer survivors [66]. The Better Exercise Adherence after Treatment for Cancer (BEAT Cancer) intervention was recently adapted to serve the needs of rural cancer survivors [66]. The primary barriers to physical activity in this population were similar to those observed in the general population of rural communities, including transportation, cost, expertise, and lack of awareness. The authors suggest that successful implementation of physical activity programs among rural cancer survivors will take a village, which illustrates the need to effectively integrate resources and identify strategies to reduce environmental barriers unique to rural communities [66].

Future Directions: Implementation Strategies and Measures for Success

There are clearly significant disparities in obesity observed in racial and ethnic minorities, rural communities, and low-income populations. Obesity prevention strategies face the significant challenge of targeting disproportionately affected populations with significant individual, community, and environmental barriers in place. So, how can we develop obesity prevention protocols that are equitably distributed, culturally sensitive, and result in sustainable positive change? Community-based interventions offer the unique opportunity to support these efforts by building on existing community capacity and resources to implement these changes.

African-Americans are disproportionately represented in the overall prevalence of overweight and obesity in the United States. Men are most likely to be overweight or obese; however, African American women have higher rates of overweight and obesity compared to other racial/ethnic groups [67]. Psychological stressors have been associated with greater risk of obesity and leads to coping behaviors such as increased higher-fat food intake, emotional eating, and poor appetite regulation [68]. Everyday experiences with racism, also a psychological stressor, has been associated with increased BMI among African American women [69]. Future research is needed to address coping strategies as well as the psychological stressors in interventions targeting obesity among African Americans.

Community-based obesity prevention efforts must first seek to measure community readiness for diet and physical activity interventions. As part of this assessment, strategies must seek to identify existing socioeconomic, environmental, and cultural barriers unique to each community. This will allow providers to identify gaps in understanding and also allow for the development of a multidisciplinary team to address the barriers identified.

The intermediate outcomes will include data obtained during early implementation phases. Measuring changes in obesity-related behavior that include diet and physical activity, and the mechanisms that contribute to these behaviors, during the intervention will establish how successful the implementation strategy is when community-based resources are fully engaged. And finally, long-term data will allow for a better assessment of the sustainability of these interventions. To be truly effective long term, obesity prevention must be equitably distributed, cost-effective, and supported by community capacity. If the strategies are not tailored to fit the unique needs of the community, it stands to reason that the existing community infrastructure will not continue to support the interventions long-term.

Thus, the goal of achieving significant positive change in an equitable manner must acknowledge the need for a team-based approach. "It takes a village." Critical barriers such as the high cost of healthy foods or the promotion of unhealthy behaviors will not disappear when the study is over unless real change is implemented. A successful community-based intervention must build on existing community capacity to improve the efficiency and integration of existing social and economic resources. It must support the goal of nutrition assistance and economic development to improve the health of the community as a whole. Ultimately, a successful community-based intervention must provide a framework and identify resources to build strategic partnerships and educate the community to help them develop real, attainable skills to promote healthy eating and physical activity. Because of the significant role that community plays on the barriers to obesity prevention, a community-based approach provides the best opportunity to achieve long-term success and reduce health disparities in high-risk communities.

References

1. Hales CM, Carroll MD, Fryar CD, Ogden CL. Prevalence of obesity and severe obesity among adults: United States, 2017–2018. NCHS Data Brief. 2020;360:1–8.
2. US DoHaH Services. Healthy People 2020 topics and objectives: nutrition and weight status. In: OoDPaH, editor. Promotion; 2020. US Department of Health and Human Services.
3. Kumanyika SK. A framework for increasing equity impact in obesity prevention. Am J Public Health. 2019;109(10):1350–7.
4. Ogden CL, Carroll MD, Fakhouri TH, Hales CM, Fryar CD, Li X, Freedman DS. Prevalence of obesity among youths by household income and education level of head of household – United States 2011–2014. MMWR Morb Mortal Wkly Rep. 2018;67:186–9.
5. Ogden CL, Fakhouri TH, Carroll MD, Hales CM, Fryar CD, Li X, Freedman DS. Prevalence of obesity among adults, by household income and education – United States, 2011–2014. MMWR Morb Mortal Wkly Rep. 2017;66:1369–73.

6. Swinburn B, Egger G, Raza F. Dissecting obesogenic environments: the development and application of a framework for identifying and prioritizing environmental interventions for obesity. Prev Med. 1999;29(6):563–70.
7. Institute of Medicine. Accelerating progress in obesity prevention: solving the weight of the nation. Washington, DC: National Academies Press; 2012.
8. Shiriki Kumanyika. Getting to equity in obesity prevention: a new framework. Washington, DC: National Academy of Medicine; 2017.
9. Kumanyika SK. Health equity is the issue we have been waiting for. J Public Helath Manag Pract. 2016;22:S8–S10.
10. Eicher-Miller HA, Fulgoni VL, Keast DR. Processed food contributions to energy and nutrient intake differ among US children by race/ethnicity. Nutrients. 2015;7(12):10076–88.
11. IFIC Foundation. Understanding our food communications tool kit. Washington, DC: IFIC Foundation. DC2014
12. Trofholz A, Tate A, Fulkerson JA, Hearst MO, Neumark-Sztainer D, Berge JM. Description of the home food environment in Black, White, Hmong, Latino, Native American and Somali homes with 5–7-year-old children. Public Health Nutr. 2019;22(5):882–93.
13. Arcan C, Larson N, Bauer K, Berge J, Story M, Neumark-Sztainer D. Dietary and weight-related behaviors and body mass index among Hispanic, Hmong, Somali, and white adolescents. J Acad Nutr Diet. 2014;114(3):375–83.
14. Arcan C, Culhane-Pera KA, Pergament S, Rosas-Lee M, Xiong MB. Somali, Latino and Hmong parents' perceptions and approaches about raising healthy-weight children: a community-based participatory research study. Public Health Nutr. 2018;21(6):1079–93.
15. Kaholokula JK, Ing CT, Look MA, Delafield R, Sinclair K. Culturally responsive approaches to health promotion for Native Hawaiians and Pacific Islanders. Ann Hum Biol. 2018;45(3):249–63.
16. Nacapoy AH, Kaholokula JK, West MR, et al. Partnerships to address obesity disparities in Hawai'i: the PILI 'Ohana project. Hawaii Med J. 2008;67(9):237–41.
17. Kaholokula JK, Look MA, Wills TA, et al. Kā-HOLO Project: a protocol for a randomized controlled trial of a native cultural dance program for cardiovascular disease prevention in Native Hawaiians. BMC Public Health. 2017;17(1):321.
18. Kirkpatrick SI, Dodd KW, Reedy J, Krebs-Smith SM. Income and race/ethnicity are associated with adherence to food-based dietary guidance among US adults and children. J Acad Nutr Diet. 2012;112(5):624–635.e626.
19. Krause C, Sommerhalder K, Beer-Borst S, Abel T. Just a subtle difference? Findings from a systematic review on definitions of nutrition literacy and food literacy. Health Promot Int. 2018;33(3):378–89.
20. Verghese A, Raber M, Sharma S. Interventions targeting diet quality of Supplemental Nutrition Assistance Program (SNAP) participants: a scoping review. Prev Med. 2019;119:77–86.
21. Bessems K, Linssen E, Lomme M, van Assema P. The effectiveness of the good affordable food intervention for adults with low socioeconomic status and small incomes. Int J Environ Res Public Health. 2020;17(7):2535.
22. Velardo S. The nuances of health literacy, nutrition literacy, and food literacy. J Nutr Educ Behav. 2015;47(4):385–389.e381.
23. Glasgow RE, Askew S, Purcell P, et al. Use of RE-AIM to address health inequities: application in a low-income community health center based weight loss and hypertension self-management program. Transl Behav Med. 2013;3(2):200–10.
24. Ritzwoller DP, Glasgow RE, Sukhanova AY, et al. Economic analyses of the Be Fit Be Well program: a weight loss program for community health centers. J Gen Intern Med. 2013;28(12):1581–8.
25. Bull ER, Dombrowski SU, McCleary N, Johnston M. Are interventions for low-income groups effective in changing healthy eating, physical activity and smoking behaviours? A systematic review and meta-analysis. BMJ Open. 2014;4(11):e006046.

26. Marcus BH, Williams DM, Dubbert PM, et al. Physical activity intervention studies: what we know and what we need to know: a scientific statement from the American Heart Association Council on Nutrition, Physical Activity, and Metabolism (Subcommittee on Physical Activity); Council on Cardiovascular Disease in the Young; and the Interdisciplinary Working Group on Quality of Care and Outcomes Research. Circulation. 2006;114(24):2739–52.
27. Hiscock R, Judge K, Bauld L. Social inequalities in quitting smoking: what factors mediate the relationship between socioeconomic position and smoking cessation? J Public Health (Oxf). 2011;33(1):39–47.
28. Niederdeppe J, Fiore MC, Baker TB, Smith SS. Smoking-cessation media campaigns and their effectiveness among socioeconomically advantaged and disadvantaged populations. Am J Public Health. 2008;98(5):916–24.
29. White M, Adams J, Heywood P. How and why do interventions that increase health overall widen inequalities within populations? In: Babones S, editor. Health, inequality and public health. Bristol: Policy Press; 2009. p. 65–81.
30. Michie S, Jochelson K, Markham WA, Bridle C. Low-income groups and behaviour change interventions: a review of intervention content, effectiveness and theoretical frameworks. J Epidemiol Community Health. 2009;63(8):610–22.
31. Calancie L, Leeman J, Jilcott Pitts SB, et al. Nutrition-related policy and environmental strategies to prevent obesity in rural communities: a systematic review of the literature, 2002–2013. Prev Chronic Dis. 2015;12:E57.
32. Barnidge EK, Radvanyi C, Duggan K, et al. Understanding and addressing barriers to implementation of environmental and policy interventions to support physical activity and healthy eating in rural communities. J Rural Health. 2013;29(1):97–105.
33. West ST, Weddell MS, Whetstone LM, Jilcott Pitts SB. Stakeholder perceptions of obesity-prevention strategies: a comparison of geographically diverse rural counties. J Public Health Manag Pract. 2013;19(6):511–20.
34. Champion JD, Collins JL. Retrospective chart review for obesity and associated interventions among rural Mexican-American adolescents accessing healthcare services. J Am Assoc Nurse Pract. 2013;25(11):604–10.
35. Edwards MB, Miller JL, Blackburn L. After-school programs for health promotion in rural communities: Ashe County Middle School 4-H After-School Program. J Public Health Manag Pract. 2011;17(3):283–7.
36. Hammons AJ, Wiley AR, Fiese BH, Teran-Garcia M. Six-week Latino family prevention pilot program effectively promotes healthy behaviors and reduces obesogenic behaviors. J Nutr Educ Behav. 2013;45(6):745–50.
37. Muzaffar H, Raffaelli M, Teran-Garcia M, Wiley A, Gonzalez M, Hannon BA. A community-based participatory assessment of the health status and obesity risks in children from rural farmworker families in the Midwest. Hisp Health Care Int. 2019;17(4):149–55.
38. Gittelsohn J, Vijayadeva V, Davison N, et al. A food store intervention trial improves caregiver psychosocial factors and children's dietary intake in Hawaii. Obesity (Silver Spring). 2010;18(Suppl 1):S84–90.
39. Mead E, Gittelsohn J, Kratzmann M, Roache C, Sharma S. Impact of the changing food environment on dietary practices of an Inuit population in Arctic Canada. J Hum Nutr Diet. 2010;23(Suppl 1):18–26.
40. Brown BD, Harris KJ, Harris JL, Parker M, Ricci C, Noonan C. Translating the diabetes prevention program for Northern Plains Indian youth through community-based participatory research methods. Diabetes Educ. 2010;36(6):924–35.
41. Vastine A, Gittelsohn J, Ethelbah B, Anliker J, Caballero B. Formative research and stakeholder participation in intervention development. Am J Health Behav. 2005;29(1):57–69.
42. Pitts SB, Vu MB, Garcia BA, et al. A community assessment to inform a multilevel intervention to reduce cardiovascular disease risk and risk disparities in a rural community. Fam Community Health. 2013;36(2):135–46.

43. Fleischhacker S, Byrd RR, Ramachandran G, et al. Tools for healthy tribes: improving access to healthy foods in Indian country. Am J Prev Med. 2012;43(3 Suppl 2):S123–9.
44. Conrey EJ, Frongillo EA, Dollahite JS, Griffin MR. Integrated program enhancements increased utilization of Farmers' Market Nutrition Program. J Nutr. 2003;133(6):1841–4.
45. Phillips MM, Raczynski JM, West DS, Pulley L, Bursac Z, Leviton LC. The evaluation of Arkansas Act 1220 of 2003 to reduce childhood obesity: conceptualization, design, and special challenges. Am J Community Psychol. 2013;51(1–2):289–98.
46. Love CV, Taniguchi TE, Williams MB, et al. Diabetes and obesity associated with poor food environments in American Indian communities: the tribal health and resilience in vulnerable environments (THRIVE) study. Curr Dev Nutr. 2019;3(Suppl 2):63–8.
47. World Health Organisation. Global action plan on physical activity 2018–2020. Geneva: WHO; 2018.
48. Nobles J, Thomas C, Banks Gross Z, et al. "Let's talk about physical activity": understanding the preferences of under-served communities when messaging physical activity guidelines to the public. Int J Environ Res Public Health. 2020;17(8):2782.
49. Williamson C, Baker G, Mutrie N, Niven A, Kelly P. Get the message? A scoping review of physical activity messaging. Int J Behav Nutr Phys Act. 2020;17(1):51.
50. Coughlin SS, Smith SA. A review of community-based participatory research studies to promote physical activity among African Americans. J Ga Public Health Assoc. 2016;5(3):220–7.
51. Evenson KR, Jones SA, Holliday KM, Cohen DA, McKenzie TL. Park characteristics, use, and physical activity: a review of studies using SOPARC (system for observing play and recreation in communities). Prev Med. 2016;86:153–66.
52. Marquet O, Hipp JA, Alberico C, et al. Use of SOPARC to assess physical activity in parks: do race/ethnicity, contextual conditions, and settings of the target area, affect reliability? BMC Public Health. 2019;19(1):1730.
53. Chadwick JQ, Tullier MA, Wolbert L, et al. Collaborative implementation of a community-based exercise intervention with a partnering rural American Indian community. Clin Trials. 2019;16(4):391–8.
54. Short KR, Chadwick JQ, Cannady TK, et al. Using financial incentives to promote physical activity in American Indian adolescents: a randomized controlled trial. PLoS One. 2018;13(6):e0198390.
55. Okamoto SK, Kulis S, Marsiglia FF, Steiker LK, Dustman P. A continuum of approaches toward developing culturally focused prevention interventions: from adaptation to grounding. J Prim Prev. 2014;35(2):103–12.
56. Look MA, Maskarinec GG, de Silva M, Seto T, Mau ML, Kaholokula JK. Kumu hula perspectives on health. Hawaii J Med Public Health. 2014;73(12 Suppl 3):21–5.
57. Shintani T, Beckham S, Tang J, O'Connor HK, Hughes C. Waianae Diet Program: long-term follow-up. Hawaii Med J. 1999;58(5):117–22.
58. Vaughan KB, Kaczynski AT, Wilhelm Stanis SA, Besenyi GM, Bergstrom R, Heinrich KM. Exploring the distribution of park availability, features, and quality across Kansas City, Missouri by Income and Race/Ethnicity: an Environmental Justice Investigation. Ann Behav Med. 2013;45(suppl_1):S28–38.
59. Umstattd Meyer MR, Prochnow T, Bridges CN, et al. Assessing physical activity in temporary spaces: application of SOPARC/iSOPARC® for Play Streets. Res Q Exerc Sport. 2020;91(2):346–53.
60. Lindsay AC, Wallington SF, Lees FD, Greaney ML. Exploring how the home environment influences eating and physical activity habits of low-income, Latino children of predominantly immigrant families: a qualitative study. Int J Environ Res Public Health. 2018;15(5):978.
61. Lutfiyya MN, Lipsky MS, Wisdom-Behounek J, Inpanbutr-Martinkus M. Is rural residency a risk factor for overweight and obesity for U.S. children? Obesity (Silver Spring). 2007;15(9):2348–56.
62. Murimi MW, Harpel T. Practicing preventive health: the underlying culture among low-income rural populations. J Rural Health. 2010;26(3):273–82.

63. Hennessy E, Kraak VI, Hyatt RR, et al. Active living for rural children: community perspectives using PhotoVOICE. Am J Prev Med. 2010;39(6):537–45.
64. Umstattd Meyer MR, Bridges Hamilton CN, Prochnow T, et al. Come together, play, be active: physical activity engagement of school-age children at Play Streets in four diverse rural communities in the U.S. Prev Med. 2019;129:105869.
65. Pollack Porter KM, Bridges Hamilton CN, Umstattd Meyer MR. Implementing play streets in low-income rural communities in the United States. Health Promot Pract. 2020; https://doi.org/10.1177/1524839920957228.
66. Rogers LQ, Goncalves L, Martin MY, et al. Beyond efficacy: a qualitative organizational perspective on key implementation science constructs important to physical activity intervention translation to rural community cancer care sites. J Cancer Surviv. 2019;13(4):537–46.
67. Ogden CL, Fryar CD, Martin CB, et al. Trends in obesity prevalence by race and Hispanic Origin-1999–2000 to 2017–2018. JAMA. 2020;324(12):1208–10.
68. Sims R, Gordon S, Garcia W, et al. Perceived stress and eating behaviors in a community-based sample of African Americans. Eat Behav. 2008;9(2):137–42.
69. Cozier YC, Palmer JR, Rosenberg L. Comparison of methods for collection of DNA samples by mail in the Black Women's Health Study. Ann Epidemiol. 2004;14(2):117–22.

Community-Based Interventions for HPV Vaccination

Shannon M. Christy, Lindsay N. Fuzzell, Paige W. Lake, Stephanie Staras, Vivian Colon Lopez, Alicia Best, Pamela C. Hull, and Susan T. Vadaparampil

Overview/Introduction

Human papillomavirus (HPV) is the most common sexually transmitted infection in the USA [1]. Spread through intimate skin-to-skin contact [2], more than 40 HPV types can infect human anogenital regions and mouths and throats of people through vaginal, anal, and oral sex [3]. Sexually transmitted HPV types are categorized as either low-risk or high-risk [2, 4]. Low-risk HPV types (e.g., HPV types 6, 11, 26, 40, 42, 53, 54, 55, 57, 66, 73, 82, 83, 84, 73) can cause anogenital warts and recurrent respiratory papillomatosis, whereas high-risk HPV types (e.g., HPV types 16, 18, 31, 33, 35, 39, 45, 51, 52, 56, 58, 59, 68) can lead to multiple types of cancers in humans [4]. The majority of HPV-related cancers are attributed to high-risk HPV

S. M. Christy (✉) · L. N. Fuzzell · P. W. Lake · S. T. Vadaparampil
H. Lee Moffitt Cancer Center and Research Institute, Tampa, FL, USA
e-mail: Shannon.Christy@moffitt.org; Lindsay.Fuzzell@moffitt.org; Paige.Lake@moffitt.org; Susan.Vadaparampil@moffitt.org

S. Staras
University of Florida, Gainesville, FL, USA
e-mail: sstaras@ufl.edu

V. Colon Lopez
University of Puerto Rico, San Juan, Puerto Rico
e-mail: vivian.colon@upr.edu

A. Best
College of Public Health, University of South Florida, Tampa, FL, USA
e-mail: abest@usf.edu

P. C. Hull
Markey Cancer Center, Community Impact Office, University of Kentucky, Lexington, KY, USA
e-mail: Pam.Hull@uky.edu

C. Hughes Halbert (ed.), *Cancer Health Disparities*,
https://doi.org/10.1007/978-3-031-37638-2_10

types 16 and 18; [5] and globally by region, the two most common HPV types are types 16 and 18 [2].

Most sexually active people will be infected with at least one HPV type at some point in their lifetime [2]. The majority of individuals are infected with HPV during or shortly after their initial sexual experience [1]. Most HPV infections are asymptomatic and resolve on their own within 2 years [2]. However, in some individuals, high-risk HPV infections persist and over the course of years can develop into oropharyngeal and anal cancers regardless of gender or biological sex at birth, penile cancer among those born male, and cervical, vaginal, and vulvar cancers among those born female [2].

In the USA, approximately 34,800 cancer cases each year are caused by HPV infections [6]. From 2012 to 2016 in the USA, 91% cases of cervical cancers and 91% of anal cancers were caused by high-risk HPV types [6]. Furthermore, most vaginal (75%), oropharyngeal (71%), vulvar (69%), and penile cancers (63%) diagnosed in the USA between 2012 and 2016 were also caused by infections from high-risk HPV types [6]. Importantly, marked disparities in HPV prevalence and/or HPV-related cancers exist based on geography, rurality, gender, race/ethnicity, and sexual and gender minority status [7–9]. HPV vaccination has the potential to significantly address HPV-related cancer incidence, mortality, and disparities.

Three vaccines against HPV infection have been licensed by the US Food and Drug Administration (FDA) [10]. The bivalent vaccine (2vHPV), which prevents HPV types 16 and 18, was approved in 2009 for females ages 10–25 initially [11] and subsequently extended to include 9-year-old females [11]. The quadrivalent vaccine (4vHPV) was approved for females ages 9–26 in 2006 [12] and males ages 9–26 in 2009 [13] and guards against HPV types 6, 11, 16, and 18. The nine-valent vaccine (9vHPV), which protect against HPV types 6, 11, 16, 18, 31, 33, 45, 52, and 58, was approved in 2014 for females ages 9–26 and males ages 9–15 years [14]. Approval of the 9vHPV vaccine was later extended to include males ages 16–26 years [15]. In October 2018, the FDA further extended its approval of the 9vHPV vaccine to those ages 27–45 [16]. Since 2016, only the nine-valent vaccine has been utilized in the USA [17]. Approximately 92% of HPV-related cancers in the USA each year are caused by one of the HPV types for which the 9vHPV vaccine offers protection; thus, more than 32,000 HPV-attributed cancers in the USA could be prevented each year if those ages 9–26 years received the HPV vaccine [6].

The US Advisory Committee on Immunization Practices (ACIP) has issued recommendations related to both adolescent and adult HPV vaccine administration [10]. ACIP recommendations have included routine vaccination for 11- and 12-year-old females and males since 2006 and 2011, respectively [18]. The HPV vaccine is recommended during early adolescence due to the strong immune response experienced among young adolescents as well as decreased likelihood that adolescents have prior exposure to HPV (i.e., vaccination is most effective when given prior to sexual debut) [18]. ACIP recommendations have stated that the vaccine can be administered starting at age 9 [18]. Current ACIP recommendations state that individuals who have not previously completed the HPV vaccine series are recommended to receive the vaccine through age 26 [18]. Among those aged 27–45 years, in June 2019, ACIP recommended shared clinical decision-making to consider benefits and limitations of vaccination in an age group where the majority will have had prior exposure to HPV [18]. Since 2016, ACIP recommendations have stated that individuals ages 9–14 receive two doses of the HPV vaccine, while individuals ages 15 years and older and those who are immunocompromised receive three doses [19].

Overall, US HPV vaccination rates have been trending upward among both adolescents and young adults (AYA) [10, 20]. HPV vaccine rates from the 2018 National Immunization Survey-Teen (NIS-Teen)—the most recent year for which data were available at the time of writing—were 68.1% for series initiation (at least one dose) of the HPV vaccine series and 51.1% for series completion (up-to-date on all recommended doses) among adolescents ages 13–17 years [21]. Like other adolescent vaccinations, HPV vaccination requires parental consent under the age of 18 years. However, it is notable that HPV vaccination receipt rates trail uptake rates for other adolescent vaccinations; rates of one or more doses of a meningococcal vaccine (MenACWY) was 86.6% and uptake of tetanus and reduced diphtheria toxoids and acellular pertussis vaccine (Tdap) was 88.9% in 2018 [21]. Among adults ages 18–26 years, HPV vaccine rates from the 2018 National Health Interview Survey (NHIS)—the most recent year for which data were available at the time of writing—were 39.9% for series initiation and 21.5% for series completion [20]. However, HPV vaccination initiation and completion rates vary across multiple factors, including geography (e.g., region, state, rural) and sociodemographic factors (e.g., biological sex, ethnicity, health insurance status) [21]. For instance, in 2018, Rhode Island had the highest HPV rate of teens ages 13–17 years receiving one or more HPV vaccine doses in the USA (89.3%), whereas Mississippi had the lowest rate of teens ages 13–17 years receiving one or more HPV vaccine doses (51.7%) [22]. Of note, as of 2019, Rhode Island was one of four locations in the USA with an HPV vaccine school entry requirement; the other locations are Virginia (females only), Puerto Rico, and Washington D.C. [23]. In 2020, an HPV vaccine school entry requirement rule will go into effect in Hawaii [24]. In addition, males have historically had lower initiation and completion rates compared to females, due in part to the delay in approval of the vaccine for males [20, 21]. Racial and ethnic minority adolescents are more likely to initiate the vaccine series but less likely to complete the series compared to non-Hispanic Whites [25]. Non-Hispanic White adults are more likely than Hispanic adults to have initiated the HPV vaccine series [20]. Variability in HPV vaccination series initiation and completion related to rural, medically underserved, and sexual and gender minority populations will be further described in subsequent sections of the current chapter, followed by a discussion of novel intervention settings to address the need for innovative strategies to increase HPV vaccine series initiation and completion.

HPV Vaccination Among Individuals Living in Rural Communities

Rural vs. Urban HPV Vaccination Rates

Rural geographic disparities in HPV vaccine coverage have persisted since the introduction of the vaccine, with lower vaccination in rural areas compared to urban and/or suburban areas, regardless of the definition of rurality used. Early studies examining HPV vaccine series initiation among females in 2006–2008, the first few years after approval for females, found significantly lower rates of initiation among girls living in rural areas compared to urban areas, based on data from self-reported surveys and Medicaid claims [26, 27]. In the first year after approval of the vaccine for males, 2011 NIS-Teen data indicated low rates for both female and male adolescents, with highest initiation ($\geq$ 1 dose) for those living in mostly urban areas (56.9% among females; 10.3% among males), followed by suburban areas (53.1% among females; 7.2% among males), and then lowest in mostly rural areas (43.1% among females; 6.4% among males) [28]. Multiple studies detected the same pattern for adolescents in subsequent years [29–31].

According to 2018 NIS-Teen data, the HPV vaccination coverage rates for adolescents reaffirmed the pattern of lower coverage with decreasing levels of urbanicity, both for series initiation (71.9% mostly urban, 66.6% suburban, 59.5% mostly rural) and completion (56.1% mostly urban, 49.1% suburban, 40.7% mostly rural) [21]. An in-depth characterization of adolescents stratified by these three metropolitan statistical area categories found that the urban-to-rural gradient pattern was consistent across all subgroups for age, gender, immigration status, and US region [32]. The pattern was also consistent for non-Hispanic Whites and Hispanics of any race; however, for non-Hispanic Blacks, there was no difference between mostly urban and suburban residents, and the difference between mostly urban and mostly rural was not significant, potentially due to a small sample size in NIS-Teen for Blacks living in mostly rural areas.

Unique Challenges, Barriers, and Facilitators for Rural Populations

Rural populations experience a number of structural, system-level barriers to accessing healthcare, such as long distance to care, lack of public transportation, shortage of healthcare providers and facilities, and limited broadband internet access [33, 34]. After accessing care, rural patients are more likely to experience provider-level barriers, such as lack of provider recommendation for HPV vaccine [35, 36] and poor-quality provider communication [37]. In 2011 NIS-Teen, rural parents were less likely than urban or suburban parents to report having a collaborative conversation with their healthcare provider about HPV vaccination, and this communication difference significantly explained, or mediated, the rural versus urban/suburban disparity in HPV vaccination rates [37].

At the individual level, rural residents delay care more often due to higher rates of poverty and unemployment, and low levels of HPV-specific knowledge compared to urban and suburban residents, as well as health beliefs [33, 36, 38–41]. An analysis of data from the 2013 to 2017 Health Information National Trends Survey (HINTS) found that rural adults were less likely than urban adults to be aware of HPV and HPV vaccine, and they were less likely to know that HPV is a sexually transmitted infection and that it causes cervical cancer [42]. Certain parental health beliefs associated with greater HPV vaccine hesitancy in rural areas include concerns about vaccine safety, beliefs that the vaccine is not necessary or that one's child is not at risk, and general fatalistic health beliefs [39, 43–46].

Interventions to Address Rural Disparities in HPV Vaccine Initiation and Completion

A limited number of interventions have been developed and tested that specifically target the unique barriers to HPV vaccination experienced by rural populations, as described below.

School-Based Interventions In 2012–2013, Vanderpool and colleagues tested a school-based intervention in two high schools located in a rural county in south-central Kentucky, developed in partnership with the local public health department [47]. The school nurses utilized multiple communication channels to inform parents/students of the opportunity to receive the HPV vaccine at school after completing the required consent form as well as promotional incentives for participation. Nurses implemented grade-specific immunization clinics on site during the school day. Free vaccines were provided to all interested students with consent forms, either through the federal Vaccines for Children (VFC) program or covered by the project, since the nurses could not bill private insurance companies. The intervention resulted in improvements in the schools' HPV vaccine initiation rate from 24% to 57% and the completion rate from 14% to 45%.

Economic Incentives for Adult Women Cost is a substantial barrier to HPV vaccination for adults ages 18 and older since they do not qualify for free vaccines under the federal VFC program. Vanderpool and colleagues assessed rural-urban differences in the effect of removing the cost barrier for young adult women [48, 49]. In 2007–2009, the team enrolled and provided free HPV vaccine vouchers to 706 women in three clinic settings in eastern Kentucky. They observed significantly higher series initiation in the urban university clinic (50.7%) compared to a rural clinic (45.1%) and a rural community college clinic (6.8%).

Multilevel Interventions In 2009, an academic-community partnership in North Carolina developed a theory-based, social culturally targeted marketing campaign for rural mothers of girls ages 11–12, as well as their healthcare providers and the media as important behavior influencers [50]. The team tested the multilevel, community-wide campaign in four rural counties, distributing materials via public and private health clinics and via a variety of community venues. High engagement of the healthcare providers, organizations, and mothers was documented. However, the study produced mixed results. Two of the four intervention counties experienced a modest increase in HPV vaccine initiation rates at 2% points above the trend observed in control counties, while the other two counties did not improve.

Another study in North Carolina assessed a multilevel, community-wide intervention in one rural county, compared to four control counties for 12 months during 2012–2013 [51]. The two-phase intervention included the following: (1) *Phase 1* (practice-/provider-level) which is a 1-hour provider/staff education session about implementing immunization registry-driven recall with postcard reminders, optional web-based registry trainings, pre-printed postcards and posters, financial incentives for sending reminders (up to $1000), and coaching phone calls every 2 weeks and (2) *Phase 2* (school-level) which is nontargeted school-generated telephone reminders sent from school to parents of adolescents. The study resulted in significant improvements in population-level HPV initiation and completion rates for adolescents, with the largest improvements among 11- and 12-year-olds (series initiation improvement of 14.2–32.1% for boys and 27.4–43.4 for girls).

In 2010–2015, an academic-community partnership designed a multilevel intervention that was culturally targeted for predominantly rural counties in the Appalachian region of Ohio [52, 53]. The intervention components included clinic-level promotion of HPV vaccine educational materials; a 1-hour provider-level training session; and parent-level education delivered via a mailed brochure, DVD video, magnet reminder, and a telephone educational session. A group-randomized trial in 24 clinics across 12 counties demonstrated that the intervention resulted in a small but significant increase in HPV vaccination series initiation by 6 months among the enrolled patients who were not vaccinated at baseline compared to the control group (13.1% versus 6.5%, respectively).

HPV Vaccination Among Medically Underserved Individuals and Those of Limited Financial Resources

HPV Vaccine Initiation and Completion Among Medically Underserved Individuals and Those of Limited Financial Resources

Individuals are defined as being part of a medically underserved population if there is "a shortage of providers for a specific group of people within a defined geographic area." [54] Commonly cited medically underserved populations include those who are Medicaid-eligible, low income, migrant farm workers, homeless, and Native Americans [54]. Among medically underserved adolescents (i.e., individuals receiving care at federally qualified health centers (FQHC), safety net clinics, or funded by Medicaid), HPV vaccine initiation estimates, without intervention, vary

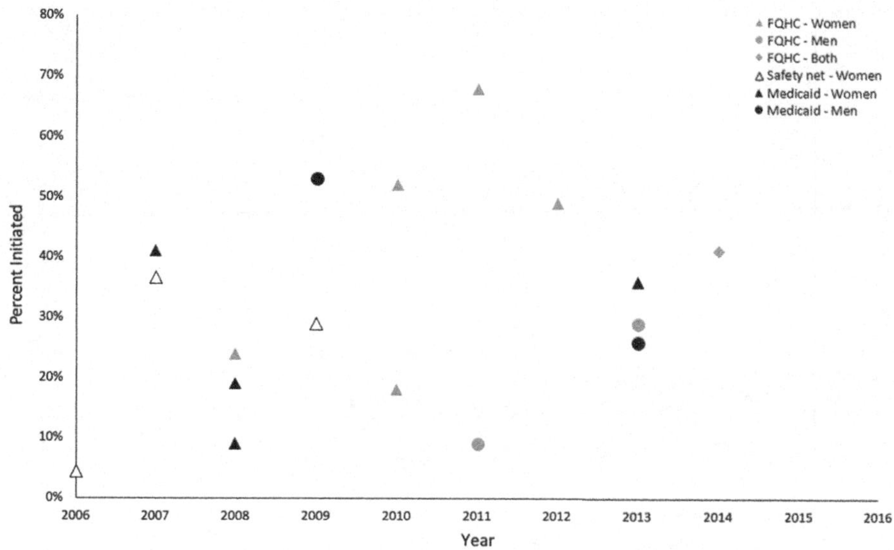

Fig. 1 HPV vaccine initiation among adolescents and young adults from 2006 to 2016

widely across studies and show a general pattern of increasing prevalence over time (Fig. 1) [27, 55–69]. HPV vaccine initiation estimates range from a low of 4.5% among 10- to 26-year-old females attending a Kansas City safety net center between 2006 and 2009 to a high of 68% among 11- to 21-year-old females attending an urban academic health center or seven affiliated FQHCs in 2011 [58, 63]. One study in 2014 found that 41% of females and males receiving care in FQHC settings initiated the HPV vaccine. [62] Compared to Medicaid and safety net populations, FQHCs have the highest HPV vaccine initiation estimates with four studies showing initiation rates at 50% or higher [57–59]. Within safety net clinics, three studies examined HPV vaccine initiation: all three included only girls and were conducted in 2009 or earlier [63–65]. While most studies included adolescents as young as 9, 10, or 11 years, one study considered only adults ages 21 to 29 years in FQHCs between 2009 and 2013 and found initiation was approximately 4% [70].

Studies of HPV vaccine series completion among medically underserved adolescents show no discernable pattern over time, between types of medical services received, or by gender (Fig. 2) [55–59, 61, 63–67, 71]. It is clear that completion rates remain below 50%. The most recent study (conducted in 2017–2018) within an FQHC found that 46% of 9- to 26-year-olds completed the recommended doses [61]. Similar baseline completion rates were found among women in eight FQHC practices in 2011 (42%) and females in four safety net clinics in 2007–2009 (among those who initiated, 40% completed the vaccine series) [58, 64]. Very low completion rates were also found across time: 2% among females ages 10 to 26 years from 2006 to 2009, 2% among Medicaid enrolled females ages 11 to 18 years in June 2008, and 1% among 11- to 21-year-old boys attending an urban academic health center or seven affiliated FQHCs in 2011 [58, 63, 67].

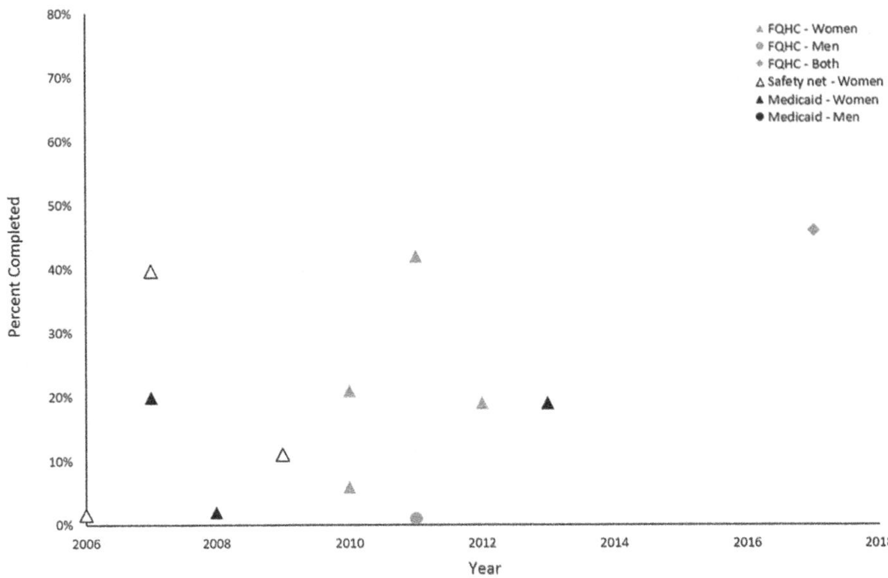

Fig. 2 HPV vaccine completion among adolescents and young adults from 2006 to 2018

Barriers and Facilitators to HPV Vaccination Among Medically Underserved Individuals and Those of Limited Financial Resources

Similar to the general population, physician recommendation, increased age, and receipt of other adolescent vaccines are common facilitators of HPV vaccination among medically underserved AYAs [56, 59–61, 65, 72, 73]. Within FQHC and Medicaid populations, the most commonly identified and strongly associated facilitator of HPV vaccination was physician discussion and recommendation of the vaccine [56, 59–61, 72]. For instance, in a study of Latina mothers with a daughter between the ages of 9 and 18 attending an FQHC, after adjusting for age, mother's education, interview language, acculturation, and HPV vaccine knowledge, a physician recommendation was associated with a 493 times increased odds of HPV vaccine initiation [56]. Older age is also associated with an increased percentage of adolescents receiving the HPV vaccine [56, 59, 60, 65, 73]. However, adolescents who initiated the series at a younger rather than older age were more likely to complete the series [55, 74]. Finally, adolescents who received the other recommended vaccines for their age, especially the non-school entry required meningococcal conjugate vaccine, had higher rates of HPV vaccine receipt [58, 64].

Medically underserved adolescents are also eligible for programs providing access to affordable vaccines that can serve as facilitators of HPV vaccination. Two mechanisms provide access to vaccines for low-income adolescents: availability of the federal universal vaccine coverage program (VFC) and participation in certain health insurance plans. States can leverage the VFC program to offer vaccines recommended by the ACIP at no cost to individuals who are 18 years of age and younger universally or only those who are Medicaid-eligible, uninsured, underinsured, or American Indian or Alaskan Native [75, 76]. Underinsured individuals have to receive vaccines at FQHCs or rural health clinics to qualify for no cost vaccinations given by a VFC provider. HPV vaccination rates are higher among providers who participate in VFC and in states that expanded VFC eligibility to all children [77, 78].

Health insurance influences HPV vaccine initiation and completion within medically underserved individuals at several levels. First, compared to those who are uninsured, insured individuals, regardless of whether through Medicaid or private insurance, are more likely to initiate the HPV vaccine [55, 70]. Among insured 11- to 18-year-old males, compared to privately insured, those with Medicaid insurance were more likely to initiate the vaccine but less likely to complete the series [68, 79]. Finally, among adolescents with Medicaid insurance, participation in different plans influences rates of vaccine initiation and completion [27, 74].

Barriers to HPV vaccination among medically underserved populations are both similar and distinct from the general population. Like the general population, parents' lack of awareness of the HPV vaccine, especially among parents of boys, can be a barrier to initiation for patients in safety net and FQHC populations [60, 65]. Practical barriers may be more important among medically underserved populations as some parents attending FQHCs worry about the cost of the vaccine and/or have competing demands of work or child care [56, 80]. Adolescent girls from households where the household income was less than 100% of the federal poverty level have been found to be less likely to complete the HPV vaccine series [55].

Interventions to Increase HPV Vaccination Among Medically Underserved Individuals and Those of Limited Financial Resources

Nine interventions have been conducted to increase HPV vaccination rates among medically underserved populations (Table 1) [57, 58, 62, 69, 73, 81–84]. Three interventions were conducted within each population of interest (i.e., FQHC, safety net, and Medicaid). Interventions have targeted parents ($n = 4$), providers ($n = 2$), parents and providers simultaneously ($n = 2$), and providers and clinics ($n = 1$). Interventions aimed to increase parents' decision to vaccinate ($n = 1$), initiation ($n = 3$), receipt of dose two or three ($n = 1$), and initiation and completion ($n = 4$). Among the nine interventions, seven showed evidence of intervention effectiveness.

Table 1 HPV vaccine interventions among medically underserved adolescents and young adults

First author	Years of study	Underserved type	Population	Intervention	Outcome	Effect
Parent-level interventions						
Baldwin [81]	2013	Safety net	11- to 17-year-olds	Self-persuasion tasks on a tablet	Parents' decision stage	81.8% (27/33) wanted child vaccinated after intervention
Rand [82]	2013–2014	Medicaid	11- to 16-year-olds	HPV vs. general text message	Initiation	30% increase
Richman [83]	2014–2016	Medicaid and uninsured	9- to 17-year-olds	Text or email reminders vs. postcard	Receipt of dose 2 and 3	No difference
Tiro [73]	2011	Safety net	Females 11- to 18-year-olds	Vaccine vs. HPV brochure, calls to declined parents, recalls for overdue	Initiation, dose 2, and dose 3	Initiation increased among Hispanics only (AOR 1.43; 95% CI 1.02–2.02) Recalls were effective for 3-dose completion (AOR 1.99; 95% CI 1.16–3.45), regardless of race/ethnicity
Provider-level interventions						
Moss [57]	2010	FQHC	Females 12- to 17-years-old	Webinar with CDC's AFIX	1-month initiation and completion	1.6% increase in initiation ($p < 0.05$) 1% increase in completion ($p < 0.01$)
Perkins [58]	2011–2013	FQHC	11- to 21-year-olds	Monthly meetings with HPV-focused education, audit/feedback, maintenance of certification part IV credit	Initiation and next needed dose completion	Initiation increased: girls OR 1.6, boys OR 11; $p < 0.001$ for both Next needed dose increased: girls OR 1.4, boys OR 23; $p < 0.05$ for both

Table 1 (continued)

First author	Years of study	Underserved type	Population	Intervention	Outcome	Effect
Multilevel interventions						
Sanderson [84]	2013–2015	Safety net	Black or Hispanic aged 9–18 years	Parent education video and flyer Provider and staff training	Initiation and completion	No difference
Staras [69]	2013	Medicaid and Children's Health Insurance Program	11- to 17-year-olds	Postcards sent to parents Provider tablet-based prompt	Initiation	Increases with interventions Postcards (girls AOR =1.6; 95% CI 1.1–2.3) Tablet (girls, AOR = 1.5; 95% CI 1.0–2.3 and boys, AOR = 1.4; 95% CI 1.0–2.0) Postcard and tablet (girls, AOR = 2.4; 95% CI 1.4–4.3 and boys, AOR = 1.6; 95% CI 1.0–2.5)
Fisher-Borne [62]	2014–2015	FQHC	11- to 12-year-olds	Provider education and recommendation training Clinic-level audit feedback Money for EHR modifications (randomized to technical assistance, \$10,000 3-month grant, or \$90,000 2-year grant).	Pre-post initiation	14.6 percentage point increase Driven by 18.4% increase in \$90,000 group

AOR adjusted odds ratio, *OR* odds ratio, *CDC* Centers for Disease Control and Prevention, *FQHC* federally qualified health center, *EHR* electronic health records

HPV Vaccination Among Individuals from Racial/Ethnic Minority Groups and/or Individuals Born Outside of the USA

HPV Vaccination Rates Among Racial/Ethnic Minority Groups and/or Individuals Born Outside of the USA

Compared to non-Hispanic Whites, racial/ethnic minority groups have demonstrated differences in HPV vaccination initiation versus completion. A systematic review indicated that Black and Hispanic adolescents were more likely to have initiated the HPV vaccine series compared to non-Hispanic White adolescents when studies were restricted to provider-verified vaccinations [25]. Despite higher vaccination initiation rates, rates of receiving subsequent doses remain significantly lower among Black and Hispanics, as compared to Whites, with disparities in vaccination completion greater among Blacks than Hispanics [25].

Unique Challenges, Barriers, and Facilitators for Racial/Ethnic Minority Groups and/or Individuals Born Outside of the USA

Several factors may influence vaccine initiation and completion rates among racial/ethnic minority groups such as differences across groups in foreign-born status, socioeconomic status, insurance coverage, healthcare access, and provider recommendation. Knowledge may also play a role in HPV vaccination among individuals from these racial/ethnic subgroups. Higher levels of knowledge about Pap testing, HPV infection, and vaccination among African American women have been associated with greater likelihood of HPV vaccination [85]. In a 2015 study, mothers of Latina, Chinese, Korean, and Black adolescent girls from low-income households, most of whom were foreign-born, had relatively low awareness of HPV and the HPV vaccine [86]. In the large, nationally representative 2013–2014 HINTS survey, non-Hispanic Black and Hispanic men and women were less likely to have heard of HPV and the HPV vaccine than non-Hispanic Whites [87]. In another study, compared to non-Hispanic White women, Black women demonstrated lower knowledge about HPV transmission and lower awareness of the HPV vaccine, but greater awareness of the link between HPV infection and cervical cancer compared to non-Hispanic White women [88]. Parents of non-Hispanic Black and Hispanic adolescents and racial/ethnic minority adolescents are significantly less likely to receive a recommendation for the HPV vaccine compared to parents of non-Hispanic White patients or non-Hispanic White patients [89, 90]. Although recommendation rates have improved among these racial/ethnic groups over time, the rate of increase in vaccine recommendation for Hispanic males ages 13–17 has remained low [91]. A systematic review conducted in 2020 identified three primary themes of barriers of vaccination among racial/ethnic minority groups when compared to non-Hispanic Whites [92]. Themes identified in articles published from July 2010 through July

2020 included differences in (1) provider recommendation and differences in patient/parent HPV/HPV vaccine knowledge and awareness, (2) mistrust in the healthcare system as well as HPV vaccine safety concerns, and (3) religious and cultural beliefs, especially among those born outside of the USA [92].

Foreign-born status may also influence disparities in HPV vaccination. In the 2011–2015 NHIS sample, 18–31-year-old foreign-born Asian and Latina women were less likely to initiate the HPV vaccine series compared to foreign-born White women, and foreign-born White, Black, Asian, and Latina women were also less likely to initiate the series than US-born White women [93]. Similarly, in 2013–2015 NHIS data of 18–35-year-old women, all foreign-born women were less likely to initiate vaccination compared with US-born women (14% vs. 30%, respectively) [94]. That same study found that foreign-born women with US citizenship status were more likely to initiate the HPV vaccine series compared to non-citizens [94]. Among young adults, vaccine initiation is often associated with having a usual source of care, OB/GYN provider, or previously receiving a Pap test, regardless of region of birth [94]. However, foreign-born women are often more likely to experience barriers related to health insurance coverage and access to care, which may account for some differences in vaccination initiation and completion among women in the AYA group [93, 94].

Trust in one's provider and the healthcare system may also play an important role in HPV vaccination among racial/ethnic minorities. Black men and women (ages 18–73) who participated in focus groups to discuss their experiences with trustworthiness of healthcare providers reported that trust was largely based upon perceived lack of physicians' interpersonal and technical competence [95]. Racism and experiences of discrimination were also cited as barriers to trust in physicians [95]. The authors of this qualitative study concluded that distrust is associated with decreased adherence to physician recommendations [95]. Indeed, Black men and women who report low levels of trust in healthcare providers are less willing to receive the HPV vaccine [96]. Compared to non-Hispanic White women, Black women report less trust in cancer-related information from media sources and charitable organizations but are more likely to trust cancer-related information from government health agencies, family members, religious organization and leaders, and television compared to non-Hispanic White women [88]. These findings provide insight into potential intervention strategies at the patient, provider, system, and community levels.

HPV Vaccine Interventions for Racial/Ethnic Minority Groups and/or Individuals Born Outside of the USA

There remains a need for culturally targeted interventions in preferred languages to increase vaccine acceptance, initiation, and completion among racially and ethnically diverse groups, including those who are born outside of the USA. Many prior interventions targeting these groups focus on increasing HPV knowledge among patients and/or parents. For instance, in a study conducted among Hispanic women and their daughters aged 11–17 from 2011 to 2013, individuals received either an HPV vaccine educational brochure coupled with a cervical cancer educational prevention program in their preferred language (English or Spanish) or the educational brochure in their preferred language only [97]. The educational program was delivered to both mothers and daughters by a community health educator and included components about HPV infection, vaccination, cervical cancer, screening, and reproductive health. Learning activities and tips for talking to daughters about sex were also included. In addition, participants were provided with a resource sheet containing information about referrals to local clinics, how to make an appointment to receive the vaccine, and vaccine cost and received follow-up phone calls [97]. Those in the intervention group were 2.24 times more likely to complete the vaccine series than the brochure-only group. Another intervention focused on the development of culturally and linguistically appropriate educational videos targeted to Latino and Korean-American parents of 11–17-year-olds [98]. The intervention was available in multiple languages and addressed the association between HPV infection and cervical cancer and important points about the HPV vaccine, with core elements across both parent groups, as well as elements targeted specifically for Korean and Latino parents. Individuals in the educational video intervention demonstrated significantly improved informed decision-making, increased knowledge, and decreased decisional conflict compared to those in the control condition. In addition, among Haitian mothers of adolescents, a brief motivational interviewing intervention resulted in significantly increased HPV-related knowledge but was not effective in improving initiation and completion rates [99].

Several interventions have demonstrated efficacy in increasing knowledge/awareness about HPV vaccination, specifically among females from racial/ethnic minority groups. An educational lecture series at colleges with predominantly Black students that aimed to improve knowledge about HPV vaccine, HPV infection, cervical cancer, and cancer screening significantly improved knowledge among Black female students and influenced intentions to receive the HPV vaccine [100]. During a study conducted among a group of Black and Hispanic women at high risk of cervical cancer, an educational video was presented during a visit to a colposcopy clinic with topics including HPV infection, prevalence, symptoms, HPV vaccine, cervical cancer screening, and cervical dysplasia. Knowledge was assessed pre- and post-video viewing and significantly increased, as did vaccine acceptability [101].

There are fewer multilevel interventions targeted toward racial/ethnic minority groups. However, one 2015–2016 multilevel intervention focused on improving vaccination among patients of an urban family medicine clinic which served primarily low-income and African American patients. The clinic incorporated consistent and positive HPV vaccine messaging targeted toward patients and focused on engaging community members, providers, and clinic staff [102]. Over time, this project significantly increased vaccine initiation (12.8 percentage point increase in males, 10.6 percentage point increase in females) and completion (16 percentage point increase in males, 10.9 percentage point increase in females) [102]. Significant increases in HPV vaccine completion rates were observed in young adult patients, but not adolescents [102].

HPV Vaccination Among Young Adults

HPV Vaccination Rates Among Young Adults

The period of young adulthood (aged 18–26) is often characterized by sexual exploration and autonomous decision-making [103]. The average age at which individuals in the USA report initiating sexual activity is age 18.1 among men and 17.8 among women [104]. Among sexually active adults, young women (ages 20–24) and young men (ages 25–29) [18, 19, 110–112] have the highest prevalence of HPV compared to other age groups [113]. Additionally, many young adults either enroll in college or begin military service, both of which impact healthcare access and related decision-making [114]. For instance, college students and military personnel are provided health insurance coverage and/or have access to designated health centers [115, 116]. In addition to increased access, the frequency of healthcare utilization often increases for young women in accordance with reproductive health guidelines [117]. For instance, the US Preventive Services Task Force recommends that women begin screening for cervical cancer starting at age 21 and continue to receive cervical cancer screenings at appropriate intervals through age 65 [118]. As individuals transition to young adulthood, they can potentially override their parents' decisions to decline the HPV vaccine during adolescence [119]. As of 2018, 39.9% of adults aged 18–26 had initiated the HPV vaccine series, and only 21.5% had completed the recommended number of doses [20]. Overall, HPV vaccine initiation and completion rates in the USA are higher for young women ages 18–26 (53.6% and 35.3%, respectively) compared to young men ages 18–26 (27.0% and 9.0%, respectively) [20]. In addition, young adults who have previously been diagnosed with cancer are at risk for developing a second cancer (including an HPV-related cancer) and thus can greatly benefit from HPV vaccination [120]. However, prior studies have demonstrated low rates of initiation and completion among AYA cancer survivors [121]. In short, young adults are a priority population in efforts to promote the HPV vaccine due to high HPV prevalence, increased healthcare utilization (among women), low HPV vaccination rates, and self-directed healthcare decision-making.

Barriers, Facilitators, and Challenges to HPV Vaccination for Young Adults

Patient-level factors associated with HPV vaccination among young adults include HPV knowledge, attitudes, and beliefs about the HPV vaccine (e.g., perceived benefits, safety concerns, etc.), education level, health literacy, religious beliefs, relationship status, sexual activity, and perceptions of HPV risk [105, 115, 122–125]. Healthcare system-level factors influencing HPV vaccination primarily include access to healthcare (e.g., health insurance status, vaccine cost, etc.) and provider recommendation [89, 105–107, 115]. In fact, provider recommendation is the strongest predictor of HPV vaccination among young adults, regardless of gender, biological sex at birth, or sexual orientation [89, 106]. Unfortunately, low HPV knowledge among many healthcare providers, along with discomfort discussing sexual behavior, may prevent providers from recommending the vaccine [108]. Additionally, providers are less likely to recommend the HPV vaccine to young men compared to women [115].

Risk perception is an important patient-level factor associated with HPV vaccination among all young adults; however, reasons underlying perceptions of risk tend to vary for men and women. Young heterosexual women who are in committed relationships are less likely to be vaccinated compared to their counterparts who are single or dating, and this is largely attributed to perceptions of monogamy as protective against HPV infection [123]. Among sexually active individuals, the prevalence of any type of HPV infection is highest among men [103], yet, HPV knowledge and risk perception are low among young heterosexual men compared to women [115]. Barnard and colleagues found that many young adults did not view themselves at risk for HPV [115]. Given that contextual factors associated with HPV vaccination can vary among young adults, targeted interventions are necessary to increase HPV vaccination initiation and completion in this population.

Targeted HPV Vaccination Interventions for Young Adults

Very few interventions focused on HPV vaccine series initiation have exclusively targeted young adults or been rigorously tested in randomized controlled trials (RCTs), and only one of these studies included men [110, 111]. In a systematic review of HPV vaccine interventions conducted among college students, Barnard and colleagues found that uptake of at least one dose of the HPV vaccine ranged from 5% to 53%; but only one intervention significantly increased vaccine uptake compared to the control condition [111]. In addition to college-based interventions, a few studies have demonstrated efficacy in increasing HPV vaccine initiation and completion in clinic and community-based samples of young adults using patient reminders [110, 111].

Most interventions tested among young adults involved patient-level strategies (e.g., HPV education and/or patient reminders). In particular, individual HPV education provided through video appears to be efficacious at increasing HPV vaccine initiation and completion among young adult women [112, 126]. In an RCT, college women (aged 18–26) shown narrative HPV educational videos featuring both peers and medical experts were twice as likely to initiate the vaccine compared to those in the control group (OR = 2.07; 95% CI = 1.05, 4.10; $p = 0.036$), whereas the peer-only and medical expert-only videos did not improve vaccination rates [126]. In another RCT, young women (aged 18–26) recruited from community settings who had received the first dose of an HPV vaccine and who were prompted to watch a 13-minute HPV education video were more than twice as likely than control participants to complete the vaccine series (OR = 2.44; 95% CI = 1.47, 4.05; $p = 0.001$) [112]. Study participants were provided vaccinations at no cost, limiting external validity [112]. Importantly, both aforementioned interventions addressed patient education alone, which is not recommended by the Community Guide to Preventive Services [127]. Additionally, reminder letters sent directly to patients or their parents have demonstrated efficacy at improving HPV vaccine completion among females aged 9–26 who had already initiated the first dose (56.4% vs. 46.6%, $p < 0.01$), although the intervention effect was not as strong among young women aged 18–26 (43.5% vs. 37.0%, $p < 0.01$) compared to girls aged 9–17 (66.2 vs. 53.5%, $p < 0.01$) [128].

Very few HPV vaccination interventions involving young adults have been rigorously tested at the provider or systems level, and only one has shown efficacy at increasing HPV vaccine series initiation and completion [110, 111]. Ruffin and colleagues found that provider prompts generated through clinics' electronic health record systems increased HPV vaccine series initiation and series completion among females aged 9–26 [129]. It is important to note that no provider or system-level interventions to date have focused exclusively on young adults, and only two included men (but only up to the age of 22) [110]. As system-level barriers related to access to healthcare may be mitigated by targeting young adults in college settings [115], interventions combining patient, provider, and system-level strategies in college health centers represent an emerging opportunity. Furthermore, Healthy Campus 2020 identified HPV vaccination as a health-related priority among college students [130]. Based on available research, college health centers could be enhanced to facilitate greater HPV vaccination series initiation and completion among young adults by incorporating digital patient education (e.g., videos) combined with health system-generated patient reminders and provider prompts [110–112, 126, 128, 129]. More research is necessary to identify intervention strategies that are most efficacious among young men, as well as to test the effectiveness of multilevel interventions specifically targeting young adult populations.

HPV Vaccination Among Sexual and Gender Minority Individuals

HPV Vaccination Rates Among Sexual and Gender Minority Individuals

As summarized from the Institute of Medicine report published in 2011 [131], researchers face three important challenges in attempting to gather valid and reliable data for describing sexual and gender minority groups in assessing their health: (1) operationally defining and measuring sexual orientation and gender identity, (2) overcoming the reluctance of some lesbian, gay, bisexual, or transgender (LGBT) individuals to identify themselves to researchers, and (3) obtaining representative samples of relatively small populations. Although there are scarce data that describe HPV vaccination rates across these vulnerable subgroups, it is well established that men who have sex with men (MSM) have a high risk for anal cancer [132], which is even greater if they are living with HIV [133]. Lesbian and bisexual women report a significant history of cervical abnormalities [135–137]; however, lesbian and bisexual women have also reported low perceived risk of HPV infection due to lack of male sexual partners [125]. Sexual minority women are less likely to receive regular Pap tests compared to heterosexual women [109, 138], placing them at risk for the development of cervical cancer. In some groups, such as the transgender community, empirical data assessing HPV-related cancer incidence and mortality are lacking primarily because of an absence of large-scale observational studies in this population [139].

Although HPV comorbidities and HPV-related cancers disparities are documented in a few sexual and gender minority groups, little research has addressed HPV vaccination among these populations. Available epidemiological studies indicate that HPV vaccine initiation and completion are low among sexual and gender minorities prior to and after the recommendation from the ACIP updated in late 2011 [140–142]. At that time, a routine recommendation was made for males at age 11 or 12, and catch-up vaccination through age 21 for all males, and through age 26 for MSM and for immunocompromised persons, including those with HIV infection [134, 142]. In 2015, recommendations for use of the nine-valent vaccine (9vHPV) were made for the same populations [143]. It is also important to note that US studies varied in their methodological approaches, some with relatively small sample sizes and variability in the year the studies were conducted (Table 2). Indeed, when interpreting the study findings, it is important to consider the temporality in which the study was conducted with regard to ACIP recommendations. Table 2 shows epidemiological studies conducted in the USA which explore HPV vaccination uptake among sexual and gender minorities. An online study of 1457 young MSM in the USA aged 18–26 reported that only 6.8% had received one or more vaccine doses [144]. During the same time period, The National HIV Behavioral Surveillance Study, a behavioral study implemented through a series of cross-sectional surveys [145], reported that for 18–26-year-old MSMs, the HPV vaccination initiation rate was 4.9% (2.7% initiation rate among MSMs 18 years and older overall) [146]. This rate increased to 17.2% among MSM aged 18–26 during the 2014 study [147]. A 2014 national sample of young adult (18–26-year-old) gay and bisexual men found that only 13% had initiated the HPV vaccine series [140]. Of those who initiated the series, more than half (56%) completed the three-dose series [140]. Conversely, a prospective study conducted from 1996 to 2014 using data from 10,663 males and females enrolled in the Growing Up Today Study reported that HPV vaccination initiation was especially low among heterosexual males, compared to bisexual or gay men [148].

In women identifying as sexual and gender minorities, similar lack of estimates for HPV vaccination initiation and completion is also observed in the literature, despite the documented burden for HPV-related comorbidities. Data from the 2006 to 2010 National Survey of Family Growth (NSFG), which used a stratified,

Table 2 HPV vaccination (initiation and completion) rates among sexual and gender minority population groups

Author (publication date)	Year study	Sample	Results
Gorbach (2017) [151]	2012–2014	Young Men's HPV study Multisite, clinic-based study Total sample (n = 808)	HPV ≥ 1 = 13.7% 4.6% completed doses
Reiter (2015) [140]	Fall 2013	National sample of gay and bisexual men Total sample: 428 (18–26 years old) 72% identified as gay	HPV ≥ 1 = 13% 54% completed doses
Meites (2014) [146]	2011	National HIV Behavioral Surveillance System Venue-based sampling Total sample: n = 9819	4.9% initiated HPV vaccine No data on HPV completion
Oliver (2017) [147]	2014	National HIV Behavioral Surveillance System Venue-based sampling Total sample = 2892	HPV ≥ 1 = 17.2% HPV ≥ 1 = 37.2% in HIV+ MSM
Cummings (2015) [144]	December 2011	Online survey YMSM 18–26 years old Total sample: n = 1457	HPV ≥ 1 = 6.7%
Polek (2017) [141]	2013–2014	National Health Interview Survey 2013–2014 Total sample n = 5695 (n = 135 lesbian)	HPV ≥ 1 = 16.8% in lesbians HPV ≥ 1 = 26.8% in bisexuals
McRee (2014) [150]	October to November 2013	Online survey: lesbian 18–26 years old N = 543	HPV ≥ 1 = 45% 70% of initiators reported completing the series
Halkitis (2019) [177]	Fall 2015	P18 Cohort Study of young gay, bisexual, and other men who have sex with men Analytic sample (n = 486)	18.1% completed doses
Charlton (2017) [148]	1996–2014	Prospective cohort study of females and males enrolled in the growing up today study (Total sample = 10,663; lesbian n = 149; gay n = 169)	HPV ≥ 1 (lesbians) = 6.8% HPV ≥ 1 (gay) = 5.9%

three-stage cluster sampling strategy to establish a national probability sample, only 8.5% of lesbians and 33.2% of bisexual individuals who had heard of the HPV vaccine had initiated the HPV vaccine [149]. In 2013, data from the National Sample of Lesbian and Bisexual Women (n = 543) reported that 45% of respondents initiated the HPV vaccine series and 70% of initiators completed the series [150]. Although studies have included transgender women in their sample [151], specific information regarding vaccine uptake in this group is limited. It is also important to note that there are no HPV vaccine recommendations specifically targeting transgender individuals [152].

Barriers and Facilitators for HPV Vaccine Series Initiation and Completion Among Sexual and Gender Minority Individuals

Several studies have examined barriers to HPV vaccination among individuals from sexual minority groups using qualitative and quantitative methods [153–155] at the patient, provider, and system levels. Despite the lower rates of HPV initiation and completion, gay and bisexual men have indicated their willingness to receive the HPV vaccine, with estimates ranging from 36% to 74% [153, 154, 156, 157]. In a national sample of lesbian and bisexual women, 32% had completed the three dose series, and among those who had initiated, but not yet completed the series, 47% intended to complete the series [150]. At a patient level, modifiable factors such as low awareness of HPV infection, HPV-related cancers (other than cervical cancer), and HPV vaccine knowledge are consistent barriers to HPV vaccination in sexual and gender minorities [155]. Other individual-level barriers are cost, lower perceived risk of infection, and perceived benefits of the vaccine [154, 158] and, among transgender women, belief that HPV/HPV vaccination was not relevant to them [155]. At the provider and system levels, the lack of LGBT-trained providers (HPV vaccine knowledge/expertise) and identity-affirming and culturally appropriate healthcare setting deter HPV vaccination uptake among these individuals [155]. The latter barriers have also been identified in the literature across a variety of LGBT health issues, representing consistent, yet modifiable barriers to overall LGBT health [159]. Notably, studies among gender and sexual minorities have reported high rates of having a routine medical checkup in the past year (ranging from 40% to 80%) [140, 146, 160], suggesting missed opportunities for HPV vaccination among this population.

Overwhelmingly, recommendation by healthcare providers is one of the most important facilitators for HPV vaccine initiation and completion [134, 144, 150, 151, 155]. Among young adult MSM, disclosure of sexual behavior to their healthcare providers is a strong mediator of HPV uptake [161]. Although limited studies explore correlates of HPV vaccine acceptability and uptake among the LGBT community, findings from studies focused on MSM address the need for targeted educational and interventional efforts among providers and healthcare systems for culturally sensitive, affirming, and effective communication in this community [155]. Moreover, an online survey conducted in 2009 among gay/bisexual ($n = 312$) and heterosexual men ($n = 296$) found that men may be more accepting of HPV vaccine when it is framed as both preventing genital warts and an HPV-related cancer, regardless of which of the three most common HPV-related cancers in men was described (anal, oral, or penile cancers) [162]. Although only 42% of men were willing to receive the HPV vaccine when framed as preventing genital warts alone, 60% were willing to get it when it was framed as preventing cancer in addition to genital warts ($p < 0.001$) [162]. In the comparison performed between groups (gay/bisexual vs. heterosexual men), their findings suggest that men respond similarly to different ways of framing HPV-related disease regardless of sexual orientation

($p = 0.35$). However, gay and bisexual men were more willing to get the HPV vaccine than their heterosexual counterparts ($p < 0.001$) [162].

Interventions to Address Disparities in HPV Vaccine Initiation and Completion Among Sexual and Gender Minority Individuals

Among young adults, despite ACIP recommendations [134], many age-eligible individuals are not receiving the HPV vaccine, making efforts to increase vaccination important in this age group. The percentage of adults aged 18–26 who received the recommended number of doses of HPV vaccine increased from 13.8% in 2013 to 21.5% in 2018 [20], however these rates remain suboptimal. Most of the epidemiological and behavioral studies among sexual and gender minorities focus on HPV uptake target young adults (older than 18 years). This approach is expected as adolescents are engaged in an ongoing process of sexual development [163]; many adolescents may be unsure of their sexual orientation, while others have been clear about it since childhood [131]. Several interventions target HPV vaccine uptake among young adults at the individual, provider, and clinic levels; however, those interventions do not address clinic- or provider-level barriers for sexual and gender minorities [126, 128, 129, 164–174].

Of the interventions addressing HPV vaccine uptake for young adults, only one addresses sexual and gender minorities (Table 3) [135, 175, 176]. The Outsmart HPV intervention (ClinicalTrials.gov identifiers: NCT04032106 and NCT02835755) is a web-based intervention targeted to young gay and bisexual men was first pilot-tested to examine the acceptability for these individuals in influencing HPV vaccination knowledge, attitudes, and beliefs using the protection-motivation theory (PMT) as the theoretical framework [135, 175, 176]. The intervention, which includes vaccine reminders, aims at increasing HPV vaccine initiation and completion among young individuals who report having a history of same-sex partners, being sexually attracted to males, or identify as gay, bisexual, or queer (i.e., sexual minority males) [135, 175, 176]. The results of the pilot study showed that HPV vaccine initiation was higher among participants in the intervention group (45%) than those in the control group (26%; $p = 0.02$) [135]. HPV vaccination completion rates in the intervention group (11%) were higher than in the control group, although the difference was not statistically significant (3%; $p = 0.07$) [135]. Findings from the posttest survey show positive effects on several attitudes and beliefs such as greater perception that MSM are at higher risk for anal cancer relative to other men; greater HPV vaccination self-efficacy; and lower perceived harms of the HPV vaccine on posttest surveys in the intervention group compared to those in the control group (all *ps* < 0.05) [176].Overall, intervention participants reported high levels of acceptability and satisfaction with the *Outsmart HPV* intervention [176]. As of the writing of this chapter, the efficacy of the *Outsmart HPV* in increasing HPV vaccination rates is currently being tested in a larger trial [175].

Table 3 HPV vaccine interventions among sexual and gender minorities

Author, year	Study design, period; intervention type	Population; venues	Modifiable factors assessed
Outcome: *Vaccine initiation and completion*			
Reiter, 2018 [135]	Randomized clinical trial conducted from July and September 2016 Web-based intervention (*outsmart HPV*) consisted of two components: (1) population-targeted, individually tailored content about HPV and HPV vaccine and (2) monthly HPV vaccination reminders sent via email and/or text message	150 young gay and bisexual men between the ages 18 and 25 years National sample recruited via Facebook advertisement	*Individual*: Attitudes and beliefs Acceptability Communication with health provider about HPV vaccine
Outcome: *Vaccine series initiation and completion*			
Reiter, 2020 [175] Fall 2019–ongoing Intervention	Three-arm prospective randomized clinical trial Web-based intervention	Young gay, bisexual, and other men who have sex with men (YGBMSM) between the ages 18 and 25 Recruitment was made through paid advertisements on social media sites USA	*Individual:* Perceived vulnerability, perceived severity, response efficacy, rewards of the maladaptive response, self-efficacy, response costs, intention, knowledge, worry, stigma

Given the higher burden of HPV infection and disease, as well as the documented lack of evidence-based interventions, culturally appropriate interventions to promote HPV vaccine uptake among sexual and gender minorities are needed. Specifically, interventions designed to improve vaccine uptake should consider a multilevel approach, to address structural and social stigma, cultural competencies, and effective patient-provider communication to support physician recommendations [131]. Further, these findings underscore a missed prevention opportunity for these at-risk and underserved population and might also suggest, in parallel, the need for proactive strategies at a clinic, provider, or policy (e.g., school-entry requirement) level, to increase HPV vaccination uptake in young SGM, particularly prior the onset of sexual behavior.

HPV Vaccination in Novel Settings

As researchers and health professionals seek to increase HPV vaccination, interventions in novel settings for implementation of interventions will become important to reach sociocultural groups with lower rates of HPV vaccination rates. Promising novel settings to improve HPV vaccination rates in the USA include pharmacies, schools, and dental practices [178]. The use of immunization registry data is also important for increasing HPV vaccination rates.

Settings

Pharmacies

HPV vaccination provision in pharmacies has potential for considerable reach given the large number of pharmacies in the USA and their locations throughout rural and underserved areas [178]. Pharmacies are widely trusted by consumers, have longer hours, and can provide similar quality of care at comparable or lower cost than HCPs [178]. This model has been leveraged to deliver vaccines to a large segment of the population for seasonal influenza vaccination. As of 2019, in 47 states, pharmacies have the capability to vaccinate adolescents and adults against HPV within their scope of practice [179], enhancing the overall accessibility of HPV vaccinations. Restrictions exist in some states, however, including the need for a prescription (3 states) and age restrictions for adolescents (22 states) [179], which reduces the ability of age-eligible individuals to obtain the vaccine at their local pharmacy. In addition, other potential barriers exist. For instance, pharmacies may not be considered an "in-network" care provider, thereby placing the financial burden/out of pocket costs of vaccination on the patient/family [178]. Similarly, one study interviewing HPV vaccination stakeholders highlighted pharmacies as a potential strategy for improving vaccination rates, although noted that lack of insurance company reimbursement to pharmacies can be a barrier [40]. The authors of that study concluded that policy changes are needed surrounding HPV vaccination at the pharmacy level, including ensuring that all healthcare providers, including pharmacists, can administer the HPV vaccine and that pharmacies are included as providers in the VFC program [40]. In one national survey of adolescent boys and their parents on comfort with alternative settings for HPV vaccine delivery, half of parents and a third of their sons reported comfort with vaccination in pharmacy or school settings [180]. In another large, national sample, 29% of parents expressed willingness to get their child's HPV vaccine at a pharmacy [181]. Pharmacists report positive perceptions of the HPV vaccination series but report barriers such as inadequate insurance coverage, low demand for the vaccine in pharmacies, and the subsequent expiration of vaccine before use in the pharmacy setting [182]. Studies examining effectiveness of pharmacy-based interventions for HPV vaccination are limited. In one program serving underinsured Hispanic college students, 89 (mostly female) students received the first HPV dose and 43 (48%) completed all three doses, demonstrating acceptability of pharmacy-based vaccine programs for this population [167]. Another "pharmacist-led" intervention in a clinic setting utilized an HPV vaccination strategy where the pharmacist led the education of clinic staff, stocking of HPV vaccine product, review of upcoming patients for HPV vaccine eligibility, and electronic medical record prompts for providers [183]. RCTs of pharmacy interventions compared with interventions in other traditional and novel settings are needed to demonstrate feasibility, acceptability, and efficacy.

Schools

Another promising setting for HPV vaccination is within schools with students ages 9–18. School health centers provide comprehensive medical care to students but exist in less than 10% of schools in the USA [178]. Despite this lower reach, school health centers may be more convenient for parents who have access to them, increasing the likelihood that all HPV doses will be completed. Compared with community health centers, adolescents who received HPV vaccination in school health centers were more likely to complete the series [184]. Barriers to vaccination in school health centers may include parent out-of-pocket costs, school health center costs to purchase vaccines, and obtaining parent consent. Schools hosting or promoting interventions implemented by others with dedicated staff are potential solutions, along with school distribution of HPV vaccine campaign materials and parent reminder letters about vaccine follow-up [185]. Large-scale, voluntary vaccination programs in school settings have been effective in other countries for increasing HPV vaccination (e.g., Canada, Australia) [186–188]. A similar program in the USA with smaller groups of schools has shown promise in rural and Appalachian Kentucky [47].

Dental Practices

Provision of HPV vaccination in dental practices may be a practical and sustainable alternative to provision in traditional settings due to the link between HPV and oral cancer. The substantial reach to adolescents who attend clinics for dental and orthodontia care may provide a large population eligible for vaccination [178]. However, feasibility of vaccination in dental practices may be lower than other novel settings given the training of dental staff [178]. Despite awareness of the link between HPV and oral cancer in the dental field, one systematic review highlighted the lack of communication about, and recommendation for, HPV vaccination by dental providers [189]. The lack of in-depth knowledge and health literacy surrounding HPV in dental providers may be a barrier to discussing the link between the virus and oral caners [190]. Dental opinion leaders reported possible facilitators of HPV vaccination in the dental setting including increasing HPV knowledge for dental providers and for parents and promoting HPV prevention as within the scope of dental care [191]. In one large, national sample of parents of adolescents, only 23% of parents indicated comfort with their teen receiving an HPV vaccination at a dentist [192]. HPV vaccination interventions in dental practices have potential for increasing vaccination rates, but both dental staff and parent comfort and knowledge must be addressed.

Using Immunization Registry and Immunization Information Systems Data

State immunization registries or immunization information systems (IIS) are computer-based systems that confidentially collect and summarize immunization data on a population level [193]. State IIS are tools that can facilitate HPV vaccination through tracking immunization doses and their timing, including series initiation, completion, up-to-date status, and missing/late doses. Registries may enable tracking HPV vaccination across multiple providers and settings (e.g., primary care providers, gynecological care, pharmacies) and enable identification of regions, health systems, or clinics with low initiation and completion rates [40]. In 2016, 49 states used IIS to track childhood immunizations [193]. IIS can potentially be integrated with electronic health records and can include decision support tools. Immunization registries are effective in increasing vaccination due to their ability to track immunizations, increase accountability for providers and practices, and support other vaccine interventions (e.g., patient and provider reminders) [194]. Currently, however, not all US providers are required to use IIS, and IIS have considerable costs in terms of necessary state-level funding, time, effort, and staff dedicated to upkeep [194, 195]. The continued use of IIS is vital for the acceleration of HPV vaccination in AYAs. The use of additional IIS capabilities has been used to improve HPV vaccination [196], including generation of patient/parent HPV vaccine reminders (via mail or phone), provider performance feedback on HPV vaccine rates, and provider reminder prompts via the electronic medical record about needed HPV doses [194].

Gaps and Future Directions

The potential for HPV vaccination to address cancer health disparities has not yet been fully realized. In general, uptake of HPV vaccination has fallen short of targets in national initiatives. Despite the potential to reduce the burden of HPV-related cancers, vaccine series initiation and completion by race/ethnicity, biological sex at birth, gender, socioeconomic status, geography, age, and sexual orientation remain suboptimal. Extensive research suggests the most effective interventions will be targeted approaches that consider multiple levels of influence, including the unique individual, interpersonal, systems, community, and policy-level factors that act as barriers and facilitators to HPV vaccine uptake. State immunization registries have the potential to identify disparities in individual states and might inform the development of targeted interventions for adolescents, parents, young adults, and providers. At the individual level, knowledge, beliefs, and attitudes can play a powerful role in understanding vaccine behaviors. As such, developing messaging and materials that are reflective of the sociocultural characteristics and language preferences of the target communities is essential. Education and messaging must consider the unique audiences involved in HPV vaccination decision-making. For instance, in the case of adolescents, parents often are the vaccine decision-makers; thus, HPV vaccination education materials must consider that parents will be a key part of the audience for this information. At the interpersonal level, communication and messaging from healthcare providers are vital. Given the well-established role of provider recommendation in HPV vaccine uptake, it is crucial that recommendation strategies are evidence-based and consider the unique context of local communities. At the systems level, leveraging well-established strategies such as reminder and recall systems can support individual and interpersonal interactions in the clinic setting. Additionally, reaching communities in settings where they are most comfortable and have established trust should also be considered in order to reduce barriers to access. Thus, at the policy level, school entry policies as well as consideration of the broader contexts or settings for vaccine delivery such as pharmacies or schools can help to remove barriers to access. Coverage for vaccination beyond age 18 through public financing mechanisms may also be an important strategy for unique populations that were not vaccinated during adolescence, such as AYA cancer survivors or LGBTQ communities.

Acknowledgments The authors of the chapter wish to thank Mary Katherine Haver, MLIS, AHIP, Medical Librarian, at the Moffitt Cancer Center Biomedical Library for conducting an initial search for articles for this chapter.

References

1. Satterwhite CL, Torrone E, Meites E, et al. Sexually transmitted infections among US women and men: prevalence and incidence estimates, 2008. Sex Transm Dis. 2013;40(3):187–93.
2. IARC. Human papillomaviruses. IARC. 2012;100:255–313.
3. Centers for Disease Control. Human Papillomavirus (HPV). 2019. https://www.cdc.gov/hpv/index.html
4. Cogliano V, Baan R, Grosse Y, Secretan B, Ghissassi F. Carcinogenicity of human papillomaviruses. Lancet Oncol. 2005;6(4):204.
5. National Cancer Institute. HPV and cancer. 2019. https://www.cancer.gov/about-cancer/causes-prevention/risk/infectious-agents/hpv-and-cancer
6. Senkomago V, Henley SJ, Thomas CC, Mix JM, Markowitz LE, Saraiya M. Human papillomavirus–attributable cancers—United States, 2012–2016. Morb Mortal Wkly Rep. 2019;68(33):724.
7. Van Dyne EA, Henley SJ, Saraiya M, Thomas CC, Markowitz LE, Benard VB. Trends in human papillomavirus–associated cancers—United States, 1999–2015. Morb Mortal Wkly Rep. 2018;67(33):918.
8. Zahnd WE, James AS, Jenkins WD, et al. Rural–urban differences in cancer incidence and trends in the United States. Cancer Epidemiol Biomarkers Prev. 2018;27(11):1265–74.
9. Sudenga SL, Nyitray AG, Torres BN, et al. Comparison of anal HPV natural history among men by country of residence: Brazil, Mexico, and the United States. J Infect. 2017;75(1):35–47.
10. Markowitz LE, Gee J, Chesson H, Stokley S. Ten years of human papillomavirus vaccination in the United States. Acad Pediatr. 2018;18(2):S3–S10.
11. U.S. Food & Drug Adminstration. Approval letter – ceravix. 2009.
12. U.S. Food & Drug Administration. Approval letter – human papillomavirus quadrivalent (Types 6, 11, 16, 18) vaccine, recombinant. 2006.

13. U.S. Food & Drug Administration. Approval letter – gardasil. 2009.
14. U.S. Food & Drug Administration. Approval letter – GARDASIL 9. 2014.
15. Services Dohah. Supplement approval for human papillomavirus 9-valent vaccine, recombinant. 2015.
16. U.S. Food & Drug Administration. Supplement approval, human papillomavirus 9-valent, recombinant, Ages 27–45. 2018.
17. Meites E, Szilagyi PG, Chesson HW, Unger ER, Romero JR, Markowitz LE. Human papillomavirus vaccination for adults: updated recommendations of the Advisory Committee on Immunization Practices. Am J Transplant. 2019;19(11):3202–6.
18. Meites E. Human papillomavirus vaccination for adults: updated recommendations of the Advisory Committee on Immunization Practices. MMWR Morb Mortal Wkly Rep. 2019;68:698–702.
19. Meites E. Use of a 2-dose schedule for human papillomavirus vaccination—updated recommendations of the Advisory Committee on Immunization Practices. MMWR Morb Mortal Wkly Rep. 2016;65
20. Boersma P, Black LI. Human papillomavirus vaccination among adults aged 18–26, 2013–2018. NCHS Data Brief. 2020;(354):1–8.
21. Walker TY, Elam-Evans LD, Yankey D, et al. National, regional, state, and selected local area vaccination coverage among adolescents aged 13–17 years—United States, 2018. Morb Mortal Wkly Rep. 2019;68(33):718.
22. Centers for Disease Control. TeenVaxView | 2018 adolescent HPV vaccination coverage report. Atlanta: CDC; 2019.
23. HPV Roundtable. School entry requirements for HPV vaccine. 2019.
24. Skinner EG, Alise. HPV vaccine: State Legislation and Regulation. 2020. https://www.ncsl.org/research/health/hpv-vaccine-state-legislation-and-statutes.aspx
25. Spencer JC, Calo WA, Brewer NT. Disparities and reverse disparities in HPV vaccination: a systematic review and meta-analysis. Prev Med. 2019;123:197–203.
26. Reiter PL, Cates JR, McRee A-L, et al. Statewide HPV vaccine initiation among adolescent females in North Carolina. Sex Transm Dis. 2010;37(9):549.
27. Staras SA, Vadaparampil ST, Haderxhanaj LT, Shenkman EA. Disparities in human papillomavirus vaccine series initiation among adolescent girls enrolled in Florida Medicaid programs, 2006–2008. J Adolesc Health. 2010;47(4):381–8.
28. Curtis CR, Dorell C, Yankey D, et al. National human papillomavirus vaccination coverage among adolescents aged 13–17 years—National Immunization Survey–Teen, United States, 2011. MMWR Surveill Summ. 2014;63(Suppl 2):61–70.
29. Henry KA, Stroup AM, Warner EL, Kepka D. Geographic factors and human papillomavirus (HPV) vaccination initiation among adolescent girls in the United States. Cancer Epidemiol Prev Biomarkers. 2016;25(2):309–17.
30. Vielot NA, Butler AM, Brookhart MA, Becker-Dreps S, Smith JS. Patterns of use of human papillomavirus and other adolescent vaccines in the United States. J Adolesc Health. 2017;61(3):281–7.
31. Henry KA, Swiecki-Sikora AL, Stroup AM, Warner EL, Kepka D. Area-based socioeconomic factors and human papillomavirus (HPV) vaccination among teen boys in the United States. BMC Public Health. 2018;18(1):19.
32. Williams CL, Walker TY, Elam-Evans LD, et al. Factors associated with not receiving HPV vaccine among adolescents by metropolitan statistical area status, United States, National Immunization Survey–Teen, 2016–2017. Hum Vaccin Immunother. 2020;16(3):562–72.
33. Douthit N, Kiv S, Dwolatzky T, Biswas S. Exposing some important barriers to health care access in the rural USA. Public Health. 2015;129(6):611–20.
34. Luque J, Raychowdhury S, Weaver M. Health care provider challenges for reaching Hispanic immigrants with HPV vaccination in rural Georgia. Rural Remote Health. 2012;12(2):1975.
35. Allison MA, Dunne EF, Markowitz LE, et al. HPV vaccination of boys in primary care practices. Acad Pediatr. 2013;13(5):466–74.

36. Boyd ED, Phillips JM, Schoenberger Y-MM, Simpson T. Barriers and facilitators to HPV vaccination among rural Alabama adolescents and their caregivers. Vaccine. 2018;36(28):4126–33.
37. Moss JL, Gilkey MB, Rimer BK, Brewer NT. Disparities in collaborative patient-provider communication about human papillomavirus (HPV) vaccination. Hum Vaccin Immunother. 2016;12(6):1476–83.
38. Buchwald D, Muller C, Bell M, Schmidt-Grimminger D. Attitudes toward HPV vaccination among rural American Indian women and urban white women in the northern plains. Health Educ Behav. 2013;40(6):704–11.
39. Reiter PL, Brewer NT, Gottlieb SL, McRee A-L, Smith JS. Parents' health beliefs and HPV vaccination of their adolescent daughters. Soc Sci Med. 2009;69(3):475–80.
40. Cartmell KB, Young-Pierce J, McGue S, et al. Barriers, facilitators, and potential strategies for increasing HPV vaccination: a statewide assessment to inform action. Papillomavirus Res. 2018;5:21–31.
41. Kepka DL, Ulrich AK, Coronado GD. Low knowledge of the three-dose HPV vaccine series among mothers of rural Hispanic adolescents. J Health Care Poor Underserved. 2012;23(2):626–35.
42. Mohammed KA, Subramaniam DS, Geneus CJ, et al. Rural-urban differences in human papillomavirus knowledge and awareness among US adults. Prev Med. 2018;109:39–43.
43. Tiggelaar SM, Rafalski M, Davidson MA, Hu Y, Burnett L. HPV knowledge and vaccine acceptability in Appalachian Tennessee and Kentucky, USA. J Fam Plann Reprod Health Care. 2014;40(1):75–6.
44. Vanderpool RC, Dressler EVM, Stradtman LR, Crosby RA. Fatalistic beliefs and completion of the HPV vaccination series among a sample of young Appalachian Kentucky women. J Rural Health. 2015;31(2):199–205.
45. Vanderpool RC, Huang B, Deng Y, et al. Cancer-related beliefs and perceptions in Appalachia: findings from 3 states. J Rural Health. 2019;35(2):176–88.
46. Thomas TL, Caldera M, Maurer J. A short report: parents HPV vaccine knowledge in rural South Florida. Hum Vaccin Immunother. 2019;15(7–8):1666–71.
47. Vanderpool RC, Breheny PJ, Tiller PA, et al. Implementation and evaluation of a school-based human papillomavirus vaccination program in rural Kentucky. Am J Prev Med. 2015;49(2):317–23.
48. Vanderpool RC, Casey BR, Crosby RA. HPV-related risk perceptions and HPV vaccine uptake among a sample of young rural women. J Community Health. 2011;36(6):903.
49. Crosby RA, Casey BR, Vanderpool R, Collins T, Moore GR. Uptake of free HPV vaccination among young women: a comparison of rural versus urban rates. J Rural Health. 2011;27(4):380–4.
50. Cates JR, Shafer A, Diehl SJ, Deal AM. Evaluating a county-sponsored social marketing campaign to increase mothers' initiation of HPV vaccine for their preteen daughters in a primarily rural area. Soc Mark Q. 2011;17(1):4–26.
51. Chung RJ, Walter EB, Kemper AR, Dayton A. Keen on teen vaccines: improvement of adolescent vaccine coverage in rural North Carolina. J Adolesc Health. 2015;56(5):S14–6.
52. Paskett ED, Krok-Schoen JL, Pennell ML, et al. Results of a multilevel intervention trial to increase human papillomavirus (HPV) vaccine uptake among adolescent girls. Cancer Epidemiol Biomarkers Prev. 2016;25(4):593–602.
53. Katz ML, Paskett ED. The process of engaging members from two underserved populations in the development of interventions to promote the uptake of the HPV vaccine. Health Promot Pract. 2015;16(3):443–53.
54. Health Resources and Services Administration. What is shortage designation? 2021. https://bhw.hrsa.gov/workforce-shortage-areas/shortage-designation
55. Cowburn S, Carlson M, Lapidus J, Heintzman J, Bailey S, DeVoe J. Insurance continuity and human papillomavirus vaccine uptake in Oregon and California federally qualified health centers. Am J Public Health. 2014;104(9):e71–9.
56. Gerend MA, Zapata C, Reyes E. Predictors of human papillomavirus vaccination among daughters of low-income Latina mothers: the role of acculturation. J Adolesc Health. 2013;53(5):623–9.

57. Moss JL, Reiter PL, Dayton A, Brewer NT. Increasing adolescent immunization by webinar: a brief provider intervention at federally qualified health centers. Vaccine. 2012;30(33):4960–3.
58. Perkins RB, Zisblatt L, Legler A, Trucks E, Hanchate A, Gorin SS. Effectiveness of a provider-focused intervention to improve HPV vaccination rates in boys and girls. Vaccine. 2015;33(9):1223–9.
59. Flores YN, Salmeron J, Glenn BA, Lang CM, Chang LC, Bastani R. Clinician offering is a key factor associated with HPV vaccine uptake among Mexican mothers in the USA and Mexico: a cross-sectional study. Int J Public Health. 2019;64(3):323–32.
60. Colon-Lopez V, Toro-Mejias LM, Conde-Toro A, et al. Views on HPV and HPV vaccination: the experience at a Federal Qualified Clinic in Puerto Rico. J Health Care Poor Underserved. 2016;27(3):1411–26.
61. VanderVeen N, Wieneke A, Tran S, Kim A, Davis K, Taubel D. Perceived barriers and trends in HPV vaccination via patient survey responses at Kalamazoo, Michigan's federally-qualified health center. J Community Health. 2020;45(1):48–54.
62. Fisher-Borne M, Preiss AJ, Black M, Roberts K, Saslow D. Early outcomes of a multilevel human papillomavirus vaccination pilot intervention in federally qualified health centers. Acad Pediatr. 2018;18(2S):S79–84.
63. Sandri KJ, Verdenius I, Bartley MJ, et al. Urban and rural safety net health care system clinics: no disparity in HPV4 vaccine completion rates. PLoS One. 2014;9(5):e96277.
64. Tiro JA, Pruitt SL, Bruce CM, et al. Multilevel correlates for human papillomavirus vaccination of adolescent girls attending safety net clinics. Vaccine. 2012;30(13):2368–75.
65. Bastani R, Glenn BA, Tsui J, et al. Understanding suboptimal human papillomavirus vaccine uptake among ethnic minority girls. Cancer Epidemiol Biomark Prev. 2011;20(7):1463–72.
66. Perkins RB, Brogly SB, Adams WG, Freund KM. Correlates of human papillomavirus vaccination rates in low-income, minority adolescents: a multicenter study. J Women's Health (2002). 2012;21(8):813–20.
67. Cook RL, Zhang J, Mullins J, et al. Factors associated with initiation and completion of human papillomavirus vaccine series among young women enrolled in Medicaid. J Adolesc Health. 2010;47(6):596–9.
68. Agawu A, Buttenheim AM, Taylor L, Song L, Fiks AG, Feemster KA. Sociodemographic differences in human papillomavirus vaccine initiation by adolescent males. J Adolesc Health. 2015;57(5):506–14.
69. Staras SA, Vadaparampil ST, Livingston MD, Thompson LA, Sanders AH, Shenkman EA. Increasing human papillomavirus vaccine initiation among publicly insured Florida adolescents. J Adolesc Health. 2015;56(5 Suppl):S40–6.
70. Heintzman J, Hatch B, Coronado G, et al. Role of race/ethnicity, language, and insurance in use of cervical cancer prevention services among low-income Hispanic women, 2009–2013. Prev Chronic Dis. 2018;15:E25.
71. Ng J, Ye F, Roth L, et al. Human papillomavirus vaccination coverage among female adolescents in managed care plans – United States, 2013. MMWR Morb Mortal Wkly Rep. 2015;64(42):1185–9.
72. Staras SA, Vadaparampil ST, Patel RP, Shenkman EA. Parent perceptions important for HPV vaccine initiation among low income adolescent girls. Vaccine. 2014;32(46):6163–9.
73. Tiro JA, Sanders JM, Pruitt SL, et al. Promoting HPV vaccination in safety-net clinics: a randomized trial. Pediatrics. 2015;136(5):850–9.
74. Inguva S, Barnard M, Ward LM, et al. Factors influencing human papillomavirus (HPV) vaccination series completion in Mississippi Medicaid. Vaccine. 2020;38(8):2051–7.
75. Centers for Disease Control and Prevention. VFC detailed questions and answers for parents. CDC. 2014 [updated Dec 17, 2014].
76. Centers for Disease Control and Prevention. VFC Childhood Vaccine Supply Policy 2009. CDC 2009.
77. Malo TL, Staras SA, Bynum SA, Giuliano AR, Shenkman EA, Vadaparampil ST. Human papillomavirus vaccine administration among Medicaid providers who consistently recommended vaccination. Sex Transm Dis. 2014;41(1):24–8.

78. Gowda C, Dempsey AF. Medicaid reimbursement and the uptake of adolescent vaccines. Vaccine. 2012;30(9):1682–9.
79. Agawu A, Hanlon AL, Buttenheim AM, Song L, Fiks AG, Feemster KA. Disparities in human papillomavirus vaccine series completion by adolescent males: a retrospective cohort study. Acad Pediatr. 2020;20(3):364–73.
80. Mills LA, Head KJ, Vanderpool RC. HPV vaccination among young adult women: a perspective from Appalachian Kentucky. Prev Chronic Dis. 2013;10:E17.
81. Baldwin AS, Denman DC, Sala M, et al. Translating self-persuasion into an adolescent HPV vaccine promotion intervention for parents attending safety-net clinics. Patient Educ Couns. 2017;100(4):736–41.
82. Rand CM, Brill H, Albertin C, et al. Effectiveness of centralized text message reminders on human papillomavirus immunization coverage for publicly insured adolescents. J Adolesc Health. 2015;56(5 Suppl):S17–20.
83. Richman AR, Torres E, Wu Q, et al. Text and email messaging for increasing human papillomavirus vaccine completion among uninsured or Medicaid-insured adolescents in rural eastern North Carolina. J Health Care Poor Underserved. 2019;30(4):1499–517.
84. Sanderson M, Canedo JR, Khabele D, et al. Pragmatic trial of an intervention to increase human papillomavirus vaccination in safety-net clinics. BMC Public Health. 2017;17(1):158.
85. Bynum SA, Brandt HM, Sharpe PA, Williams MS, Kerr JC. Working to close the gap: identifying predictors of HPV vaccine uptake among young African American women. J Health Care Poor Underserved. 2011;22(2):549–61.
86. Glenn BA, Tsui J, Singhal R, et al. Factors associated with HPV awareness among mothers of low-income ethnic minority adolescent girls in Los Angeles. Vaccine. 2015;33(2):289–93.
87. Adjei Boakye E, Tobo BB, Rojek RP, Mohammed KA, Geneus CJ, Osazuwa-Peters N. Approaching a decade since HPV vaccine licensure: racial and gender disparities in knowledge and awareness of HPV and HPV vaccine. Hum Vaccin Immunother. 2017;13(11):2713–22.
88. Ojeaga A, Alema-Mensah E, Rivers D, Azonobi I, Rivers B. Racial disparities in HPV-related knowledge, attitudes, and beliefs among African American and white women in the USA. J Cancer Educ. 2019;34(1):66–72.
89. Gilkey MB, McRee A-L. Provider communication about HPV vaccination: a systematic review. Hum Vaccin Immunother. 2016;12(6):1454–68.
90. Ylitalo KR, Lee H, Mehta NK. Health care provider recommendation, human papillomavirus vaccination, and race/ethnicity in the US National Immunization Survey. Am J Public Health. 2013;103(1):164–9.
91. Burdette AM, Webb NS, Hill TD, Jokinen-Gordon H. Race-specific trends in HPV vaccinations and provider recommendations: persistent disparities or social progress? Public Health. 2017;142:167–76.
92. Amboree TL, Darkoh C. Barriers to human papillomavirus vaccine uptake among racial/ethnic minorities: a systematic review. J Racial Ethn Health Disparities. 2020;8:1–16.
93. Agénor M, Abboud S, Delgadillo JG, Pérez AE, Peitzmeier SM, Borrero S. Intersectional nativity and racial/ethnic disparities in human papillomavirus vaccination initiation among US women: a national population-based study. Cancer Causes Control. 2018;29(10):927–36.
94. Cofie LE, Hirth JM, Guo F, Berenson AB, Markides K, Wong R. HPV vaccination among foreign-born women: examining the National Health Interview Survey 2013–2015. Am J Prev Med. 2018;54(1):20–7.
95. Jacobs EA, Rolle I, Ferrans CE, Whitaker EE, Warnecke RB. Understanding African Americans' views of the trustworthiness of physicians. J Gen Intern Med. 2006;21(6):642.
96. Otanez S, Torr BM. Ethnic and racial disparities in HPV vaccination attitudes. J Immigr Minor Health. 2018;20(6):1476–82.
97. Parra-Medina D, Morales-Campos DY, Mojica C, Ramirez AG. Promotora outreach, education and navigation support for HPV vaccination to Hispanic women with unvaccinated daughters. J Cancer Educ. 2015;30(2):353–9.
98. Valdez A, Stewart SL, Tanjasari SP, Levy V, Garza A. Design and efficacy of a multilingual, multicultural HPV vaccine education intervention. J Commun Healthc. 2015;8(2):106–18.

99. Joseph NP, Bernstein J, Pelton S, et al. Brief client-centered motivational and behavioral intervention to promote HPV vaccination in a hard-to-reach population: a pilot randomized controlled trial. Clin Pediatr. 2016;55(9):851–9.
100. Staples JN, Wong MS, Rimel B. An educational intervention to improve human papilloma virus (HPV) and cervical cancer knowledge among African American college students. Gynecol Oncol. 2018;149(1):101–5.
101. Mora AS, Madrigal JM, Jordan L, Patel A. Effectiveness of an educational intervention to increase human papillomavirus knowledge in high-risk minority women. J Low Genit Tract Dis. 2018;22(4):288–94.
102. McGaffey A, Lombardo NP, Lamberton N, et al. A "sense"-ational HPV vaccination quality improvement project in a family medicine residency practice. J Natl Med Assoc. 2019;111(6):588–99.
103. Mulye TP, Park MJ, Nelson CD, Adams SH, Irwin CE Jr, Brindis CD. Trends in adolescent and young adult health in the United States. J Adolesc Health. 2009;45(1):8–24.
104. Finer LB, Philbin JM. Trends in ages at key reproductive transitions in the United States, 1951–2010. Womens Health Issues. 2014;24(3):e271–9.
105. Newman PA, Logie CH, Doukas N, Asakura K. HPV vaccine acceptability among men: a systematic review and meta-analysis. Sex Transm Infect. 2013;89(7):568–74.
106. Rosenthal S, Weiss TW, Zimet GD, Ma L, Good M, Vichnin M. Predictors of HPV vaccine uptake among women aged 19–26: importance of a physician's recommendation. Vaccine. 2011;29(5):890–5.
107. Laz TH, Rahman M, Berenson AB. Human papillomavirus vaccine uptake among 18-to 26-year-old women in the United States: National Health Interview Survey, 2010. Cancer. 2013;119(7):1386–92.
108. Leung SOA, Akinwunmi B, Elias KM, Feldman S. Educating healthcare providers to increase human papillomavirus (HPV) vaccination rates: a qualitative systematic review. Vaccine: X. 2019;3:100037.
109. Agénor M, Krieger N, Austin SB, Haneuse S, Gottlieb BR. Sexual orientation disparities in Papanicolaou test use among US women: the role of sexual and reproductive health services. Am J Public Health. 2014;104(2):e68–73.
110. Smulian EA, Mitchell KR, Stokley S. Interventions to increase HPV vaccination coverage: a systematic review. Hum Vaccin Immunother. 2016;12(6):1566–88.
111. Barnard M, Cole AC, Ward L, Gravlee E, Cole ML, Compretta C. Interventions to increase uptake of the human papillomavirus vaccine in unvaccinated college students: a systematic literature review. Prev Med Rep. 2019;14:100884.
112. Vanderpool RC, Cohen EL, Crosby RA, et al. "1-2-3 Pap" intervention improves HPV vaccine series completion among Appalachian women. J Commun. 2013;63(1):95–115.
113. Lewis RM, Markowitz LE, Gargano JW, Steinau M, Unger ER. Prevalence of genital human papillomavirus among sexually experienced males and females aged 14–59 years, United States, 2013–2014. J Infect Dis. 2018;217(6):869–77.
114. Park MJ, Mulye TP, Adams SH, Brindis CD, Irwin CE Jr. The health status of young adults in the United States. J Adolesc Health. 2006;39(3):305–17.
115. Barnard M, George P, Perryman ML, Wolff LA. Human papillomavirus (HPV) vaccine knowledge, attitudes, and uptake in college students: implications from the Precaution Adoption Process Model. PLoS One. 2017;12(8):e0182266.
116. Hoerster KD, Lehavot K, Simpson T, McFall M, Reiber G, Nelson KM. Health and health behavior differences: US military, veteran, and civilian men. Am J Prev Med. 2012;43(5):483–9.
117. Martinez G. Use of family planning and related medical services among women aged 15–44 in the United States: National Survey of Family Growth, 2006–2010. Washington, DC: US Department of Health and Human Services, Centers for Disease Control and …; 2013.
118. Curry SJ, Krist AH, Owens DK, et al. Screening for cervical cancer: US Preventive Services Task Force recommendation statement. JAMA. 2018;320(7):674–86.
119. Hopfer S, Clippard JR. College women's HPV vaccine decision narratives. Qual Health Res. 2011;21(2):262–77.

120. Klosky JL, Hudson MM, Chen Y, et al. Human papillomavirus vaccination rates in young cancer survivors. J Clin Oncol. 2017;35(31):3582.
121. Castellino SM, Allen KE, Pleasant K, Keyes G, Poehling KA, Tooze JA. Suboptimal uptake of human papillomavirus (HPV) vaccine in survivors of childhood and adolescent and young adult (AYA) cancer. J Cancer Surviv. 2019;13(5):730–8.
122. Preston SM, Darrow WW. Are men being left behind (or catching up)? Differences in HPV awareness, knowledge, and attitudes between diverse college men and women. Am J Mens Health. 2019;13(6):1557988319883776.
123. Thompson EL, Vamos CA, Piepenbrink R, et al. Human papillomavirus risk perceptions and relationship status: a barrier to HPV vaccination? J Behav Med. 2019;42(5):991–7.
124. Best AL, Thompson EL, Adamu AM, et al. Examining the influence of religious and spiritual beliefs on HPV vaccine uptake among college women. J Relig Health. 2019;58(6):2196–207.
125. Agénor M, Jahn JL, Kay E, et al. Human papillomavirus risk perceptions among young adult sexual minority cisgender women and nonbinary individuals assigned female at birth. Perspect Sex Reprod Health. 2019;51(1):27–34.
126. Hopfer S. Effects of a narrative HPV vaccination intervention aimed at reaching college women: a randomized controlled trial. Prev Sci. 2012;13(2):173–82.
127. The Community Guide. Vaccination programs: community-based interventions implemented in combination. 2015.
128. Chao C, Preciado M, Slezak J, Xu L. A randomized intervention of reminder letter for human papillomavirus vaccine series completion. J Adolesc Health. 2015;56(1):85–90.
129. Ruffin MT, Plegue MA, Rockwell PG, Young AP, Patel DA, Yeazel MW. Impact of an electronic health record (EHR) reminder on human papillomavirus (HPV) vaccine initiation and timely completion. J Am Board Fam Med. 2015;28(3):324–33.
130. American College Health Association. Healthy Campus. Student objectives. 2020. https://www.acha.org/HealthyCampus/HealthyCampus/Student_Objectives.aspx
131. IOM (Institute of Medicine). 2011. The Health of Lesbian, Gay, Bisexual, and Transgender People: Building a Foundation for Better Understanding. Washington, DC: The National Academies Press.
132. Palefsky J. Human papillomavirus and anal neoplasia. Curr HIV/AIDS Rep. 2008;5(2):78.
133. Colón-López V, Shiels MS, Machin M, et al. Anal cancer risk among people with HIV infection in the United States. J Clin Oncol. 2018;36(1):68.
134. Gerend MA, Madkins K, Gregory Phillips I, Mustanski B. Predictors of human papillomavirus vaccination among young men who have sex with men. Sex Transm Dis. 2016;43(3):185.
135. Reiter PL, Katz ML, Bauermeister JA, Shoben AB, Paskett ED, McRee A-L. Increasing human papillomavirus vaccination among young gay and bisexual men: a randomized pilot trial of the outsmart HPV intervention. LGBT Health. 2018;5(5):325–9.
136. Eaton L, Kalichman S, Cain D, et al. Perceived prevalence and risks for human papillomavirus (HPV) infection among women who have sex with women. J Women's Health. 2008;17(1):75–84.
137. Chido-Amajuoyi OG, Shete S, Talluri R. Prevalence of abnormal cervical cancer screening outcomes among women in the United States: results from the National Health Interview Survey, 2018. Am J Obstet Gynecol. 2020;223(6):938–41.
138. Grasso C, Goldhammer H, Brown RJ, Furness B. Using sexual orientation and gender identity data in electronic health records to assess for disparities in preventive health screening services. Int J Med Inform. 2020;142:104245.
139. Braun H, Nash R, Tangpricha V, Brockman J, Ward K, Goodman M. Cancer in transgender people: evidence and methodological considerations. Epidemiol Rev. 2017;39(1):93–107.
140. Reiter PL, McRee A-L, Katz ML, Paskett ED. Human papillomavirus vaccination among young adult gay and bisexual men in the United States. Am J Public Health. 2015;105(1):96–102.
141. Polek C, Hardie T. Changing HPV vaccination rates in bisexual and lesbian women. J Am Assoc Nurse Pract. 2017;29(6):333–9.

142. Control CfD, Prevention. Recommendations on the use of quadrivalent human papillomavirus vaccine in males – advisory committee on immunization practices (ACIP), 2011. MMWR Morb Mortal Wkly Rep. 2011;60(50):1705–8.
143. Petrosky E, Bocchini JA Jr, Hariri S, et al. Use of 9-valent human papillomavirus (HPV) vaccine: updated HPV vaccination recommendations of the advisory committee on immunization practices. MMWR Morb Mortal Wkly Rep. 2015;64(11):300.
144. Cummings T, Kasting ML, Rosenberger JG, Rosenthal SL, Zimet GD, Stupiansky NW. Catching up or missing out? Human papillomavirus vaccine acceptability among 18-to 26-year-old men who have sex with men in a US national sample. Sex Transm Dis. 2015;42(11):601–6.
145. Centers for Disease Control. National HIV Behavioral Surveillance (NHBS) | Surveillance Systems | Statistics Center | HIV/AIDS | CDC. 2020.
146. Meites E, Markowitz LE, Paz-Bailey G, Oster AM, Group NS. HPV vaccine coverage among men who have sex with men – National HIV Behavioral Surveillance System, United States, 2011. Vaccine. 2014;32(48):6356–9.
147. Oliver SE, Hoots BE, Paz-Bailey G, Markowitz LE, Meites E, Group NS. Increasing human papillomavirus vaccine coverage among men who have sex with men—National HIV Behavioral Surveillance, United States, 2014. J Acquir Immune Defic Syndr (1999). 2017;75(Suppl 3):S370.
148. Charlton BM, Reisner SL, Agénor M, Gordon AR, Sarda V, Austin SB. Sexual orientation disparities in human papillomavirus vaccination in a longitudinal cohort of US males and females. LGBT Health. 2017;4(3):202–9.
149. Agénor M, Peitzmeier S, Gordon AR, Haneuse S, Potter JE, Austin SB. Sexual orientation identity disparities in awareness and initiation of the human papillomavirus vaccine among US women and girls: a national survey. Ann Intern Med. 2015;163(2):99–106.
150. McRee A-L, Katz ML, Paskett ED, Reiter PL. HPV vaccination among lesbian and bisexual women: findings from a national survey of young adults. Vaccine. 2014;32(37):4736–42.
151. Gorbach PM, Cook R, Gratzer B, et al. Human papillomavirus vaccination among young men who have sex with men and transgender women in 2 US cities, 2012–2014. Sex Transm Dis. 2017;44(7):436.
152. Brown B, Poteat T, Marg L, Galea JT. Human papillomavirus-related cancer surveillance, prevention, and screening among transgender men and women: neglected populations at high risk. LGBT Health. 2017;4(5):315–9.
153. Gutierrez B Jr, Leung A, Jones KT, et al. Acceptability of the human papillomavirus vaccine among urban adolescent males. Am J Mens Health. 2013;7(1):27–36.
154. Wheldon CW, Daley EM, Buhi ER, Nyitray AG, Giuliano AR. Health beliefs and attitudes associated with HPV vaccine intention among young gay and bisexual men in the southeastern United States. Vaccine. 2011;29(45):8060–5.
155. Apaydin KZ, Fontenot HB, Shtasel D, et al. Facilitators of and barriers to HPV vaccination among sexual and gender minority patients at a Boston community health center. Vaccine. 2018;36(26):3868–75.
156. Reiter PL, Brewer NT, McRee A-L, Gilbert P, Smith JS. Acceptability of HPV vaccine among a national sample of gay and bisexual men. Sex Transm Dis. 2010;37(3):197.
157. Gilbert P, Brewer NT, Reiter PL, Ng TW, Smith JS. HPV vaccine acceptability in heterosexual, gay, and bisexual men. Am J Mens Health. 2011;5(4):297–305.
158. Daley EM, Vamos CA, Zimet GD, Rosberger Z, Thompson EL, Merrell L. The feminization of HPV: reversing gender biases in US human papillomavirus vaccine policy. Am J Public Health. 2016;106(6):983.
159. Smalley KB, Warren JC, Barefoot KN. LGBT health: meeting the needs of gender and sexual minorities. Cham: Springer; 2017.
160. Meites E, Krishna NK, Markowitz LE, Oster AM. Health care use and opportunities for human papillomavirus vaccination among young men who have sex with men. Sex Transm Dis. 2013;40(2):154.

161. Stupiansky NW, Liau A, Rosenberger J, et al. Young men's disclosure of same sex behaviors to healthcare providers and the impact on health: results from a US national sample of young men who have sex with men. AIDS Patient Care STDs. 2017;31(8):342–7.
162. McRee A-L, Reiter PL, Chantala K, Brewer NT. Does framing human papillomavirus vaccine as preventing cancer in men increase vaccine acceptability? Cancer Epidemiol Prev Biomarkers. 2010;19(8):1937–44.
163. Rosario M, Schrimshaw EW, Hunter J. Predicting different patterns of sexual identity development over time among lesbian, gay, and bisexual youths: a cluster analytic approach. Am J Community Psychol. 2008;42(3–4):266–82.
164. Preston SM, Darrow WW. Improving human papillomavirus-related knowledge and attitudes among ethnically diverse young adults. Health Equity. 2019;3(1):254–63.
165. Juraskova I, Bari RA, O'Brien MT, McCaffery KJ. HPV vaccine promotion: does referring to both cervical cancer and genital warts affect intended and actual vaccination behavior? Womens Health Issues. 2011;21(1):71–9.
166. Moore GR, Crosby RA, Young A, Charnigo R. Low rates of free human papillomavirus vaccine uptake among young women. Sex Health. 2010;7(3):287–90.
167. Navarrete JP, Padilla ME, Castro LP, Rivera JO. Development of a community pharmacy human papillomavirus vaccine program for underinsured university students along the United States/Mexico border. J Am Pharm Assoc. 2014;54(6):642–7.
168. Pahud B, Clark S, Herigon JC, et al. A pilot program to improve vaccination status for hospitalized children. Hosp Pediatr. 2015;5(1):35–41.
169. Gerend MA, Shepherd JE. Predicting human papillomavirus vaccine uptake in young adult women: comparing the health belief model and theory of planned behavior. Ann Behav Med. 2012;44(2):171–80.
170. Szilagyi PG, Humiston SG, Gallivan S, Albertin C, Sandler M, Blumkin A. Effectiveness of a citywide patient immunization navigator program on improving adolescent immunizations and preventive care visit rates. Arch Pediatr Adolesc Med. 2011;165(6):547–53.
171. Kharbanda EO, Stockwell MS, Fox HW, Andres R, Lara M, Rickert VI. Text message reminders to promote human papillomavirus vaccination. Vaccine. 2011;29(14):2537–41.
172. Matheson EC, Derouin A, Gagliano M, Thompson JA, Blood-Siegfried J. Increasing HPV vaccination series completion rates via text message reminders. J Pediatr Health Care. 2014;28(4):e35–9.
173. Patel A, Stern L, Unger Z, et al. Staying on track: a cluster randomized controlled trial of automated reminders aimed at increasing human papillomavirus vaccine completion. Vaccine. 2014;32(21):2428–33.
174. Perkins R, Zisblatt L, Legler A, Trucks E, Hanchate A, Gorin S. Effectiveness of a provider-focused intervention to improve HPV vaccination rates in boys and girls. Vaccine. 2015;33(9):7.
175. Reiter PL, Gower AL, Kiss DE, et al. A web-based human papillomavirus vaccination intervention for young gay, bisexual, and other men who have sex with men: protocol for a randomized controlled trial. JMIR Res Protoc. 2020;9(2):e16294.
176. McRee A-L, Shoben A, Bauermeister JA, Katz ML, Paskett ED, Reiter PL. Outsmart HPV: acceptability and short-term effects of a web-based HPV vaccination intervention for young adult gay and bisexual men. Vaccine. 2018;36(52):8158–64.
177. Halkitis PN, Valera P, LoSchiavo CE, et al. Human papillomavirus vaccination and infection in young sexual minority men: the P18 cohort study. AIDS Patient Care STDs. 2019;33(4):149–56.
178. Shah PD, Gilkey MB, Pepper JK, Gottlieb SL, Brewer NT. Promising alternative settings for HPV vaccination of US adolescents. Expert Rev Vaccines. 2014;13(2):235–46.
179. Brewer NT, Chung JK, Baker HM, Rothholz MC, Smith JS. Pharmacist authority to provide HPV vaccine: novel partners in cervical cancer prevention. Gynecol Oncol. 2014;132:S3–8.
180. McRee A-L, Reiter PL, Pepper JK, Brewer NT. Correlates of comfort with alternative settings for HPV vaccine delivery. Hum Vaccin Immunother. 2013;9(2):306–13.

181. Calo WA, Gilkey MB, Shah P, Marciniak MW, Brewer NT. Parents' willingness to get human papillomavirus vaccination for their adolescent children at a pharmacy. Prev Med. 2017;99:251–6.
182. Hastings TJ, Hohmann LA, McFarland SJ, Teeter BS, Westrick SC. Pharmacists' attitudes and perceived barriers to human papillomavirus (HPV) vaccination services. Pharmacy. 2017;5(3):45.
183. Cebollero J, Walton SM, Cavendish L, Quairoli K, Cwiak C, Kottke MJ. Evaluation of human papillomavirus vaccination after pharmacist-led intervention: a pilot project in an ambulatory clinic at a large academic urban medical center. Public Health Rep. 2020;135(3):313–21.
184. Federico SG, Abrams L, Everhart RM, Melinkovich P, Hambidge SJ. Addressing adolescent immunization disparities: a retrospective analysis of school-based health center immunization delivery. Am J Public Health. 2010;100(9):1630–4.
185. Moss JL, Feld AL, O'Malley B, et al. Opportunities for increasing human papillomavirus vaccine provision in school health centers. J Sch Health. 2014;84(6):370–8.
186. Cheffins T, De La Rue S, Reeve C, Culpan M. School-based vaccinations delivered by general practice in rural North Queensland: an evaluation of a new human papillomavirus vaccination program. Commun Dis Intell Q Rep. 2008;32(1):94.
187. Ogilvie G, Anderson M, Marra F, et al. A population-based evaluation of a publicly funded, school-based HPV vaccine program in British Columbia, Canada: parental factors associated with HPV vaccine receipt. PLoS Med. 2010;7(5):e1000270.
188. Watson M, Shaw D, Molchanoff L, McInnes C. Challenges, lessons learned and results following the implementation of a human papilloma virus school vaccination program in South Australia. Aust N Z J Public Health. 2009;33(4):365–70.
189. Walker KK, Jackson RD, Sommariva S, Neelamegam M, Desch J. USA dental health providers' role in HPV vaccine communication and HPV-OPC protection: a systematic review. Hum Vaccin Immunother. 2019;15(7–8):1863–9.
190. Vázquez-Otero C, Vamos CA, Thompson EL, et al. Assessing dentists' human papillomavirus-related health literacy for oropharyngeal cancer prevention. J Am Dent Assoc. 2018;149(1):9–17.
191. Griner SB, Thompson EL, Vamos CA, et al. Dental opinion leaders' perspectives on barriers and facilitators to HPV-related prevention. Hum Vaccin Immunother. 2019;15(7–8):1856–62.
192. Lazalde GE, Gilkey MB, Kornides ML, McRee A-L. Parent perceptions of dentists' role in HPV vaccination. Vaccine. 2018;36(4):461–6.
193. Murthy N, Rodgers L, Pabst L, Fiebelkorn AP, Ng T. Progress in childhood vaccination data in immunization information systems—United States, 2013–2016. MMWR Morb Mortal Wkly Rep. 2017;66(43):1178.
194. Groom H, Hopkins DP, Pabst LJ, et al. Immunization information systems to increase vaccination rates: a community guide systematic review. J Public Health Manag Pract. 2015;21(3):227–48.
195. Centers for Disease Control and Prevention. 2013–2018 immunization information functional standards 2019. https://www.cdc.gov/vaccines/programs/iis/functional-standards/func-stds-2013-2018.html
196. Szilagyi P, Albertin C, Gurfinkel D, et al. Effect of state immunization information system centralized reminder and recall on HPV vaccination rates. Pediatrics. 2020;145(5):e20192689.

Opportunities, Challenges, and Priorities for Achieving Equity in Cancer Outcomes

John D. Carpten and Mariana C. Stern

Introduction

The understanding of the causes of cancer health disparities, and strategies for their elimination, faces many challenges but also provides unexpected opportunities to increase our understanding of cancer development, treatment, and survivorship. We summarize below some of these opportunities and highlight key challenges.

Opportunities

Reducing Disparities in Minority Populations Will Help Lower the Cancer Burden

The burden of cancer is declining [1], thanks to many decades of progress toward understanding cancer etiology, implementation of successful prevention strategies, development of novel and better treatments, and improvement of survivorship outcomes. The future holds much promise for continuous significant reductions of the cancer burden and transitioning cancer to a chronic disease instead of a terminal death sentence. Unfortunately, these great improvements have not benefitted all individuals equally, and disparities persist within the USA and globally for many

J. D. Carpten
Comprehensive Cancer Center, Beckman Research Institute, City of Hope, Duarte, CA, USA

M. C. Stern (✉)
Department of Population and Public Health Sciences, Department of Urology, Norris Comprehensive Cancer Center, Keck School of Medicine, University of Southern California, Los Angeles, CA, USA
e-mail: marianas@usc.edu

C. Hughes Halbert (ed.), *Cancer Health Disparities*,
https://doi.org/10.1007/978-3-031-37638-2_11

cancer types, for specific populations defined by race/ethnicity, age, socioeconomic status, gender, geography, or immigration status. Whereas racial/ethnic disparities in the USA are in a shrinking trajectory, much work remains to be done among racial/ethnic minorities and other underserved populations to ensure health equity for all.

As described in previous chapters, there are multiple determinants of cancer health disparities. It is unknown how many cancer deaths could be prevented if all those determinants were removed. But a study from the American Cancer Society gives us a glimpse into the magnitude of the problem. For instance, focusing on one single determinant, such as level of education, it was estimated that an average of 22% of all cancer deaths in the USA could be prevented if everyone had a college-level education [2]. In 2018, this figure represented 134,000 cancer deaths that could have been prevented in the USA alone. The range varied by cancer, with estimates of prevention up to 55% for cervical cancer, a cancer known to be caused by infection with the human papilloma virus, and 100% preventable through screening. Thus, no woman should ever have to be diagnosed with, or die of, this cancer. Yet, disparities in socioeconomic status, health literacy about prevention for this disease through screening and vaccination, and access to care lead to disparities among racial/ethnic minority women, as well as among women of low socioeconomic status, women living in rural areas, and transgender individuals [3–7].

The persistence of cancer disparities not only has a toll on the communities who suffer the greatest cancer burden but also has an impact on the economy of the countries where disparities occur. The economic burden of cancer has been estimated to be 1.8% and 1.07% of the gross domestic product (GPD) for the USA and the European Union, respectively (canceratlas.cancer.org). And in the USA alone, the cost associated with cancer disparities among racial and ethnic minorities is in the order of several hundred billions of dollars a year [8]. Around the world, the cost of lost productivity due to cancer ranges from 0.25% to 0.5% of the GPD (canceratlas.cancer.org).

Studies Among Minority Populations Can Help Understand Cancer Etiology

Studies of racial/ethnic minority migrant populations have helped elucidate the etiology of some cancers and the relative contribution of environmental versus individual risk factors. These findings can help understand cancer etiology for all racial/ethnic groups. For instance, the observation several decades ago that Japanese living in Japan have lower incidence of prostate, colon, and breast cancers compared to Japanese living in the USA was instrumental in highlighting the contribution of changes in lifestyle and/or environmental risk factors for these cancers and paved the way for future studies to identify them [9]. Similarly, the observation that migrants from regions with high stomach cancer incidence continue to have an elevated cancer risk in the USA compared to the majority population has suggested that intrinsic factors relevant for these minority populations that have not changed with immigration, such as infection with *Helicobacter pylori*, and/or dietary factors, may play a role in contributing to the observed disparities [10]. Therefore, studies to understand the etiology of cancer disparities among minorities may help uncover cancer determinants that might be relevant for many other populations, not just those who suffer a greater burden.

Another example of the impact of cancer disparities research on understanding cancer etiology is offered by the lessons learned from studies focused on understanding the molecular underpinnings of disparities. An example is the striking disparity suffered by Black men, who have close to 80% higher change of developing prostate cancer than White men [11] and who face higher chances of developing more aggressive disease and dying from it [12, 13]. African genetic ancestry was identified early on as a key risk factor for prostate cancer, alongside age and family history of prostate cancer [14–16]. This observation led to a series of studies that resulted in the discovery of multiple genetic variants at the 8q24 locus and other loci, which are more common among Black men and could partially account for the observed disparities [17–19]. Interestingly, these findings led to the discovery of associations between these variants and prostate cancer risk among other non-Black populations [18], as well as associations with other cancer types [17], which led to uncovering novel cancer biology and the role of noncoding RNAs [20].

A final example of the impact of cancer disparities research illustrates the potential convergence of environmental and genetic factors, and it is given by the increased incidence of acute lymphoblastic leukemia among Hispanic/Latino(x) children. Whereas genetic risk factors have been identified, the rapidly increasing rates among this minority population in a short time suggest other factors are at play. Among them, infection with cytomegaloviruses was identified as a risk factor, along with type of birth delivery, which may interact with inherited factors [12, 21, 22]. These novel risk factors and potential interactions would not have been uncovered if studies of cancer disparities among racial/ethnic minorities had not been conducted. The findings of these studies have illuminated novel cancer development mechanisms that may impact all populations and can be prevented with adequate strategies.

Addressing disparities among minorities in the USA can help guide research and interventions in developing countries where those minorities or their ancestors came from.

As discussed, the field of cancer disparities research uses both self-identified race and genetic ancestry as descriptors for individuals participating in research studies. This is especially the case in the USA. As we consider the latter, genetic ancestry, we relate proportions of inherited variation from trunk populations with specific geographic roots, namely, African, Asian, European, and American Indian [23]. In turn, we can begin to ask the question about whether addressing disparities among minorities in the USA can help guide research and interventions in ancestral countries of origin or across the diaspora. Importantly, considering minorities in the USA, examples would include African American individuals and their ancestral

African origins, or Hispanic/Latinos/a(x) individuals and their admixed ancestral origins, which include European, Indigenous American, and African backgrounds. It is also of note that many of the countries that comprise trunk populations in Africa and Latin America are low- to middle-income or developing countries. Thus, we can also assess relationships between inherited ancestral contributions and certain phenotypes, including diseases such as cancer across these broad and diverse populations [14, 24].

Pertaining to the question at hand (can studies in US minorities guide research in these ancestral populations?), there is mounting evidence that it can. There are several examples in support of this. As mentioned previously, the most significant genetic variation that is associated with increased risk of prostate cancer is reflected by a number of single nucleotide polymorphisms that map the 8q24 locus [14, 19]. Also as stated, these prostate cancer risk variants reside on haplotypes that are derived from and enriched among Sub-Saharan African populations. It is not a surprise therefore that prostate cancer ranks among the most common male-specific cancers in Sub-Saharan Africa [25]. It should also be stated that current epidemiological data in Africa suggests that the incidence rate is higher among White men, for instance, in South Africa; however, access to diagnostic facilities is significantly lower for Black African individuals across the continent and there is limited access to screening [25]. Despite complications in truly understanding the actual incidence rate of prostate cancer among Black African men, another important consideration is treatment and outcomes. Recent data suggest that hormonal therapies targeting androgen and the androgen receptor that might include enzalutamide and abiraterone are more effective in African American men compared to White men with castration resistance prostate cancer [26]. This could provide rationale for testing the utilization and efficacy of androgen-based therapeutic regimens for treating prostate cancer in Sub-Saharan African men.

The study of breast cancer, particularly triple-negative breast cancer (TNBC) among young African American women, serves another example of how studies in US minorities can guide research into ancestral populations or across a diaspora. Breast cancer rates in the USA are higher among White women compared to African American women; however, the age-adjusted incidence specifically of TNBC is higher among young African American women compared to their White peers [27]. Moreover, the rates of TNBC are also high among women across aspects of the African diaspora including Black Sub-Saharan African women (SSWA) and Afro Caribbean women [28, 29]. Interestingly, studies assessing hereditary susceptibility and the utility of a breast cancer polygenic risk score showed a higher genetic contribution in African American and SSWA and AA cases versus White cases, specifically among the hormone receptor-negative or otherwise triple-negative breast cancers [30]. Taken together, these and other studies support a potential role for shared genetic ancestry in the increase of TNBC diagnoses among Black women in the USA and Sub-Saharan Africa. Finally, among the most striking and obvious links relates to the Duffy allele, which is highly enriched among individuals of SSWA ancestry, arising from selective pressure from malaria infection, and that is significantly associated with TNBC [31]. Overall, the underlying genetic ancestry relationships among SSWA and AA women may provide clues to shared etiological links for TNBC diagnoses in these women. Thus, as new approaches for the diagnosis or treatment of TNBC that have been tailored from optimized effectiveness among AA women, these approaches could perhaps be generalized across SSWA women and women from other parts of the SSWA diaspora (i.e., Afro-Caribbean nations) to improve outcomes more broadly.

Yet another example of how studies in US minorities can guide research into ancestral populations is in pediatric acute lymphoblastic leukemia (ALL). Researchers performed a pharmacogenetic analysis of ALL patients where all subjects were genotyped with a high-density single-nucleotide polymorphism (SNP) array [32]. This allowed for association studies to be performed for genetic correlations with disease characteristics but also allowed for the research team to determine the genetic ancestral proportions for each patient. Their research findings revealed that ALL patients who had 10% or greater Indigenous American ancestry had a significantly higher probability of relapse following standard of care chemotherapy [32]. Interestingly, the association was also observed among patients who self-identified as White but had great than 10% Indigenous American ancestry, strongly supporting a genetic ancestry contribution. Of critical importance was that when they further stratified patients by those that received delayed intensification as part of their therapeutic regimen, they could normalize the disparity in probability of relapse [32]. The overall results of that study might suggest that pediatric ALL patients living in countries with higher Indigenous American ancestry should possibly have delayed intensification be a part of standard of care. Further, these findings might suggest that all pediatric ALL patients, regardless of self-identified race, should be assessed for specific genetic markers that describe Indigenous American ancestry to ensure that delayed intensification is applied in the appropriate setting.

As we continue to unearth additional biological links that may at least in part be explained by genetic ancestry, we also must look at potential reciprocal models, where knowledge gained first in ancestral regions can perhaps guide research and interventions in minorities in the USA. A strong example of this reciprocal model is a study of the molecular features of non-small cell lung cancers (NSCLC) in Latin American populations. Researchers performed molecular analysis of NSCLC from over 1100 patients from Latin American countries including Columbia, Costa Rica, and Mexico [24]. The results of their study revealed significant association between Indigenous American ancestry and somatic tumor mutations in key NSCLC oncogenes including EGFR and KRAS. Specifically, they demonstrated that oncogenic EGFR mutations were strongly correlated with Indigenous American ancestry, whereas mutations in KRAS were less frequent in this population of patients [24]. These results have strong translational impact, as there are specific targeted therapies for EGFR-mutated NSCLC. Moreover, the presence of concomitant KRAS mutation in EGFR mutated NSCLC reduces the efficacy of EGFR-targeting therapies. Thus, the lower rate of KRAS mutation in this population would further support the rationale for more EGFR-based treatment approaches. Ultimately, these data suggest that NSCLC patients with Indigenous American ancestral components, including the growing population here in the USA, may benefit from EGFR-based therapeutic regimens.

Challenges

The National Institute of Minority Health and Health Disparities (NIMHD) has developed a research framework to conceptualize the multilevel domains of influence that contribute to health among minorities (biological, behavioral, physical/built environment, sociocultural environment, healthcare system) and, thus, are key to understand to achieve health equity. For each of the five domains of influence identified (see figure below), there are four levels of influence that consider the whole range from individual to societal determinants (individual, interpersonal, community, societal). We can use this framework to identify key challenges across the different domains of influence, with specific focus on cancer disparities across minority populations.

Challenges That Affect Understanding of the Contribution of Biology to Health Disparities

As has been discussed previously in this chapter, there is mounting evidence over the last decade that support a role of biology related to genetic ancestry and/or race in cancer health disparities. However, overall, the amounts of resources, reagents, and data from underrepresented populations pale in comparison to what is available or has been developed from NHW individuals. This dearth of biological investigation of and data from underrepresented minority populations is evident in cohort studies to assess genetic risk of human diseases including cancer [33, 34, 35, 36]. Specifically for cancer genome-wide association studies, over 80% of individuals participating in those cohort studies were non-Hispanic White individuals [35, 36]. As described above, some of the most significant genetic variants associated with prostate cancer are specific to Sub-Saharan African ancestral genomic regions [36]. Among the challenges that limited representation could create is reduced sensitivity and specificity of polygenic risk scores, where the variants that comprise the PRS panels were discovered in largely NHW individuals. Studies are underway to measure the generalizability of currently developed cancer PRS tests. However, without ensuring that variants of most significant association in well-powered highly diverse cohorts are included in these tests, we cannot know the true accuracy and precision of these tests.

National Institute on Minority Health and Health Disparities Research Framework

Domains of Influence (Over the Lifecourse)	Levels of Influence*			
	Individual	**Interpersonal**	**Community**	**Societal**
Biological	Biological Vulnerability and Mechanisms	Caregiver–Child Interaction Family Microbiome	Community Illness Exposure Herd Immunity	Sanitation Immunization Pathogen Exposure
Behavioral	Health Behaviors Coping Strategies	Family Functioning School/Work Functioning	Community Functioning	Policies and Laws
Physical/Built Environment	Personal Environment	Household Environment School/Work Environment	Community Environment Community Resources	Societal Structure
Sociocultural Environment	Sociodemographics Limited English Cultural Identity Response to Discrimination	Social Networks Family/Peer Norms Interpersonal Discrimination	Community Norms Local Structural Discrimination	Social Norms Societal Structural Discrimination
Health Care System	Insurance Coverage Health Literacy Treatment Preferences	Patient–Clinician Relationship Medical Decision-Making	Availability of Services Safety Net Services	Quality of Care Health Care Policies
Health Outcomes	**Individual Health**	**Family/ Organizational Health**	**Community Health**	**Population Health**

National Institute on Minority Health and Health Disparities, 2018
*Health Disparity Populations: Race/Ethnicity, Low SES, Rural, Sexual and Gender Minority
Other Fundamental Characteristics: Sex and Gender, Disability, Geographic Region

Lack of Representation in Tumor Sequencing Studies

The Cancer Genome Atlas (TCGA) represents among the largest and most comprehensive cancer molecular characterization studies, encompassing 33 tumor types across over 11,000 patients. TCGA was established to provide the research community with the molecular taxonomy of various cancer types to help understand the heterogeneity and complexity of cancer. Several studies have now been performed to better understand the representation of the actual patient population from which TCGA tumors were derived. In one study, Spratt et al. (2016) analyzed self-identified race data from over 5700 cases from 10 of the 31 tumor types included in the TCGA dataset [37]. Importantly, they revealed that 77% of the cases were NHW and 12% were African American. In another study, scientists deduced the genetic ancestral proportions of each of 11,122 cases from TCGA [38]. Results from that study revealed that 80.5% of cases were predominant European ancestry, while 9.2% were predominantly Sub-Saharan West African ancestry. One could argue that if African Americans comprise 12.4% of the US population based upon the Census Bureau, 2021, then the TCGA would be close to representative. However, there are several caveats to consider. First, although we may get representation in a cohort of patients to be close to population rates for specific populations, several cancer types have significantly higher rates among underrepresented minority populations; thus, we should consider oversampling to correct for the disparate rates. Secondly, although the percentage is close to population representation, we do not have the power to make statistically significant discoveries among these tumors from under-represented minority populations. A great example of this was revealed through the discovery of *ERF* gene mutations in prostate tumors derived from African American men, where genomic sequencing was performed on over 100 tumors from African American men [39]. These gene mutations were not identified or reported in the initial TCGA prostate cancer study, likely due to the fact that of the 333 cases described in that study, only 25 (7.5%) self-identified as African American [40].

Lack of Representation in Biospecimen Efforts to Foster New Mechanistic Studies

Cancer model systems are foundational in our understanding of the cancer etiology but are also the foundation of preclinical testing in the development of new cancer drugs [41]. Expanding on the consideration of the complexity of cancer, there is also a significant lack of representation among most model systems that are routinely used in cancer research. This includes cell lines that are grown in culture and patient-derived xenograft models (PDX) that are implanted into animals (i.e., mice) allowing for systemic studies of cancer. By increasing representation in patients providing biospecimens for the creation of model systems, we can potentially gain important insights into the importance of genetic background on cancer etiology, cancer progression, drug metabolism, and drug effectiveness. However, several studies show the limitation in representation in most of the available cancer models.

In one study, researchers were able to collect racial/ethnicity information on patient donors for a large collection of cell lines from the National Cancer Institute Patient Derived Model Repository (PDMR) [42]. There were a total of 689 cell lines and models included in this collection, of which 46.1% did not have race or ethnicity data. Of the 318 cell lines where race/ethnicity data was available from the donor, 37.7% were from donors who self-identified as NHW and 11.6% were from donors who self-identified as Asian. However, only 4.2% were from donors who self-identified as African American, and only 0.4% were from those who self-identified as Hispanic [42]. In a separate independent study, researchers set out to comprehensively characterize 536 PDX models from 511 donor patients to aid in the prioritization of candidate targeted therapies [43]. These PDX models represented 25 different cancer types. Race of the donor was described for 511 of the donor patients of which 147 were unknown. Of the 364 donor patients for which self-reported race was described, 319 (88%) were reported as NHW, 39 (11%) were reported as African American, and 6 (2%) were reported as Asian [43]. It should be stated that these PDX models were also included within the PDMR, and there is likely an overlap between these studies; however, both point to a significant under-representation and lack of diversity within the major collections of model systems available for study. Importantly, recent studies have provided interesting insights into potential differences in cancer biology through the study of diverse cancer model systems [44].

It should also be noted that researchers have also performed genetic ancestry analysis of a small subset (n = 15) of cancer cell lines that are commonly used in cancer research studies and have shown that the actual racial designation for some cell lines may not be aligned with ancestry proportions [45]. The primary example was the reporting that one prostate cancer cell line, E006AA-hT, described as being derived from an African American donor, has 92% European ancestral proportion [45]. Thus, we should also ensure to consider genetic ancestry to ensure that we have a complete understanding of the actual genetic background from which models are derived to aid in interpretation of results from that study of these cell lines.

Lack of Representation in Clinical Trials

There could be no more relevant limitation in representation than what we have learned about clinical trials. Several recent studies and articles have pointed to the significant lack of diversity in clinical trials, especially for clinical trials that are performed for drug development for cancers that disproportionately affect under-represented minorities. Several glaring examples exist. For instance, African American men are roughly twofold more likely to be diagnosed with prostate cancer and greater than twofold more likely to die from this disease [46]. However, an analysis of demographics data from 59 prostate cancer trials conducted between 1987 and 2016 showed that 96% of participants were NHW men [47]. Specifically for treatment trials during this period, Black or African American men made up ~7% of participants. In terms of ethnicity, only 1.6% of men were Hispanic/Latino. Considering the large pivotal phase III clinical trial for metastatic castration resistant prostate cancer comparing the efficacy of abiraterone/prednisone versus placebo/prednisone for patients, only 2.6% of the men were Black or African American [48]. Interestingly, a retrospective analysis of outcomes data from this trial where patients were stratified by self-identified race revealed that although abiraterone was equally effective in Black and White patients, Black patients showed more durable PSA response than White patients [48]. Other similar examples exist where there is a historical lack of representation and diversity in clinical trials for cancer disparities such as multiple myeloma, which is among the most significant cancer disparities among African American men and women [46]. A study that assessed demographics for all multiple myeloma clinical trials from 2000 to 2016 revealed that Black or African American individuals represented only 8.6% of participants, and less than 2% were Hispanic/Latino [49]. This lack of representation limits our ability to truly understand the broader context of drug toxicity and efficacy as a function of race and genetic ancestry, where specific genetic haplotypes that may be enriched in some populations could modulate the overall impact of a given therapy.

Behavioral Challenges in Achieving Health Equity

There are several well established behaviors that can contribute to cancer development, such as smoking, lack of physical activity, drinking too much alcohol, or having an unhealthy diet [50]. Moreover, cancer screening behaviors can impact the lethality of cancers by contributing to earlier detection and improved outcomes, or in some instances, such as is the case with cervical cancer and colorectal cancer, avoiding the development of cancer altogether. Disparities have been reported for all these behaviors across multiple minority groups [8]. For instance, whereas rates of smoking among African American individuals are comparable levels to White individuals, African American men have higher tobacco-related cancer rates, as well as other tobacco-related diseases than other racial/ethnic groups [46]. Moreover, compared to White individuals, African American individuals are less successful at quitting tobacco products and are less likely to receive prescriptions for tobacco cessation therapies [51, 52]. Unfortunately, these disparities do not seem to be taken into consideration in a consistent manner in population risk assessments and policy [53].

Challenges exist for other cancer risk behaviors. For instance, breastfeeding has been established as one of the few known and convincing preventative factors for breast cancer development, including triple-negative breast cancer, which is associated with poorer outcomes and is more common among Black and Hispanic/Latina women [54–56]. In spite of this disparity, African American women in the USA have the lowest rates of breastfeeding compared to all other racial/ethnic groups [57, 58]. Several reasons converge to determine this disparity, including cultural perceptions and a history of discrimination, lack of access to resources to ensure support initiating and sustaining breastfeeding, the need to work without a supportive environment at work to continue breastfeeding, access to free formula through assistance programs among low income women, lack of knowledge about the benefits of breastfeeding, and resources to ensure success, among others [57].

Altogether, these examples illustrate the need to address not only the causes of disparities in cancer risk behaviors among minorities but also to ensure that policies that regulate cancer risk behaviors consider existing disparities and their determinants as well as cultural and social differences. Moreover, an important challenge to address is ensuring that all minority populations have equal access to resources that facilitate uptake of behaviors that lower cancer risk, such as effective tobacco cessation therapies, breastfeeding support, adoption of physical activity and healthy diets, information about the risks of alcohol consumption, obesity reduction, and cancer screening behaviors.

Challenges with Biomedical Research Infrastructure and Environments

Among the most significant issues plaguing cancer disparities research is the persistent limited number of underrepresented minorities in science, technology, engineering, math, and medicine (STEMM).

A key determinant of minority representation in the scientific workforce is the ability of underrepresented minorities to obtain funding to support and grow their research programs. Several factors contribute to disparities in funding for underrepresented minorities, thus contributing to lack of representation. Among these factors are biases in the scientific review process, lack of representation of minorities among those who put forth funding opportunities, and lack of prioritization of cancer disparity research, which is more commonly conducted by underrepresented minorities who want to help their own communities [59]. Moreover, there is growing concern about what has been coined "health equity tourism," [60] referring to the growing number of senior and experienced scientists who do not belong to underrepresented minority groups, who may have little training or track record of cancer health equity research yet may compete for the still limited, but growing funding opportunities for cancer disparity research funding, given the increased awareness about lack of health equity, and increasing opportunities launched to address this need [59, 60].

Another challenge faced by underrepresented minorities are biases they face as they navigate their scientific careers. Among them is what has been coined as the "diversity-innovation paradox," [61] which is based on the observation that discoveries and innovations produced by racial/ethnic minorities, particularly Black, Hispanic/Latin(x), and American Indian scientists, or by women, are more likely to be ignored or devalued than if they come from racial majorities or males, which, in turn, can impact their career development.

Challenges in the Sociocultural Environment

Chief among the challenges in addressing cancer health disparities is the impact of racism and discrimination, which are important sociocultural and psychosocial determinants of health [62], yet their effects remain understudied in cancer research. The tragic murders of Black individuals at the hands of the police during 2020 in the USA, as well as the discrimination Asian individuals experienced worldwide during the COVID-19 pandemic [63] are just a few recent examples of the persistence of racism and discrimination in our societies and have raised awareness about the need to eliminate these stressors, as well as increase our understanding of their effects. Perceived racial discrimination has been documented to contribute to the cancer burden, particularly among underrepresented minorities [64–66].

Additional psychosocial stressors that have been identified to contribute to cancer health disparities, and deserve more investigation, are discrimination, stressful life experiences, emotional distress, residential segregation, and gentrification, many of which have been linked to some cancers [67, 68].

A key challenge in understanding the contribution of the sociocultural environment domain on cancer health disparities is untangling the direct effects of social stressors and psychosocial factors, from their influence on cancer risk behaviors, such as tobacco use, alcohol consumption, unhealthy diets, obesity, or sedentary lifestyles. Stress and social interactions have been found to impact biological processes, including many of those linked to cancer biology; therefore, they could contribute to cancer development independently of their effect on cancer risk behaviors [69–73]. More work needs to be done to identify the specific processes by which social determinants impact the cancer burden and contribute to health disparities. Not only would this emphasize the urgency and importance of the role of social and psychosocial determinants on cancer disparities, but it may also provide opportunities to develop appropriate interventions designed to ameliorate the impact of social stressors among those who have already experienced them.

Another important challenge presented by the sociocultural environment is the fact that many cancer prevention interventions, and dissemination efforts about opportunities to participate in cancer research and clinical trials, are developed with the majority population in mind. Thus, due to cultural differences, language barriers, structural barriers, and/or fears or misconceptions, individuals of different racial/ethnic backgrounds and/or other underrepresented minorities might not benefit from these interventions or dissemination efforts, and this may impact their cancer burden, as well as their opportunities to benefit from participating in cancer research and clinical trials. Culturally tailored interventions, developed in partnership with the communities that can benefit from them, have shown to be a powerful approach to improve the effectiveness of cancer prevention interventions and engagement of underrepresented minorities [74–83].

Challenges with the Healthcare System

There are multiple challenges in the healthcare system that fail underrepresented minority communities and lead to disparities in access to appropriate preventative and treatment care and adherence to recommended treatments and lead to disparities in health-related quality of life during the survivorship years.

Many existing differences in cancer burden among underrepresented minorities can be eliminated if individuals get access to appropriate screening or treatment. For instance, cervical cancer is caused by one single agent, the human papillomavirus; and its presence, as well as premalignant lesions of the cervix, can be detected early through regular Pap smears. However, underrepresented minority women, both racial/ethnic minorities and women living in rural areas, women of low socioeconomic status, and transgender individuals often lag regular screening, which increases the burden of this preventable cancer [4, 76, 77, 79, 84, 85]. Eliminating barriers to access to care, with appropriate messaging adapted to each specific population, considering the unique needs and challenges that prevent access to care, is critical to reduce cancer disparities.

An important consideration to improve earlier detection of premalignant lesions or malignant cancer is the fact that for some cancers of higher burden among underrepresented minorities, there is no routine screening, and there may not be any screening tools available, which contributes to a higher burden of advanced cancers among those affected populations. An example of this is stomach cancer, which has an incidence rate among US Hispanic/Latino/a(x) individuals and Asian individuals that is two to five times higher than non-Hispanic White individuals, with Korean Americans having the highest incidence in the USA [86, 87]. Among Hispanic/Latino/a(x) individuals, there is the additional burden of suffering from a greater proportion of younger diagnoses and late-stage diagnoses [86, 88]. Given that stomach cancer is of relatively low incidence in the majority population in the USA, there are currently no guidelines for screening programs for the general population or for at-risk individuals. This is compounded by the fact that patients with early-stage cancer may not have many specific symptoms, thus contributing to late-stage diagnosis among those patients with less frequent access to care. If diagnosed early, the survival rate of this cancer is high but drops to <10% among those with metastatic disease. In Asian countries of high incidence, such as South Korea, there are screening guidelines in place, which have improved earlier detection and lowered mortality [89, 90]. However, no such guidelines exist in the USA, contributing to disparities for this cancer.

Underrepresented minorities, such as racial/ethnic populations, as well as individuals living in rural areas and those without insurance or of low socioeconomic status, suffer disparities in cancer treatment and posttreatment outcomes [8, 91–94]. Importantly, despite many advances achieved with new drugs and treatments, typically offered through participation in clinical trials, fewer underrepresented minorities participate in them [95, 96]. Key determinants of these disparities include barriers to access care, having health insurance, transportation, financial burdens, as well as language and cultural differences, and/or lower health literacy, which are not addressed at the provider and institutional level, thus presenting strong barriers for patient participation [8, 97, 98]. To address these disparities, there is a need to develop culturally appropriate approaches for patient engagement, at the provider and institutional level, as well as providing engagement approaches in the community to assist with information dissemination and patient navigation [80, 99–101]. Patient navigation or clinical care coordinators have shown to be effective tools to improve outcomes among cancer patients, particularly those underserved [101–104].

Priorities

To eliminate cancer health disparities and address the challenges described above, and at the same time leverage the many opportunities presented by achieving health equity in cancer outcomes, the following priorities need to be addressed:

1. Increase research to elucidate the determinants of disparities, and their mechanism of action, for the top cancer burdens among underrepresented minority groups, including racial/ethnic minorities, individuals of low income, individuals living in rural areas, and LGBTQ individuals. Achieving this will require the following priorities:

    (a) Enhancing resources to conduct disparities research, including novel cohorts that include underrepresented minorities, biospecimen biobanks with appropriate representation, and augmenting cancer registry data to appropriately capture data on underrepresented minorities, social determinants, and clinical outcomes.

(b) Increasing funding opportunities focusing on addressing cancer health disparities, with special focus on understudied populations and cancers.
(c) Increasing representation of underrepresented minorities among those who decide on priorities for research funding, as well as during the review process, to avoid biases and ensure that issues relevant for specific minorities are not deemed of low significance if they do not affect the majority population.
(d) Promoting inclusion of underrepresented minorities in teams focused on studying research questions that affect the populations they belong to, to insure they have a voice and can contribute their unique point of view, for the benefit of the research.

2. Improving screening and early detection among underrepresented minorities, through the following efforts:

   (a) Developing culturally tailored approaches to inform and engage the community about the benefits of timely screening and follow-up.
   (b) Developing educational interventions to train providers about the needs and characteristics of the communities they serve, to reduce mismatch between providers and patients and increase uptake of recommended interventions.
   (c) Partnering with the community to train community health educators who can disseminate information in the community about the importance of screening, as well as developing patient navigation strategies that can facilitate access to care and follow-up of screening findings.

3. Developing screening guidelines that consider the unique burdens of underrepresented minorities and not just the cancer burden of the majority population.

   Increasing representation of underrepresented minorities in research and clinical trials and increasing and facilitating access to care through the following approaches:

   (a) Developing culturally tailored approaches to educate patients about the benefits of participating in cancer research and clinical trials, which consider fears, disbeliefs, and cultural values.
   (b) Implementing patient navigation strategies that facilitate participation of patients who face financial, transportation, and health literacy barriers.
   (c) Implementing strategies at the institution level that address financial toxicity and structural barriers to care, such as bringing care to the community, instead of patients having to travel long distance to receive care. This can be achieved through partnerships between comprehensive cancer centers and community clinics and hospitals, as well as through satellites or healthcare hubs that can work in the community.
   (d) Ensuring that available resources for cancer research include representation of racial/ethnic minority populations to accelerate discoveries that can benefit all individuals.

References

1. ACS. Cancer facts and figures. Atlanta: American Cancer Society; 2021.
2. Siegel RL, et al. An assessment of progress in cancer control. CA Cancer J Clin. 2018;68:329–39. https://doi.org/10.3322/caac.21460.
3. Olusola P, Banerjee HN, Philley JV, Dasgupta S. Human papilloma virus-associated cervical cancer and health disparities. Cell. 2019;8 https://doi.org/10.3390/cells8060622.
4. Dhillon N, Oliffe JL, Kelly MT, Krist J. Bridging barriers to cervical cancer screening in transgender men: a scoping review. Am J Mens Health. 2020;14:1557988320925691. https://doi.org/10.1177/1557988320925691.
5. Amboree TL, Darkoh C. Barriers to human papillomavirus vaccine uptake among racial/ethnic minorities: a systematic review. J Racial Ethn Health Disparities. 2020; https://doi.org/10.1007/s40615-020-00877-6.
6. Peterson CE, et al. Barriers and facilitators to HPV vaccine uptake among US rural populations: a scoping review. Cancer Causes Control. 2020;31:801–14. https://doi.org/10.1007/s10552-020-01323-y.
7. Buskwofie A, David-West G, Clare CA. A review of cervical cancer: incidence and disparities. J Natl Med Assoc. 2020;112:229–32. https://doi.org/10.1016/j.jnma.2020.03.002.
8. AACR. American Association of Cancer Research CancerDisparitiesProgressReport.org [Internet]. Available from http://www.CancerDisparitiesProgressReport.org/. Philadelphia: American Association for Cancer Research; 2020).
9. Tominaga S. Cancer incidence in Japanese in Japan, Hawaii, and western United States. Natl Cancer Inst Monogr. 1985;69:83–92.
10. Pabla BS, Shah SC, Corral JE, Morgan DR. Increased incidence and mortality of gastric cancer in immigrant populations from high to low regions of incidence: a systematic review and meta-analysis. Clin Gastroenterol Hepatol. 2020;18:347–59 e345. https://doi.org/10.1016/j.cgh.2019.05.032.
11. Siegel RL, Miller KD, Jemal A. Cancer statistics, 2020. CA Cancer J Clin. 2020;70:7–30. https://doi.org/10.3322/caac.21590.
12. Zavala VA, et al. Cancer health disparities in racial/ethnic minorities in the United States. Br J Cancer. 2021;124:315–32. https://doi.org/10.1038/s41416-020-01038-6.
13. ACS. Cancer facts and figures for African Americans 2019–2021. Atlanta: American Cancer Society; 2018.
14. Freedman ML, et al. Admixture mapping identifies 8q24 as a prostate cancer risk locus in African-American men. Proc Natl Acad Sci U S A. 2006;103:14068–73.
15. Merrill RM, Brawley OW. Prostate cancer incidence and mortality rates among white and black men. Epidemiology. 1997;8:126–31. https://doi.org/10.1097/00001648-199703000-00001.
16. Powell IJ, et al. African-American heredity prostate cancer study: a model for genetic research. J Natl Med Assoc. 2001;93:120–3.
17. Haiman CA, et al. A common genetic risk factor for colorectal and prostate cancer. Nat Genet. 2007;39:954–6. https://doi.org/10.1038/ng2098.
18. Haiman CA, et al. Multiple regions within 8q24 independently affect risk for prostate cancer. Nat Genet. 2007;39:638–44. https://doi.org/10.1038/ng2015.
19. Han Y, et al. Prostate cancer susceptibility in men of African ancestry at 8q24. J Natl Cancer Inst. 2016;108 https://doi.org/10.1093/jnci/djv431.
20. Wilson C, Kanhere A. 8q24.21 locus: a paradigm to link non-coding RNAs, genome polymorphisms and cancer. Int J Mol Sci. 2021;22 https://doi.org/10.3390/ijms22031094.
21. Francis SS, et al. In utero cytomegalovirus infection and development of childhood acute lymphoblastic leukemia. Blood. 2017;129:1680–4. https://doi.org/10.1182/blood-2016-07-723148.
22. Francis SS, et al. Mode of delivery and risk of childhood leukemia. Cancer Epidemiol Biomark Prev. 2014;23:876–81. https://doi.org/10.1158/1055-9965.EPI-13-1098.

23. Shriver MD, Kittles RA. Genetic ancestry and the search for personalized genetic histories. Nat Rev Genet. 2004;5:611–8. https://doi.org/10.1038/nrg1405.
24. Carrot-Zhang J, et al. Genetic ancestry contributes to somatic mutations in lung cancers from admixed Latin American populations. Cancer Discov. 2021;11:591–8. https://doi.org/10.1158/2159-8290.CD-20-1165.
25. Bahnassy AA, Abdellateif MS, Zekri AN. Cancer in Africa: is it a genetic or environmental health problem? Front Oncol. 2020;10:604214. https://doi.org/10.3389/fonc.2020.604214.
26. George DJ, et al. Survival by race in men with chemotherapy-naive enzalutamide- or abiraterone-treated metastatic castration-resistant prostate cancer. Prostate Cancer Prostatic Dis. 2021; https://doi.org/10.1038/s41391-021-00463-9.
27. Kohler BA, et al. Annual report to the nation on the status of cancer, 1975–2011, featuring incidence of breast cancer subtypes by race/ethnicity, poverty, and state. J Natl Cancer Inst. 2015;107:djv048. https://doi.org/10.1093/jnci/djv048.
28. Der EM, et al. Triple-negative breast cancer in Ghanaian women: the Korle Bu teaching hospital experience. Breast J. 2015;21:627–33. https://doi.org/10.1111/tbj.12527.
29. Hercules SM, et al. High triple-negative breast cancer prevalence and aggressive prognostic factors in Barbadian women with breast cancer. Cancer. 2020;126:2217–24. https://doi.org/10.1002/cncr.32771.
30. Huo D, et al. Comparison of breast cancer molecular features and survival by African and European ancestry in the cancer genome atlas. JAMA Oncol. 2017;3:1654–62. https://doi.org/10.1001/jamaoncol.2017.0595.
31. Martini R, et al. Investigation of triple-negative breast cancer risk alleles in an international African-enriched cohort. Sci Rep. 2021;11:9247. https://doi.org/10.1038/s41598-021-88613-w.
32. Yang JJ, et al. Ancestry and pharmacogenomics of relapse in acute lymphoblastic leukemia. Nat Genet. 2011;43:237–41. https://doi.org/10.1038/ng.763.
33. Sirugo G, Williams SM, Tishkoff SA. The missing diversity in human genetic studies. Cell. 2019;177:26–31. https://doi.org/10.1016/j.cell.2019.02.048.
34. Haga SB. Impact of limited population diversity of genome-wide association studies. Genet Med. 2010;12:81–4. https://doi.org/10.1097/GIM.0b013e3181ca2bbf.
35. Peterson RE, et al. Genome-wide association studies in ancestrally diverse populations: opportunities, methods, pitfalls, and recommendations. Cell. 2019;179:589–603. https://doi.org/10.1016/j.cell.2019.08.051.
36. Park SL, Cheng I, Haiman CA. Genome-wide association studies of cancer in diverse populations. Cancer Epidemiol Biomark Prev. 2018;27:405–17. https://doi.org/10.1158/1055-9965.EPI-17-0169.
37. Spratt DE, et al. Racial/ethnic disparities in genomic sequencing. JAMA Oncol. 2016;2:1070–4. https://doi.org/10.1001/jamaoncol.2016.1854.
38. Yuan J, et al. Integrated analysis of genetic ancestry and genomic alterations across cancers. Cancer Cell. 2018;34:549–60 e549. https://doi.org/10.1016/j.ccell.2018.08.019.
39. Huang FW, et al. Exome sequencing of African-American prostate cancer reveals loss-of-function ERF mutations. Cancer Discov. 2017;7:973–83. https://doi.org/10.1158/2159-8290.CD-16-0960.
40. Cancer Genome Atlas Research Network. The molecular taxonomy of primary prostate cancer. Cell. 2015;163:1011–25. https://doi.org/10.1016/j.cell.2015.10.025.
41. Martinez-Pacheco S, O'Driscoll L. Pre-clinical in vitro models used in cancer research: results of a worldwide survey. Cancers (Basel). 2021;13 https://doi.org/10.3390/cancers13236033.
42. Guerrero S, et al. Analysis of racial/ethnic representation in select basic and applied cancer research studies. Sci Rep. 2018;8:13978. https://doi.org/10.1038/s41598-018-32264-x.
43. Westerman MP, Bruetman M, Pfitzer E. Lead poisoning and multiple sclerosis. Arch Environ Health. 1974;29:355–6. https://doi.org/10.1080/00039896.1974.10666615.

44. Jiagge EM, et al. Multiethnic PDX models predict a possible immune signature associated with TNBC of African ancestry. Breast Cancer Res Treat. 2021;186:391–401. https://doi.org/10.1007/s10549-021-06097-8.
45. Hooker SE Jr, et al. Genetic ancestry analysis reveals misclassification of commonly used cancer cell lines. Cancer Epidemiol Biomark Prev. 2019;28:1003–9. https://doi.org/10.1158/1055-9965.EPI-18-1132.
46. DeSantis CE, Miller KD, Goding Sauer A, Jemal A, Siegel RL. Cancer statistics for African Americans, 2019. CA Cancer J Clin. 2019;69:211–33. https://doi.org/10.3322/caac.21555.
47. Rencsok EM, et al. Diversity of enrollment in prostate cancer clinical trials: current status and future directions. Cancer Epidemiol Biomark Prev. 2020;29:1374–80. https://doi.org/10.1158/1055-9965.EPI-19-1616.
48. George DJ, et al. A prospective trial of abiraterone acetate plus prednisone in Black and White men with metastatic castrate-resistant prostate cancer. Cancer. 2021;127:2954–65. https://doi.org/10.1002/cncr.33589.
49. Duma N, et al. Representation of minorities and elderly patients in multiple myeloma clinical trials. Oncologist. 2018;23:1076–8. https://doi.org/10.1634/theoncologist.2017-0592.
50. WCRF. Diet, nutrition, physical activity, and stomach cancer. London: World Cancer Research Fund. American Institute for Cancer Research; 2018.
51. Babb S, Malarcher A, Schauer G, Asman K, Jamal A. Quitting smoking among adults – United States, 2000–2015. MMWR Morb Mortal Wkly Rep. 2017;65:1457–64. https://doi.org/10.15585/mmwr.mm6552a1.
52. Tibuakuu M, et al. National trends in cessation counseling, prescription medication use, and associated costs among US adult cigarette smokers. JAMA Netw Open. 2019;2:–e194585. https://doi.org/10.1001/jamanetworkopen.2019.4585.
53. Cwalina SN, et al. Advancing racial equity and social justice for Black communities in US tobacco control policy. Tob Control. 2021; https://doi.org/10.1136/tobaccocontrol-2021-056704.
54. Lambertini M, et al. Reproductive behaviors and risk of developing breast cancer according to tumor subtype: a systematic review and meta-analysis of epidemiological studies. Cancer Treat Rev. 2016;49:65–76. https://doi.org/10.1016/j.ctrv.2016.07.006.
55. Scott LC, Mobley LR, Kuo TM, Il'yasova D. Update on triple-negative breast cancer disparities for the United States: a population-based study from the United States cancer statistics database, 2010 through 2014. Cancer. 2019;125:3412–7. https://doi.org/10.1002/cncr.32207.
56. Newman LA, Kaljee LM. Health disparities and triple-negative breast cancer in African American women: a review. JAMA Surg. 2017;152:485–93. https://doi.org/10.1001/jamasurg.2017.0005.
57. Jones KM, Power ML, Queenan JT, Schulkin J. Racial and ethnic disparities in breastfeeding. Breastfeed Med. 2015;10:186–96. https://doi.org/10.1089/bfm.2014.0152.
58. Johnson A, Kirk R, Rosenblum KL, Muzik M. Enhancing breastfeeding rates among African American women: a systematic review of current psychosocial interventions. Breastfeed Med. 2015;10:45–62. https://doi.org/10.1089/bfm.2014.0023.
59. Odedina F, Stern MC. Role of funders in addressing the continued lack of diversity in science and medicine. Nat Med; 2021;27(11):1859–1861. https://doi.org/10.1038/s41591-021-01555-8
60. McFarling L. https://www.statnews.com/2021/09/23/health-equity-tourists-white-scholars-colonizing-health-disparities-research/ (2021).
61. Hofstra B, et al. The diversity-innovation paradox in science. Proc Natl Acad Sci U S A. 2020;117:9284–91. https://doi.org/10.1073/pnas.1915378117.
62. Williams DR, Yan Y, Jackson JS, Anderson NB. Racial differences in physical and mental health: socio-economic status, stress and discrimination. J Health Psychol. 1997;2:335–51. https://doi.org/10.1177/135910539700200305.
63. Addo IY. Double pandemic: racial discrimination amid coronavirus disease 2019. Soc Sci Humanit Open. 2020;2:100074. https://doi.org/10.1016/j.ssaho.2020.100074.

64. Williams DR, Collins C. Racial residential segregation: a fundamental cause of racial disparities in health. Public Health Rep. 2001;116:404–16. https://doi.org/10.1093/phr/116.5.404.
65. Taylor TR, et al. Racial discrimination and breast cancer incidence in US Black women: the Black Women's Health Study. Am J Epidemiol. 2007;166:46–54. https://doi.org/10.1093/aje/kwm056.
66. Coughlin SS. Social determinants of colorectal cancer risk, stage, and survival: a systematic review. Int J Color Dis. 2020;35:985–95. https://doi.org/10.1007/s00384-020-03585-z.
67. Cuevas AG, et al. Placing prostate cancer disparities within a psychosocial context: challenges and opportunities for future research. Cancer Causes Control. 2019;30:443–56. https://doi.org/10.1007/s10552-019-01159-1.
68. Chida Y, Hamer M, Wardle J, Steptoe A. Do stress-related psychosocial factors contribute to cancer incidence and survival? Nat Clin Pract Oncol. 2008;5:466–75. https://doi.org/10.1038/ncponc1134.
69. Trainor BC, Sweeney C, Cardiff R. Isolating the effects of social interactions on cancer biology. Cancer Prev Res (Phila). 2009;2:843–6. https://doi.org/10.1158/1940-6207.CAPR-09-0167.
70. Gidron Y, et al. Life events, cortisol and levels of prostate specific antigen: a story of synergism. Psychoneuroendocrinology. 2011;36:874–80. https://doi.org/10.1016/j.psyneuen.2010.11.011.
71. Price LH, Kao HT, Burgers DE, Carpenter LL, Tyrka AR. Telomeres and early-life stress: an overview. Biol Psychiatry. 2013;73:15–23. https://doi.org/10.1016/j.biopsych.2012.06.025.
72. Vick AD, Burris HH. Epigenetics and health disparities. Curr Epidemiol Rep. 2017;4:31–7. https://doi.org/10.1007/s40471-017-0096-x.
73. Cacioppo JT, Hawkley LC. Social isolation and health, with an emphasis on underlying mechanisms. Perspect Biol Med. 2003;46:S39–52.
74. Shah SK, Nakagawa M, Lieblong BJ. Examining aspects of successful community-based programs promoting cancer screening uptake to reduce cancer health disparity: a systematic review. Prev Med. 2020;141:106242. https://doi.org/10.1016/j.ypmed.2020.106242.
75. Palmer KNB, et al. Health promotion interventions for African Americans delivered in U.S. barbershops and hair salons- a systematic review. BMC Public Health. 2021;21:1553. https://doi.org/10.1186/s12889-021-11584-0.
76. Baezconde-Garbanati L, et al. Barriers and innovative interventions for early detection of cervical cancer. Salud Publica Mex. 2019;61:456–60. https://doi.org/10.21149/10425.
77. Ochoa CY, Murphy ST, Frank LB, Baezconde-Garbanati LA. Using a culturally tailored narrative to increase cervical cancer detection among Spanish-speaking Mexican-American women. J Cancer Educ. 2020;35:736–42. https://doi.org/10.1007/s13187-019-01521-6.
78. Baezconde-Garbanati L, et al. Advancing the science of cancer in Latinos, Ramirez AG, Trapido EJ, editors. Cham: Springer; 2020. p. 179–86.
79. Baezconde-Garbanati L, et al. Implementation of HPV vaccination guidelines in a diverse population in Los Angeles: results from an environmental scan of local HPV resources and needs. Vaccine. 2017;35:4930–5. https://doi.org/10.1016/j.vaccine.2017.07.080.
80. Mesa RA, Ramirez AG. Advancing the science of cancer in Latinos, Ramirez AG, Trapido EJ, editors. Cham: Springer; 2020. p. 125–31.
81. Ramirez AG, et al. Advancing the role of participatory communication in the diffusion of cancer screening among Hispanics. J Health Commun. 1999;4:31–6. https://doi.org/10.1080/108107399127075.
82. Van Duyn MA, et al. Adapting evidence-based strategies to increase physical activity among African Americans, Hispanics, Hmong, and Native Hawaiians: a social marketing approach. Prev Chronic Dis. 2007;4:A102.
83. Sentell T, Braun KL. Low health literacy, limited English proficiency, and health status in Asians, Latinos, and other racial/ethnic groups in California. J Health Commun. 2012;17(Suppl 3):82–99. https://doi.org/10.1080/10810730.2012.712621.

84. Carnahan LR, et al. Rural cancer disparities: understanding implications for breast and cervical cancer diagnoses. Clin J Oncol Nurs. 2021;25:10–6. https://doi.org/10.1188/21.CJON.S1.10-16.
85. Connolly D, Hughes X, Berner A. Barriers and facilitators to cervical cancer screening among transgender men and non-binary people with a cervix: a systematic narrative review. Prev Med. 2020;135:106071. https://doi.org/10.1016/j.ypmed.2020.106071.
86. ACS. Cancer facts and figures for Hispanics/Latinos 2018–2020. Atlanta: American Cancer Society; 2018.
87. Lee E, et al. Stomach cancer disparity among Korean Americans by tumor characteristics: comparison with Non-Hispanic Whites, Japanese Americans, South Koreans, and Japanese. Cancer Epidemiol Biomark Prev. 2017;26:587–96. https://doi.org/10.1158/1055-9965.EPI-16-0573.
88. Islami F, DeSantis CE, Jemal A. Incidence trends of esophageal and gastric cancer subtypes by race, ethnicity, and age in the United States, 1997–2014. Clin Gastroenterol Hepatol. 2019;17:429–39. https://doi.org/10.1016/j.cgh.2018.05.044.
89. Choi KS, et al. Effect of endoscopy screening on stage at gastric cancer diagnosis: results of the National Cancer Screening Programme in Korea. Br J Cancer. 2015;112:608–12. https://doi.org/10.1038/bjc.2014.608.
90. Jun JK, et al. Effectiveness of the Korean National Cancer Screening Program in reducing gastric cancer mortality. Gastroenterology. 2017;152:1319–28 e1317. https://doi.org/10.1053/j.gastro.2017.01.029.
91. Farias AJ, Du XL. Ethnic differences in initiation and timing of adjuvant endocrine therapy among older women with hormone receptor-positive breast cancer enrolled in Medicare Part D. Med Oncol. 2016;33:19. https://doi.org/10.1007/s12032-016-0732-1.
92. Farias AJ, Wu WH, Du XL. Racial differences in long-term adjuvant endocrine therapy adherence and mortality among Medicaid-insured breast cancer patients in Texas: findings from TCR-Medicaid linked data. BMC Cancer. 2018;18:1214. https://doi.org/10.1186/s12885-018-5121-z.
93. Farias AJ, et al. Racial/ethnic differences in patient experiences with health care in association with earlier stage at breast cancer diagnosis: findings from the SEER-CAHPS data. Cancer Causes Control. 2020;31:13–23. https://doi.org/10.1007/s10552-019-01254-3.
94. Falcone M, et al. Evidence for racial/ethnic disparities in emergency department visits following breast cancer surgery among women in California: a population-based study. Breast Cancer Res Treat. 2021;187:831–41. https://doi.org/10.1007/s10549-021-06119-5.
95. Chen MS Jr, Lara PN, Dang JH, Paterniti DA, Kelly K. Twenty years post-NIH Revitalization Act: enhancing minority participation in clinical trials (EMPaCT): laying the groundwork for improving minority clinical trial accrual: renewing the case for enhancing minority participation in cancer clinical trials. Cancer. 2014;120(Suppl 7):1091–6. https://doi.org/10.1002/cncr.28575.
96. Wendler D, et al. Are racial and ethnic minorities less willing to participate in health research? PLoS Med. 2006;3:e19. https://doi.org/10.1371/journal.pmed.0030019.
97. Barrett NJ, et al. Factors associated with biomedical research participation within community-based samples across 3 National Cancer Institute-designated cancer centers. Cancer. 2020;126:1077–89. https://doi.org/10.1002/cncr.32487.
98. Niranjan SJ, et al. Perceived institutional barriers among clinical and research professionals: minority participation in oncology clinical trials. JCO Oncol Pract. 2021;17:e666–75. https://doi.org/10.1200/OP.20.00970.
99. Denicoff AM, et al. The National Cancer Institute-American Society of Clinical Oncology Cancer Trial Accrual Symposium: summary and recommendations. J Oncol Pract. 2013;9:267–76. https://doi.org/10.1200/JOP.2013.001119.
100. Napoles A, Cook E, Ginossar T, Knight KD, Ford ME. Applying a conceptual framework to maximize the participation of diverse populations in cancer clinical trials. Adv Cancer Res. 2017;133:77–94. https://doi.org/10.1016/bs.acr.2016.08.004.

101. Hu B, et al. Equal access to care and nurse navigation leads to equitable outcomes for minorities with aggressive large B-cell lymphoma. Cancer. 2021; https://doi.org/10.1002/cncr.33779.
102. Williams CP, et al. Impact of lay navigation on utilization and Medicare spending for cancer survivors in the "Deep South". J Cancer Surviv. 2021; https://doi.org/10.1007/s11764-021-01064-0.
103. Del Vecchio NJ, et al. Relationships between health literacy, having a cancer care coordinator, and long-term health-related quality of life among cancer survivors. Support Care Cancer. 2021; https://doi.org/10.1007/s00520-021-06356-w.
104. Freund KM, et al. Standardized activities for lay patient navigators in breast cancer care: recommendations from a citywide implementation study. Cancer. 2019;125:4532–40. https://doi.org/10.1002/cncr.32432.

Index

C. Hughes Halbert (ed.), *Cancer Health Disparities*,
https://doi.org/10.1007/978-3-031-37638-2

SPRINGER NATURE

GPSR Compliance

The European Union's (EU) General Product Safety Regulation (GPSR) is a set of rules that requires consumer products to be safe and our obligations to ensure this.

If you have any concerns about our products, you can contact us on ProductSafety@springernature.com

In case Publisher is established outside the EU, the EU authorized representative is:

Springer Nature Customer Service Center GmbH
Europaplatz 3
69115 Heidelberg, Germany

The manufacturer's authorised representative in the EU is Springer Nature Customer Service Centre GmbH, Europaplatz 3, 69115 Heidelberg, Germany. If you have any concerns regarding our products, please contact ProductSafety@springernature.com

Printed and bound by CPI Group (UK) Ltd, Croydon, CR0 4YY
28/09/2026
02224075-0002